The Health Professions

Trends and Opportunities
in U.S. Health Care

Stephanie Chisolm, PhD

Director of Patient Education
American Urological Association Foundation
Linthicum, MD

JONES AND BARTLETT PUBLISHERS

Sudbury, Massachusetts

BOSTON   TORONTO   LONDON   SINGAPORE

World Headquarters

Jones and Bartlett Publishers
40 Tall Pine Drive
Sudbury, MA 01776
978-443-5000
info@jbpub.com
www.jbpub.com

Jones and Bartlett Publishers
Canada
6339 Ormindale Way
Mississauga, Ontario L5V 1J2
CANADA

Jones and Bartlett Publishers
International
Barb House, Barb Mews
London W6 7PA
UK

Jones and Bartlett's books and products are available through most bookstores and online book-sellers. To contact Jones and Bartlett Publishers directly, call 800-832-0034, fax 978-443-8000, or visit our website www.jbpub.com.

Substantial discounts on bulk quantities of Jones and Bartlett's publications are available to cor-porations, professional associations, and other qualified organizations. For details and specific discount information, contact the special sales department at Jones and Bartlett via the above contact information or send an email to specialsales@jbpub.com.

The author has made every effort to ensure the accuracy of the information herein. However, appro-priate information sources should be consulted, especially for new or unfamiliar procedures. It is the responsibility of every practitioner to evaluate the appropriateness of a particular opinion in the context of actual clinical situations and with due considerations to new developments. The author(s) and publisher disclaim all responsibility for any liability, loss, injury, or damage incurred as a con-sequence, directly or indirectly, of the use and application of any of the contents of this volume.

Library of Congress Cataloging-in-Publication Data
Chisolm, Stephanie.
    The health professions : trends and opportunities in U.S. health care / Stephanie Chisolm.
        p. ; cm.
    Includes bibliographical references and index.
    ISBN-13: 978-0-7637-3520-3 (pbk.)
    ISBN-10: 0-7637-3520-5 (pbk.)
    1. Medical personnel--Vocational guidance--United States. I. Title.
    [DNLM: 1. Delivery of Health Care--United States. 2. Health Care Costs--United States. 3. Health Occupations--United States. 4. Health Policy--United States. W 84 AA1 C542h 2007]
    R690.C448 2007
    610.69--dc22

                                    2006037971

6048

Production Credits
Executive Editor: David Cella
Editorial Assistant: Lisa Gordon
Production Director: Amy Rose
Production Editor: Tracey Chapman
Associate Marketing Manager: Jennifer Bengtson
Manufacturing Buyer: Therese Connell
Composition: Arlene Apone
Cover Design: Kate Ternullo
Senior Photo Researcher and Photographer: Kimberly Potvin
Cover Image: © Photos.com; © Andrew Gentry/ShutterStock, Inc.; © AbleStock; © Photodisc
Printing and Binding: Malloy, Inc.
Cover Printing: Malloy, Inc.

Printed in the United States of America
11 10 09 08 07   10 9 8 7 6 5 4 3 2 1

Contents

Acknowledgments

I would like to dedicate this book to two groups of individuals. First, to the students I have worked with: their knowledge, skill, dedication, and enthusiasm make me feel secure that the health care I may need in the future will be the best it can be! Next, to the faculty I have worked with: Your tireless efforts ensure these young people are prepared to take care of all of us in the future.

Contributors

Ann Nancy Fogel, MA, CCLS
Senior Child Life Specialist
The Joseph M. Sanzari
  Children's Hospital
Hackensack University
  Medical Center
Hackensack, NJ

Ellen Goldring, LPC, ATR-BC, CCLS
Supervisor Child Life/Creative
  Arts Therapy
Hackensack University
  Medical Center
Hackensack, NJ

James B. Hammond, MA, PA-C
Professor
James Madison University
Harrisonburg, VA

Mizuho Kanazawa, ROT, LCAT, CCLS
Hackensack University
  Medical Center
Hackensack, NJ

Jeff G. Konin, PhD, ATC, PT
Visiting Associate Professor
Department of Orthopaedic Surgery
College of Medicine
University of South Florida
Executive Director
Sports Medicine and Athletic Related
  Trauma (SMART) Institute
Tampa, FL

Erika Leeuwenburgh, LPC,
  ATR-BC, CCLS
Chief Child Life/Creative
  Arts Therapy
Hackensack University
  Medical Center
Hackensack, NJ

Kristi L. Lewis, PhD, MPH
Assistant Professor
James Madison University
Harrisonburg, VA

Theresa M. Lynch, CCLS
Child Life Specialist
Pediatric Emergency Services
The Joseph M. Sanzari
  Children's Hospital
Hackensack University
  Medical Center
Hackensack, NJ

S. Margaret Maloney,
  MOT, OTR/L
Assistant Professor
Master of Occupation
  Therapy Program
Department of Health Sciences
Cleveland State University
Cleveland, OH

Vicki C. Martin, RN, BSN, MSN, PhD
Associate Professor of Nursing
James Madison University
Harrisonburg, VA

Jennifer McCabe, MLIS
Health and Human Services Librarian
James Madison University
Harrisonburg, VA

John Mondanaro, MA, MT-BC,
   LCAT, CCLS
Music Therapist
Senior Child Life Specialist
Hackensack University
   Medical Center
Hackensack, NJ

Stephanie Omens, MA-RDT,
   LCT, CCLS
Drama Therapist
Senior Child Life Specialist
Hackensack University
   Medical Center
Hackensack, NJ

Connie L. Peterson, PhD,
   MS, ATC
Assistant Professor
Department of Health Services
James Madison University
Harrisonburg, VA

R. Theresa Prodoehl, PhD
Assistant Professor
Health Sciences Department
James Madison University
Harrisonburg, VA

Jon M. Thompson, PhD
Professor & Director
Health Services
   Administration Program
James Madison University
Harrisonburg, VA

Tammy Wagner, RD, PhD
Associate Professor
James Madison University
Harrisonburg, VA

Introduction

C hances are, if you are reading this book, you have an interest in some aspect of health care. If you are a student, you may know exactly what you want to do when you finish your undergraduate years. Did you always want to be a doctor when you grew up? Some people just know they want to do something, and then work tirelessly to achieve that goal. Maybe you were influenced by a wonderful healthcare professional when you were sick or injured as a child. Perhaps the occupational or speech therapist that helped your grandmother after her stroke inspired you to think about careers in those fields. You may come from a long line of healthcare providers and know this is your destiny. However, you may not be so clear in your career aspirations. Many students take courses in health as part of the requirements for a general liberal arts education. In those classes, they discover they love learning about their bodies and how to keep them healthy. Others are not sure what they want for a career, but they know they "just want to help people."

Regardless of how you got to this stage, learning about different health professions and the foundations of health care in the United States will be helpful for whatever career path you choose. Understanding the changes in health care over the past century gives us a better perspective of why we do what we do in primary, secondary, and tertiary prevention today. The Healthy People 2010 objectives described in Chapter 2 will continue to influence the research and reimbursement for healthcare services into the next decade. Respect for patient privacy and how we pay for health care are other key elements driving the changes we constantly see in the health field. Government and voluntary health agencies provide valuable resources for research and even career opportunities in health care.

None of the health professionals highlighted in this book work entirely alone in taking care of a patient's every need. With the advances in knowledge and technology surrounding health care in recent decades, it is impossible to be an expert in *every* aspect of health care. There just isn't time to keep up-to-date on every element of patient care. While you may only want to know about your chosen career path, it is valuable to understand the other professionals you will work side by side with on your future healthcare team. They have different educational preparation, skills, and perhaps even a different philosophy guiding their approach to patient care. Not to mention, sometimes plans change. You may want to be one type of healthcare professional, but perhaps you need to have a plan B, or C, or even D, E, or F for your future. Have you ever tried a sample of a product in one of those "big box" stores that you never thought you would like, but now it is a favorite item? Or have you always wanted to own something, bought it, and then realized it was not as wonderful as you thought it would be? Many career options are available within the healthcare field. Learning about different healthcare professionals and what they do just might introduce you to a new possible career path.

Educational requirements and certification expectations are included for each of the professions profiled in this text. The competition for acceptance in some programs offering these advanced healthcare degrees can be fairly stiff. You are competing for a limited number of seats in graduate programs with other students who are equally qualified. Some of the programs, such as those for physician assistants, require you to demonstrate, through many hours of patient contact, that you are serious about wanting to pursue the career path. If a graduate program admits you, only to find you drop out because you don't like touching patients, the program has wasted a spot in that class and a great deal of energy on your education.

To set yourself apart from the rest of the applicant pool for health professional programs, it helps to show, through volunteer or paid experience, that you are committed to the pursuit of an advanced degree in the profession. Look for opportunities over the summer, or even during the school year, to start gaining valuable healthcare experience. Join the preprofessional student groups at your college or university. Keep track of your experiences, as well as those professionals you work with in those pursuits. They can provide invaluable advice on your chosen career, in addition to serving as mentors. They may also offer to write the letter of recommendation that sets you apart from the rest of the applicants with the same GPA and prerequisite course work.

Health care is provided in and out of hospitals and neighborhood clinics. Health care is open for business 24 hours a day, 7 days a week. Some professionals limit their availability to regular working hours. Others work beyond 9-to-5 shifts to ensure health care is available when needed by millions of men, women, and children, every day and night.

Health care is a stable career path with a bright future. As you read through this book, you will see that as a population, we are living longer. There are new techniques for prevention, diagnosis, and treatment of diseases and injuries under development every day. Each of the health professionals highlighted here plays an important role in helping people live longer, healthier lives.

Chapter 1

In Sickness and in Health

Stephanie Chisolm

OBJECTIVES

After studying this chapter, the student should be able to

1. Explain the spectrum of health.
2. Identify the various domains of health and the factors that influence health status.
3. Explain life expectancy.
4. Describe factors that influence life expectancy, especially as related to health care over the last century.
5. Explain and identify primary, secondary, and tertiary prevention efforts to maintain health.

INTRODUCTION

Health is not valued till sickness comes.
Dr. Thomas Fuller (1654–1734)

Discussions of health issues and the healthcare system dominate political and media debate as well as individual conversations across the nation. Health, defined as the absence of illness, suggests a negative connotation. A functional definition of health is the ability to cope with everyday activities. A more positive perspective on health implies fitness and well-being. In any living organism, health is a form of homeostasis, a relatively stable state of equilibrium or a tendency toward such a state between the different but interdependent elements or groups of elements of an organism.

Health implies good prospects for continued survival. In humans, health encompasses broader concepts, as evidenced in the definition of health in the original mission of the World Health Organization (WHO), headquartered in Geneva, Switzerland. Established by the United Nations in 1948, WHO defines health as "a state of complete physical, mental, and social well-being, and does not consist only of the absence of disease or infirmity."

While most consider the WHO perspective the core explanation of health in humans, this definition does not provide a clear and quantifiable measure of actual health. How do you assess a "state of complete physical, mental, and social well-being?" Often, observable illness, disease, or disabilities become measures of degrees of health. The spectrum of health ranges from good to poor; one can be in a state of good health, a state of poor health, or anywhere in between. A person can function adequately from the perspective of physical and physiological abilities yet have poor mental health. Individuals can at once be relatively healthy in some aspects of life (for example, normal blood pressure of 120/80 mmHg), but unhealthy in others (for example, suffering from depression or diabetes). Thus, being healthy is not an "all-or-nothing" principle.

Health Influences

There are many facets to being healthy and many influences on our health. Some we can control, such as our diet, and others we cannot, such as our gender or genetic predisposition to illness. Factors that influence health may come from the *individual*, the *community* the individual lives in, or the *environment*. *Interpersonal factors* and even the *health care system* may also have some bearing on health.

Individual factors influencing health status include lifestyle and behaviors. Since 1964, the US Surgeon General has warned that smoking is hazardous to health. Poor dietary habits and lack of physical exercise influence obesity, a risk factor for diabetes. Engaging in sexual intercourse without using contraception places a couple at risk for unintended pregnancy. Acute and chronic physical or emotional stress may affect other risk factors and behaviors, such as high blood pressure and cholesterol levels, smoking, physical inactivity, and overeating. Individuals may inherit risk factors genetically, such as sickle cell anemia, the most common inherited blood disorder in the United States, affecting about 72,000 Americans or 1 in 500 African Americans.

Communities influence health status through available resources such as parks, jogging trails, or safe places for pedestrians to walk or ride a bike, thus increasing exercise opportunities. Community programs such as mental health services may also influence health. Many community agencies offer youth programs, elderly care, exercise or fitness classes, stress management, or other health education services to improve the health of the populations they serve. Local pharmacies or grocery stores may provide opportunities for screening for conditions such as high blood pressure or cholesterol.

Air, water, temperature, pollution, and other hazards may create environmental factors that influence health. The Environmental Protection Agency (EPA) together with other government agencies report daily Air Quality Index (AQI) values. The AQI is an index for reporting daily air quality. It tells you how clean or polluted the air is, and what associated health effects might be a concern for individuals in those communities. The AQI focuses on health effects experienced within a few hours or days after breathing polluted air. EPA calculates the AQI for five major air pollutants regulated by the Clean Air Act: ground-level ozone, particle pollution (also known as particulate matter), carbon monoxide, sulfur dioxide, and nitrogen dioxide. For each of these pollutants, EPA has established national air quality standards to protect public health. Think of the AQI as a yardstick that runs from 0 to 500 with higher AQI values indicating greater levels of air pollution and subsequently greater health concerns. An AQI value of 100 generally corresponds to the national air quality standard for the pollutant, which is the level EPA has set to protect public health. AQI values below 100 are satisfactory. When AQI values are above 100, air quality is unhealthy—first for sensitive groups of people such as asthmatics or the elderly, then for everyone as AQI values get higher (see Figure 1.1). Air quality, announced to communities through

Air Quality Index (AQI) Values	*Levels of Health Concern*	*Colors*
When the AQI is in this range:	**...air quality conditions are:**	**...as symbolized by this color:**
0 to 50	Good	Green
51 to 100	Moderate	Yellow
101 to 150	Unhealthy for Sensitive Groups	Orange
151 to 200	Unhealthy	Red
201 to 300	Very Unhealthy	Purple
301 to 500	Hazardous	Maroon

Figure 1.1 *Air Quality Index Values*
Source: Environmental Protection Agency *Air Now*. 40 CFR Part 58 Air Quality Index Reporting; Final Rule Federal Register Vol. 64, No. 149/Wednesday, August 4, 1999/Rules & Regulations, http://www.epa.gov/fedrgstr/EPA-AIR/1999/August/Day-04/a19433.pdf. Retrieved 11/04/06.

public information channels, usually utilizes a color scale of air quality hazards, green representing good AQI, maroon for hazardous AQI.

Another aspect of our environment that can influence health is the water. Standing water in communities or even in your own backyard provides breeding ground for mosquitoes, known carriers of West Nile Virus and other diseases that impact humans and other animals. Swallowing recreational water, including water in swimming pools, hot tubs, fountains, lakes, rivers, or streams contaminated with sewage or feces from humans or animals may cause Giardiasis (GEE-are-DYE-uh-sis), a diarrheal illness caused by a one-celled, microscopic parasite, *Giardia intestinalis* (also known as *Giardia lamblia*). The United States has one of the safest water supplies in the world. However, drinking water quality varies from place to place, depending on the condition of the source from which it is drawn and the treatment it receives. Every community water supplier must provide an annual report (sometimes called a consumer confidence report) to its customers. The report provides information on local drinking water quality, including the water's source, the contaminants found in the water, and an explanation of how consumers can get involved in protecting drinking water.

Extreme heat, another environmental condition, occurs when temperatures hover 10 degrees Fahrenheit or more above the average high temperature for the region and last for several weeks. Humid or muggy conditions, which add to the discomfort of high temperatures, occur when a "dome" of high atmospheric pressure traps hazy, damp air near the ground. Excessively dry and hot conditions can provoke dust storms and low visibility. Droughts occur when a long period passes without substantial rainfall. A heat wave combined with a drought is a very dangerous situation. Even short periods of high temperatures can cause serious health problems. Doing too much on a hot day, spending too much time in the sun, or staying too long in an overheated place can cause heat-related illnesses. Heat-related deaths and illness are preventable, yet annually many people succumb to extreme heat. Historically, from 1979 to 1999, excessive heat exposure caused 8,015 deaths in the United States. During this period, more people in this country died from extreme heat than from hurricanes, lightning, tornadoes, floods, and earthquakes combined. People suffer heat-related illness when their bodies are unable to compensate and properly cool themselves. Elderly people (that is, people aged 65 years and older) are more prone to heat stress because they do not adjust as well as young people to sudden changes in temperature. The elderly are more likely to have chronic medical conditions that respond to heat and are more likely to take prescription medicines that impair the body's ability to regulate its temperature. Nearly 15,000 elderly people died in France in August 2003 when temperatures reached record levels.

Interpersonal factors that may influence health include relationships and support systems. Social support received from friends, family, and coworkers can help or hinder health. Support may take objective and tangible forms, such as money, or rides to a doctor's office, or be more subjective, as in the case of close, high-quality relationships, which encourage the perception that you can count on others. Family ties, friendships, and involvement in social activities can offer a psychological buffer against stress, anxiety, and depression. People with social ties—regardless of their source—live longer than people who are isolated. People with a close network of ties with others seem to maintain better health, resist disease, and deal more successfully with problems they encounter. A study by Dr. Sheldon Cohen (2001) through the National Institutes of Health Office of Behavioral and Social Sciences Research found that diverse ties to friends, family, work, and community help to reduce susceptibility to upper respiratory illness. Chicken soup may provide relief to cold symptoms, but the friend who brings you the soup appears to be important in maintaining health.

The healthcare system itself can even influence the health of individuals if there are problems accessing quality health care. Health care refers to the industry related to the health of an individual. Various aspects of the health-care system are associated with the prevention, diagnosis, therapeutic treatment, and management of illness, along with the promotion of mental, physical, and spiritual well-being through the services offered by the medical and allied health professions discussed in detail in this text. Health care is one of the world's largest and fastest-growing industries, consuming over 10% of the gross domestic product of most developed nations. Research and technologies have improved our knowledge about disease causality and expanded treatment options, thus enabling individuals to live longer, healthier lives. In fact, life expectancy has dramatically increased over the last few centuries of human history, largely the result of improvements in public health, medicine, and nutrition.

Living a Long and Healthy Life: Life Expectancy in the United States

Life expectancy is the average number of years of life remaining to a person at a particular age, as based on a given set of age-specific death rates, generally the mortality conditions existing in the period mentioned. Life expectancy may be determined by race, gender, or other characteristics using age-specific death rates for the population with that characteristic. Life expectancy can

Table 1.1 *Life Expectancy at Birth, Age 65, and Age 75, According to Race and Sex: Selected Years, 1900-2003*

(Data are based on death certificates)

Specified age and year	All Races			White			Black or African American[1]		
	Both sexes	Male	Female	Both sexes	Male	Female	Both sexes	Male	Female
At birth				Remaining life expectancy in years					
1900[2,3]...........	47.3	46.3	48.3	47.6	46.6	48.7	33.0	32.5	33.5
1950[3]...........	68.2	65.6	71.1	69.1	66.5	72.2	60.8	59.1	62.9
1960[3]...........	69.7	66.6	73.1	70.6	67.4	74.1	63.6	61.1	66.3
1970...........	70.8	67.1	74.7	71.7	68.0	75.6	64.1	60.0	68.3
1975...........	72.6	68.8	76.6	73.4	69.5	77.3	66.8	62.4	71.3
1980...........	73.7	70.0	77.4	74.4	70.7	78.1	68.1	63.8	72.5
1981...........	74.1	70.4	77.8	74.8	71.1	78.4	68.9	64.5	73.2
1982...........	74.5	70.8	78.1	75.1	71.5	78.7	69.4	65.1	73.6
1983...........	74.6	71.0	78.1	75.2	71.6	78.7	69.4	65.2	73.5
1984...........	74.7	71.1	78.2	75.3	71.8	78.7	69.5	65.3	73.6
1985...........	74.7	71.1	78.2	75.3	71.8	78.7	69.3	65.0	73.4
1986...........	74.7	71.2	78.2	75.4	71.9	78.8	69.1	64.8	73.4
1987...........	74.9	71.4	78.3	75.6	72.1	78.9	69.1	64.7	73.4
1988...........	74.9	71.4	78.3	75.6	72.2	78.9	68.9	64.4	73.2
1989...........	75.1	71.7	78.5	75.9	72.5	79.2	68.8	64.3	73.3
1990...........	75.4	71.8	78.8	76.1	72.7	79.4	69.1	64.5	73.6

Table 1.1 *Life Expectancy at Birth, Age 65, and Age 75, According to Race and Sex: Selected Years, 1900-2003 (continued)*

Specified age and year	All Races			White			Black or African American[1]		
	Both sexes	Male	Female	Both sexes	Male	Female	Both sexes	Male	Female
At birth				Remaining life expectancy in years					
1991............	75.5	72.0	78.9	76.3	72.9	79.6	69.3	64.6	73.8
1992............	75.8	72.3	79.1	76.5	73.2	79.8	69.6	65.0	73.9
1993............	75.5	72.2	78.8	76.3	73.1	79.5	69.2	64.6	73.7
1994............	75.7	72.4	79.0	76.5	73.3	79.6	69.5	64.9	73.9
1995............	75.8	72.5	78.9	76.5	73.4	79.6	69.6	65.2	73.9
1996............	76.1	73.1	79.1	76.8	73.9	79.7	70.2	66.1	74.2
1997............	76.5	73.6	79.4	77.1	74.3	79.9	71.1	67.2	74.7
1998............	76.7	73.8	79.5	77.3	74.5	80.0	71.3	67.6	74.8
1999............	76.7	73.9	79.4	77.3	74.6	79.9	71.4	67.8	74.7
2000............	77.0	74.3	79.7	77.6	74.9	80.1	71.9	68.3	75.2
2001............	77.2	74.4	79.8	77.7	75.0	80.2	72.2	68.6	75.5
2002............	77.3	74.5	79.9	77.7	75.1	80.3	72.3	68.8	75.6
2003............	77.5	74.8	80.1	78.0	75.3	80.5	72.7	69.0	76.1
At 65 years									
1950[3].........	13.9	12.8	15.0	—	12.8	15.1	13.9	12.9	14.9
1960[3].........	14.3	12.8	15.8	14.4	12.9	15.9	13.9	12.7	15.1

continues

Table 1.1 *Life Expectancy at Birth, Age 65, and Age 75, According to Race and Sex: Selected Years, 1900-2003 (continued)*

Specified age and year	All Races			White			Black or African American[1]		
	Both sexes	Male	Female	Both sexes	Male	Female	Both sexes	Male	Female
At 65 years	Remaining life expectancy in years								
1970............	15.2	13.1	17.0	15.2	13.1	17.1	14.2	12.5	15.7
1975............	16.1	13.8	18.1	16.1	13.8	18.2	15.0	13.1	16.7
1980............	16.4	14.1	18.3	16.5	14.2	18.4	15.1	13.0	16.8
1981............	16.6	14.3	18.6	16.7	14.4	18.7	15.5	13.4	17.2
1982............	16.8	14.5	18.7	16.9	14.5	18.8	15.7	13.5	17.5
1983............	16.7	14.4	18.6	16.8	14.5	18.7	15.4	13.2	17.2
1984............	16.8	14.5	18.6	16.8	14.6	18.7	15.4	13.2	17.2
1985............	16.7	14.5	18.5	16.8	14.5	18.7	15.2	13.0	16.9
1986............	16.8	14.6	18.6	16.9	14.7	18.7	15.2	13.0	17.0
1987............	16.9	14.7	18.7	17.0	14.8	18.8	15.2	13.0	17.0
1988............	16.9	14.7	18.6	17.0	14.8	18.7	15.1	12.9	16.9
1989............	17.1	15.0	18.8	17.2	15.1	18.9	15.2	13.0	16.9
1990............	17.2	15.1	18.9	17.3	15.2	19.1	15.4	13.2	17.2
1991............	17.4	15.3	19.1	17.5	15.4	19.2	15.5	13.4	17.2
1992............	17.5	15.4	19.2	17.6	15.5	19.3	15.7	13.5	17.4
1993............	17.3	15.3	18.9	17.4	15.4	19.0	15.5	13.4	17.1
1994............	17.4	15.5	19.0	17.5	15.6	19.1	15.7	13.6	17.2

Table 1.1 *Life Expectancy at Birth, Age 65, and Age 75, According to Race and Sex: Selected Years, 1900-2003 (continued)*

Specified age and year	All Races			White			Black or African American[1]		
	Both sexes	Male	Female	Both sexes	Male	Female	Both sexes	Male	Female
	Remaining life expectancy in years								
At 65 years									
1995............	17.4	15.6	18.9	17.6	15.7	19.1	15.6	13.6	17.1
1996............	17.5	15.7	19.0	17.6	15.8	19.1	15.8	13.9	17.2
1997............	17.7	15.9	19.2	17.8	16.0	19.3	16.1	14.2	17.6
1998............	17.8	16.0	19.2	17.8	16.1	19.3	16.1	14.3	17.4
1999............	17.7	16.1	19.1	17.8	16.1	19.2	16.0	14.3	17.3
2000............	18.0	16.2	19.3	18.0	16.3	19.4	16.2	14.2	17.7
2001............	18.1	16.4	19.4	18.2	16.5	19.5	16.4	14.4	17.9
2002............	18.2	16.6	19.5	18.2	16.6	19.5	16.6	14.6	18.0
2003............	18.4	16.8	19.8	18.5	16.9	19.8	17.0	14.9	18.5
At 75 years									
1980............	10.4	8.8	11.5	10.4	8.8	11.5	9.7	8.3	10.7
1981............	10.6	9.0	11.7	10.6	9.0	11.7	10.4	9.0	11.4
1982............	10.7	9.1	11.9	10.7	9.0	11.9	10.6	9.1	11.6
1983............	10.6	9.0	11.7	10.6	8.9	11.7	10.3	8.9	11.4
1984............	10.7	9.0	11.8	10.7	9.0	11.8	10.3	8.9	11.4
1985............	10.6	9.0	11.7	10.6	9.0	11.7	10.1	8.7	11.1

continues

Table 1.1 *Life Expectancy at Birth, Age 65, and Age 75, According to Race and Sex: Selected Years, 1900-2003 (continued)*

Specified age and year	All Races			White			Black or African American[1]		
	Both sexes	Male	Female	Both sexes	Male	Female	Both sexes	Male	Female
At 75 years				Remaining life expectancy in years					
1986............	10.7	9.1	11.7	10.7	9.1	11.8	10.1	8.6	11.1
1987............	10.7	9.1	11.8	10.7	9.1	11.8	10.1	8.6	11.1
1988............	10.6	9.1	11.7	10.7	9.1	11.7	10.0	8.5	11.0
1989............	10.9	9.3	11.9	10.9	9.3	11.9	10.1	8.6	11.0
1990............	10.9	9.4	12.0	11.0	9.4	12.0	10.2	8.6	11.2
1991............	11.1	9.5	12.1	11.1	9.5	12.1	10.2	8.7	11.2
1992............	11.2	9.6	12.2	11.2	9.6	12.2	10.4	8.9	11.4
1993............	10.9	9.5	11.9	11.0	9.5	12.0	10.2	8.7	11.1
1994............	11.0	9.6	12.0	11.1	9.6	12.0	10.3	8.9	11.2
1995............	11.0	9.7	11.9	11.1	9.7	12.0	10.2	8.8	11.1
1996............	11.1	9.8	12.0	11.1	9.8	12.0	10.3	9.0	11.2
1997............	11.2	9.9	12.1	11.2	9.9	12.1	10.7	9.3	11.5
1998............	11.3	10.0	12.2	11.3	10.0	12.2	10.5	9.2	11.3
1999............	11.2	10.0	12.1	11.2	10.0	12.1	10.4	9.2	11.1
2000............	11.4	10.1	12.3	11.4	10.1	12.3	10.7	9.2	11.6
2001............	11.5	10.2	12.4	11.5	10.2	12.3	10.8	9.3	11.7
2002............	11.5	10.3	12.4	11.5	10.3	12.3	10.9	9.5	11.7
2003............	11.8	10.5	12.6	11.7	10.5	12.6	11.4	9.8	12.4

Table 1.1 *Life Expectancy at Birth, Age 65, and Age 75, According to Race and Sex: Selected Years, 1900-2003 (continued)*

—Data not available.

[1]Data shown for 1900–60 are for the nonwhite population.

[2]Death registration area only. The death registration area increased from 10 States and the District of Columbia in 1900 to the coterminous United States in 1933. See Appendix II, Registration area.

[3]Includes deaths of persons who were not residents of the 50 States and the District of Columbia.

NOTES: Populations for computing life expectancy for 1991–99 are 1990-based postcensal estimates of U.S. resident population. See Appendix I, Population Census and Population Estimates.

In 1997, life table methodology was revised to construct complete life tables by single years of age that extend to age 100 (Anderson RN. Method for Constructing Complete Annual U.S. Life Tables. National Center for Health Statistics. Vital Health Stat 2(129). 1999). Previously abridged life tables were constructed for 5-year age groups ending with 85 years and over.

Life table values for 2000 and later years were computed using a slight modification of the new life table method due to a change in the age detail of populations received from the U.S. Census Bureau. Beginning in 2003, California, Hawaii, Idaho, Maine, Montana, New York, and Wisconsin reported multiple-race data. The multiple-race data for these states were bridged to the single race categories of the 1977 Office of Management and Budget standards for comparability with other states.

Data for additional years are available. See Appendix III.

SOURCES: Grove & Hetzel (1968); Hoyert et al. (2006); NCHS (2004).

change over the lifecycle. For example, at birth, we expect a person to live for 75 years, but if they survive to 75, they may be expected to live for another 10 years. According to the National Vital Statistics report, a child born in 1900 had a life expectancy of 47.3 years. A baby born in 2002 can expect to live to 77.3 years. Extremely high infant and childhood mortality distorted the lower life expectancy in the early 1900s. If a person did make it to age 40 a century ago, they had an average of another 20 years to live. Improvements in health care have therefore mainly increased the numbers of people living beyond childhood, with less effect on overall average lifespan.

There are great variations in life expectancy worldwide, and variations between groups within single countries. In the United States in the early 20th century, large differences in life expectancy existed between people of different races; those differences have since lessened. There remain significant differences in life expectancy between men and women in the United States and other developed countries, with women outliving men. Historically in the United States, young women ran a high risk of dying during or after childbirth. Thanks to improved prenatal and obstetric care, death rates from pregnancy-related causes have fallen to very low levels. Today, women have lower mortality rates at every age. Men are three times as likely as women to die from injuries (unintentional injuries, suicide, or homicide) and progress against those causes of death has been much slower than against other causes in the last 50 years. There is also evidence that men at all ages are less likely to seek medical care and less likely to comply with medical instructions than are women.

Infant mortality and mortality from heart disease, stroke, and unintentional injuries are all substantially lower than in the 1950s, contributing to increased life expectancy. Most of the last century's improvements in life expectancy have resulted from reductions in infectious diseases among infants and children. The decline in mortality rates for these major killers is attributed to improvements in public health efforts, medical technologies, and standards of living and hygiene. In spite of advances in medicine and health care over the past century, while we have increased lifespan, we have greater rate of incidence of a disease, or *morbidity*, today because greater numbers of the population are living longer lives. Today, the leading causes of death are cardiovascular disease (heart disease), malignant neoplasms (cancer), and cerebrovascular disease (stroke). Many influencing or determining elements and factors contribute to these leading causes of morbidity and mortality. With more individuals living longer lives, the opportunity for exposure to disease-causing agents in the environment or through risky behaviors such as smoking or poor dietary choices in addition to age-related health factors, increase the need for health care in later years. As a result, we become more dependent on the medical system to keep us healthy.

| | | Deaths (per 100,000 people) |
Male	*Number of Deaths*	*Death Rates*
All Causes	1,777,578	1,043
Heart disease	344,807	315
Cancer	286,082	247
Stroke	64,769	61
Accidents	63,817	50
CLRD*	60,004	55
Diabetes	31,602	28
Pneumonia	28,658	28
Suicide	23,618	18
Kidney disease	17,811	17
Cirrhosis of the liver	17,214	14
Female	*Number of Deaths*	*Death Rates*
All Causes	1,225,773	739
Heart disease	365,953	213
Cancer	267,009	170
Stroke	102,892	60
CLRD*	62,005	38
Diabetes	37,655	23
Pneumonia	36,655	21
Alzheimer's disease	35,120	20
Accidents	34,083	22
Kidney disease	19,440	12
Septicemia	17,687	11

Note: CLRD refers to chronic lower respiratory diseases, which included chronic bronchitis and emphysema.

Source: (Minino et al., 2002)

Figure 1.2   *Age-adjusted Death Rates for Ten Leading Causes of Death in the United States, by Gender, 2000*

Miracles and Modern Medicine

Medicine, often considered something that treats, prevents, or alleviates the symptoms of disease, has contributed significant advances over time. Hippocrates, known as the Father of Modern Medicine (460 BC to 380 BC), was the first physician to use a scientific approach to the study and treatment of disease. In a time when people attributed illness to evil spirits and angering the gods, Hippocrates rejected the superstition and magic of primitive "medicine" and laid the foundations of medicine as a branch of science. Many of the descriptions of disease that he wrote more than two thousand years ago are still accurate.

Today, medicine often refers specifically to matters dealt with by physicians and surgeons. However, scientific advances in the last century have improved the prognosis for many health conditions beyond the traditional role of physicians in preventing and curing diseases. Modern medicine encompasses a wide array of treatments with a diverse assortment of professions to address an enormous variety of conditions across the lifespan. Yet some illnesses defy the best medical interventions. There are ailments that develop for no apparent reason, others that occur due to lifestyle or behaviors of the individual. Some chronic diseases require lifelong medical intervention and others disappear without any treatments, as if by magic. According to Dr. Thomas Stephen Szasz (1973), "Formerly, when religion was strong and science weak, men mistook magic for medicine; now, when science is strong and religion weak, men mistake medicine for magic." Today, we expect that modern medicine, the branch of science concerned with restoring and maintaining health, can cure most conditions. We are constantly in search of new and better treatments and therapies to improve the quality of life for those who are ill or disabled.

Caring for Our Health

People use healthcare services for many reasons: to cure illnesses and health conditions, to mend breaks and tears, to prevent or delay future healthcare problems, to reduce pain, to increase quality of life, and sometimes merely to obtain information about their health status and prognosis. The healthcare delivery system has undergone tremendous change, even over the past decade. New and emerging technologies, including drugs, devices, procedures, tests, and imaging have changed patterns of care and the sites in which that care is provided. Greater understanding of the origin and development or pathogenesis of diseases has suggested intervening treatments that may prevent disease, stop it from progressing, or rehabilitate individuals with a variety of health conditions. Most patients diagnosed with life-threatening conditions or diseases receive care from a team of healthcare providers, each with advanced training and education in his/her own area of expertise. With the vast array of new knowledge related to health being discovered every year, it would be difficult for one person to respond adequately to every health need for patients. Thus, a team approach allows experts in specific areas to work collaboratively to provide the best care to individuals who may be ill.

The various branches of the science of medicine correspond to specialized medical professions dealing with particular organs or diseases. The science of medicine is the knowledge of body systems and diseases, while the profession of medicine refers to the social structure of the group of people formally trained to apply that knowledge to treat disease. Allied health professionals work closely with medical professionals to aid the prevention, diagnosis, treatment, and rehabilitation of diseases in a variety of settings. The remaining chapters of this text describe a variety of medical and allied health professional careers. Allied healthcare professionals can include physical therapists, psychologists, occupational therapists, and dietitians, to name a few. Each of the professionals described in this text can work with individuals or even communities to prevent, diagnose, or treat many different health conditions.

Levels of Prevention for Healthy Lives

An ounce of prevention is a ton of work.
Paul Frame, MD

Treatments or measures used to prevent diseases from occurring in the first place are *primary prevention*. The US Preventative Services Task Forces' Guide to Clinical Preventive Services (USPSTF, 1996) defines primary prevention measures as "those provided to individuals to prevent the onset of a targeted condition." Primary prevention occurs in the "pre-pathogenesis period," which means before the development of a disease. Primary prevention efforts identify behavioral, genetic, environmental, and other risk factors that increase the individual's likelihood of contracting a disease or condition. Primary prevention measures include activities that help avoid a given healthcare problem. Examples of primary prevention include immunizations, the process of inducing immunity by administering an antigen (vaccine) that is derived from the infecting (or similar) agent, in order to allow the immune system to prevent infection or illness when it subsequently encounters the infectious agent. Primary prevention also encompasses health-protecting education and counseling, for example, promoting the use of automobile passenger restraints and bicycle helmets. Since successful primary prevention helps avoid the suffering, cost, and burden associated with disease; it is typically considered the most cost-effective form of health care.

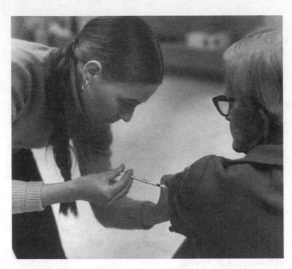

Figure 1.3
Source: Courtesy of CDC.

The US Preventative Services Task Force describes *secondary prevention* measures as those that "identify and treat asymptomatic persons who have already developed risk factors or preclinical disease but in whom the condition is not clinically apparent." These activities are focused on early case finding of asymptomatic disease that occurs commonly and has significant risk for negative outcome without treatment. Screening tests are examples of secondary prevention activities, as these are done on individuals without clinical presentation of a disease that has a significant latency period, such as hyperlipidemia, hypertension, and breast and prostate cancer. Secondary prevention activities target those who are more susceptible to health problems because of family history, age, lifestyle, health condition, or environmental factors. With early diagnosis, the natural history of disease, or how the course of an illness unfolds over time without treatment, can often be altered to maximize well-being and minimize suffering.

Medical science is working to improve the ability to diagnose disease earlier. Treatments provided before diseases manifest in noticeable health conditions may halt the progression of a disease and improve the prognosis for a

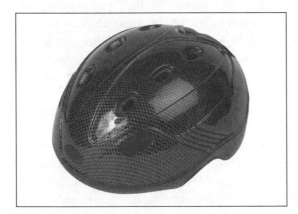

Figure 1.4
Source: © Photos.com.

longer, healthier life. One of the most aggressively marketed, potentially lucrative and perhaps controversial procedures in medicine is the full-body scanning of symptom-free patients. Used to detect presymptomatic diseases, a full-body CT scan, also known as computerized tomography, offers individuals a 3-dimensional diagnostic image of their inner body, from the brain to the pelvis. This technology provides a non-invasive procedure that checks for benign and malignant tumors, aneurysms, polyps, emphysema, and many other health conditions. Early detection provides time to optimize the treatment of the patient by detecting a disease before it manifests and can uncover life-threatening diseases not detectable during annual physicals. Some advocates welcome this procedure because it allows for treatment that is less costly and less invasive. Free-standing scanning centers, some located in shopping malls and many owned by radiologists, have sprung up in affluent metropolitan areas and offer a comprehensive, painless, noninvasive, head-to-pelvis examination of the body's internal organs—including the brain, heart, liver, lungs, prostate, and ovaries—for a $700 to $1,300 fee that is rarely covered by insurance. Critics say the practice is unproven, ill-advised, and potentially dangerous. There is concern that the procedure would lead to the discovery of numerous findings that would not ultimately affect patients' health, but would result in increased patient anxiety, unnecessary follow-up examinations and treatments, and wasted expense. Critics also worry that radiation exposure could increase the risk of developing cancer, especially in those who undergo repeated scans. Another drawback to the technology is inaccuracy in the form of false negatives and positives, which could trigger further tests that could be risky and expensive.

Full-body CT scans aside, there are many secondary prevention procedures that can and do save pain and suffering by identifying diseases early in their most treatable stages. The American Heart Association supports secondary prevention efforts to identify and treat persons with established disease or those at very high risk of developing cardiovascular disease. Providing comprehensive risk factor interventions may improve clinical outcomes, extend overall survival, and improve quality of life.

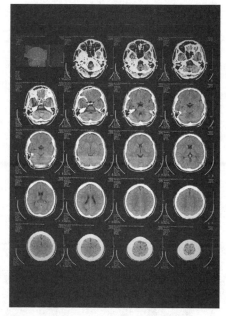

Tertiary prevention activities involve the care of established disease, with attempts made to restore to highest function, minimize the negative effects of disease, and prevent disease-related complications. Since the disease is now established, primary prevention activities may have been unsuccessful. Early detection through secondary prevention may

Figure 1.5
Source: © Trout55/ShutterStock, Inc.

have minimized the impact of the disease. Tertiary prevention is directed at managing and rehabilitating persons with diagnosed health conditions to reduce complications, improve their quality of life, and extend their years of productivity. Examples of tertiary prevention include post-operative physical therapy to regain mobility, surgery, or routine eye and foot exams for people who have diabetes.

As mentioned earlier, many health professionals play a role in all levels of prevention—primary, secondary, and tertiary. Others who are primarily involved in primary prevention activities may spend most of their time in one prevention phase, such as public health educators.

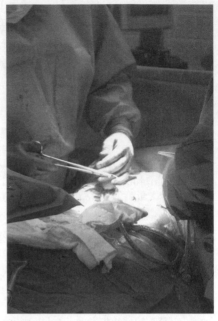

Figure 1.6
Source: © Dewayne Flowers/ShutterStock, Inc.

Trends in the Health of Americans

Monitoring the health of the nation is essential for identifying and prioritizing health policy, program, and research initiatives. Examining the current health status of a population, as well as the determinants of health, provides critical information to assess how healthcare resources are best utilized to improve the health of the people. By examining emerging trends, it is possible to identify diseases, conditions, and risk factors that warrant the attention of those providing health care in this country. Over the past 50 years, many diseases have been controlled or their morbidity and mortality substantially reduced. The improvements in health have occurred in part because of the resources that have been devoted to health education, public health programs, health research, and health care. A decline in the death rate from heart disease is an example of a major public health achievement and is partly due to public health education campaigns emphasizing healthy lifestyle (primary prevention) and the increased use of cholesterol-lowering medications (secondary prevention). The percentage of mothers receiving prenatal care in the first trimester of pregnancy has continued to edge upward. The percentage of children 19–35 months of age vaccinated for many childhood infectious diseases is at a high level. Decreased cigarette smoking in adults is a prime example of a trend in a risk factor for disease and death that has contributed to declines in mortality. Yet even with decreases in smoking since the Surgeon General's Report in 1964, about 25% of men and 20% of women were current smokers in 2002. Public health and private efforts to improve motor vehicle safety, as well as to increase safety in homes and workplaces, have contributed to lower death rates for children and adults. New medical treatments for diseases (tertiary prevention) can dramatically delay or decrease the number of deaths caused by HIV or other diseases. Infant mortality as well as mortality from heart disease, stroke, and unintentional injuries are all substantially lower than in 1950, contributing to the upward trend in life expectancy. However, the aging population is associated with increased prevalence of chronic conditions. The number of adults and children who are overweight, obese, or physically inactive has reached epidemic proportions in this country. Excessive weight places individuals at significant risk for several chronic diseases, including diabetes and cardiovascular disease.

Efforts to improve health care, and ultimately the quality and length of life for our citizens, present many challenges in a nation that is growing older and becoming more racially and ethnically diverse. As health services move further into the 21st century and new opportunities to improve health are discovered, the prospects for careers helping people to be well continue to expand.

SUMMARY

Many individuals do not think about their health much—until something goes wrong. Threats to health may come from within the individual (for example, genetic risk factors), but also from the people you interact with, the communities you live in, and the behaviors you practice. Likewise, the people you interact with, the communities you live in, and the behaviors you practice can do much to improve your health and quality of life!

Major medical advances over the past century have done a great deal to improve the length and quality of life for many individuals in this country. Medical breakthroughs such as immunizations enable us through primary prevention to avoid life-threatening health conditions such as tetanus. New diagnostic tests present opportunities and dilemmas for finding diseases early. Advances in tertiary prevention treat diseases and injuries that decades ago saw high rates of morbidity and mortality. The knowledge base of biological and behavioral causes of disease and disability continues to expand. The need for advanced training and specialization to create the greatest skills in healthcare providers also continues to expand. The following chapters will highlight additional information about health care in the United States, as well as provide in-depth information about various career education, training, and practice options in medicine and allied health care.

REFERENCES

Cohen, S. (2001). Social relationships and susceptibiity to the common cold. In C. D. Ryff & B. H. Singer (Eds.) *Emotion, Social Relationships, and Health* (pp. 221–242). NY: Oxford University Press.

Grove, R. D. & Hetzel, A. M. (1968). *Vital statistics rates in the United States: 1940–1960*. Washington, DC: US Government Printing Office.

Hoyert, D. L., Heron, M. P., Murphy, S. L., & Kung, H. (2006). Deaths: Final data for 2003. *National Vital Statistics Reports 2006, 54*(13), Hyattsville, MD: NCHS Publications.

Minino, A. M., Arias, E., Kochanek, K. D., Murphy, S. L., & Smith, B. (2002). Deaths: Final data for 2000. *National Vital Statistics Reports, 50*(15), Tables 12 and 16.

National Center for Health Statistics (NCHS). (2004). *Health, United States, 2004 with chartbook on trends in the health of Americans*. Hyattsville, MD: NCHS Publications.

Szasz, T. (1973). *The Second Sin.* Garden City, NY: Anchor/Doubleday.

U.S. Preventative Services Task Force (USPSTF). (1996). *Guide to clinical preventive services* (2nd ed.). Baltimore: Williams & Wilkins.

ADDITIONAL RESOURCES

World Health Organization (WHO)	http://www.who.int
Centers for Disease Control and Prevention	http://www.cdc.gov/
National Center for Health Statistics	http://www.cdc.gov/nchs
Health, United States 2004 Chartbook on Trends in the Health of Americans	http://www.cdc.gov/nchs/hus.htm

Chapter 2

Promoting Health for a Nation: Healthy People 2010

Stephanie Chisolm

OBJECTIVES

After studying this chapter, the student should be able to

1. Explain the historical development process of Healthy People 2010.
2. Describe the goals, objectives, and function of Healthy People 2010.
3. Identify the 10 leading health indicators used to monitor progress toward Healthy People 2010 objectives.
4. Describe the processes used to evaluate the impact of Healthy People 2010 objectives.

INTRODUCTION

> *Healthy citizens are the greatest asset any country can have.*
> Winston Churchill (1874–1965)

Modern medical miracles offer the hope of long and healthy lives to many Americans. Along with the increase in life expectancy, a host of allied health professionals have expanded the scope and practice of health care in the United States. We have seen an increase in professional specialization, as healthcare providers strive to achieve a diverse, culturally competent health workforce that provides the highest quality health care for all, especially the underserved populations. The prevention, diagnosis, and treatment of disease and injury and the rehabilitation and maintenance of individuals challenged by acute and chronic health conditions support a trillion-dollar industry. In fact, US health expenditures grew to $1.7 trillion in 2003, accounting for 15.3% of the Gross Domestic Product, and outpacing growth in the overall economy by 3 percentage points (CMS, 2003). Rising medical costs are frequently topics of debate, around dinner tables, political circles, and within the healthcare industry itself.

While over a trillion dollars seems like a huge sum, especially when compared to poorer countries, higher spending on health care does not necessarily prolong lives. In 2000, the United States spent more on health care than any other country in the world: an average of $4,500 per person. Switzerland was second highest, at $3,300 or 71%. Nevertheless, average US life expectancy ranks 27th in the world, at 77 years. Many countries achieve higher life expectancy rates with significantly lower spending. With a life expectancy of 76.9 years, Cuba ranks 28th in the world. However, Cuba's spending per person on health care is one of the lowest in the world, at $186, about one twenty-fifth of the spending of the United States (UC Atlas, 2005). Comparing Cuba with the United States, vastly increased spending does not necessarily enable significantly longer life expectancies.

In addition to spending more per capita, over 45 million Americans lack basic health insurance, and are therefore less likely to receive preventive care. In contrast, Cuba has universal health care and one of the highest doctor-to-patient ratios in the world. While health care in the United States is among the best in the world, the technologies and treatments available are not accessible to all. People of color and other vulnerable populations are more likely to experience healthcare barriers and to suffer from high rates of disease and early death.

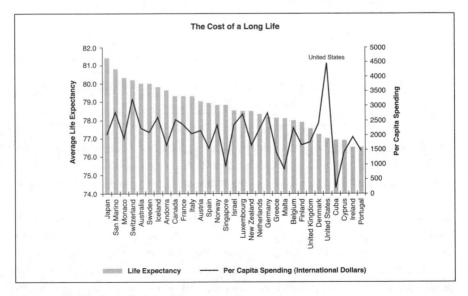

Figure 2.1 *The Cost of a Long Life*
Source: UC Atlas of Global Inequality (http://ucatlas.ucsc.edu/spend.php)

Healthy People 2010

Even as the size, complexity, and technological sophistication of health care have expanded in recent years, more and more Americans are experiencing limited access to services, inconsistent quality of services, and uncontrolled expenses. Reducing the disparities to improve the quality and quantity of life for *all* Americans is the goal of Healthy People 2010, a framework for prevention for the nation. Healthy People 2010 is a statement of national health objectives. The Office of Disease Prevention and Health Promotion, within the US Department of Health and Human Services, manages these objectives to strengthen the disease prevention and health promotion priorities.

Designed to identify the most significant preventable threats to health, and establish national goals to reduce these threats, Healthy People 2010 objectives build on initiatives pursued over the past two decades. The 1979 Surgeon General's Report, *Healthy People,* laid the foundation for a national prevention agenda. The 1980 *Promoting Health/Preventing Disease: Objectives for the Nation,* and *Healthy People 2000: National Health Promotion and Disease Prevention Objectives,* established national health objectives and served as the basis for the development of state and community plans.

> *The new century brings new challenges and opportunities to improve the health of everyone in the United States. People not only want to live a long life, but they also want to enjoy a healthy life. As the baby boom becomes the senior boom, quality of life will become a central issue for our health system. With Healthy People 2010, we want to add years to your life and health to your years.*
> —HHS Secretary Donna E. Shalala, January 2000

States, communities, professional organizations, and others use these objectives to help develop programs to improve health. Developed through a broad consultation process, Healthy People 2010 built on the best scientific knowledge, designed to measure programs over time. The first of two overarching goals of Healthy People 2010 is to *help individuals of all ages increase life expectancy and improve their quality of life.* Life expectancy is the average number of years people born in a given year can expect to live based on a set of age-specific death rates. Life expectancy for persons at every age group has increased during the past century. Based on today's age-specific death rates, an individual who was 75 in 2002 could expect to live another 11.5 years. Living longer with chronic or debilitating illness may decrease the quality of the individual's life. Quality of life reflects the value assigned to duration of life as modified by the impairments, functional status, and social opportunities, influenced by disease, injury, and treatment or social and political policy. It highlights a general sense of happiness and satisfaction with our lives and environment. Quality of life may encompass all aspects of life, including health, recreation, culture, rights, values, beliefs, and aspirations. Health-related quality of life is an overall sense of well-being with a strong relation to a person's health perceptions and ability to function. On a larger scale, quality of life can be viewed as including all aspects of community life that have a direct and quantifiable influence on the physical and mental health of its members.

Globally, the constitution of the World Health Organization states that the enjoyment of the highest attainable standard of health is one of the fundamental rights of every human being without distinction of race, religion, political beliefs, or economic or social condition. Yet even in North America, where technological advances in the healthcare field have made significant improvements in the quantity and quality of lives, there remain disparities between groups based on these very distinctions. There are large differences in health status by race and ethnic origin. Several factors may account for this, including socioeconomic status, health practices, psychosocial issues, limited resources (that is, housing, food, etc.), environmental exposures, discrimination, and access to health care. Socioeconomic and cultural differences among racial and ethnic groups in the United States will likely continue to influence patterns of disease, disability, and health care use in the future.

However, the second overarching goal of Healthy People 2010 is to *eliminate health disparities among different segments of the population.* Differences in health, life expectancy, and quality of life can occur by gender, race, or ethnicity, education or income, disability, geographic location, or even sexual orientation.

Documented repeatedly across a broad range of medical conditions, racial and ethnic disparities in health status continue to exist. This is true despite major health improvements for the nation as a whole. In response, government agencies and organizations are sponsoring research, collecting data, and developing resources to close the gaps in the health of, and the health services provided to, the minority and majority populations. Understanding the trends in disparities between different segments of the population enables healthcare programs to address the prevention needs of those groups. It is possible to split the US population along many different lines—racial and ethnic, gender, age, socioeconomic, and geographic. When determining whom a particular type of illness or injury affects, it is important to consider all of these characteristics. They shape a person's beliefs, values, preferences, and life experiences. Those factors, in turn, strongly affect how a person responds to prevention efforts. Research by the Agency for Healthcare Research and Quality (AHRQ) focuses on identifying and understanding how inequities in health care contribute to disparities, and how to eliminate those disparities. For example

- Cancer mortality rates are 35% higher in blacks than whites, however much can be done to reduce or eliminate this disparity by administering population- and community-based prevention programs and improving the effective delivery of both preventive and treatment services in the clinical setting.
- Cervical cancer, a disease that can be greatly reduced by effective health care, is 5 times higher in Vietnamese women in the United States than white women.
- Infant mortality is nearly 2.5 times higher in African-Americans than in whites.
- Before age 75, women are more likely to die in the hospital after a heart attack, yet studies suggest that women typically receive fewer high-technology cardiac procedures than men do.
- African-American diabetics are 7 times more likely to have amputations and develop kidney failure than white diabetics.

Within Healthy People 2010, leading federal agencies with the most relevant scientific experience developed 28 different focus areas. The Healthy People Consortium—an alliance of more than 350 national membership organizations and 250 state health, mental health, substance abuse, and environmental agencies—also informed the development process for these objectives. In addition, a series of regional and national meetings and an interactive Web site, received more than 11,000 public comments on the draft objectives. Within those 28 focus areas, Healthy People 2010 features 467 science-based objectives and 10 Leading Health Indicators, which are a smaller set of objectives chosen to track progress toward meeting Healthy People 2010 goals. The Leading Health Indicators represent the important determinants of health for the full range of issues in the 28 focus areas of Healthy People 2010.

Both public and private organizations have made great strides in identifying causes of disease and disability, discovering treatments and cures, and working with practitioners to educate the public to reduce the incidence and prevalence of major diseases as well as the functional limitations and discomfort or premature death they may cause. Healthy People 2010 and the Leading Health Indicators provide a means to assess where we are in health care today, and what steps we can improve for the future. The Healthy People 2010 objectives seek to increase life expectancy and quality of life for all Americans by helping individuals gain the knowledge, motivation, and opportunities needed to make informed decisions about their health.

Table 2.1 *Healthy People 2010 Focus Areas*

1. Access to Quality Health Services	15. Injury and Violence Prevention
2. Arthritis, Osteoporosis, and Chronic Back Conditions	16. Maternal, Infant, and Child Health
3. Cancer	17. Medical Product Safety
4. Chronic Kidney Disease	18. Mental Health and Mental Disorders
5. Diabetes	19. Nutrition and Overweight
6. Disability and Secondary Conditions	20. Occupational Safety and Health
7. Educational and Community-Based Programs	21. Oral Health
8. Environmental Health	22. Physical Activity and Fitness
9. Family Planning	23. Public Health Infrastructure
10. Food Safety	24. Respiratory Diseases
11. Health Communication	25. Sexually Transmitted Diseases
12. Heart Disease and Stroke	26. Substance Abuse
13. HIV	27. Tobacco Use
14. Immunization and Infectious Diseases	28. Vision and Hearing

The Leading Health Indicators (LHIs) are measures of the health of the nation over the next 10 years. The process of selecting the Leading Health Indicators mirrored the collaborative and extensive efforts undertaken to develop Healthy People 2010. The process, led by an interagency work group within the US Department of Health and Human Services, allowed individuals and organizations to provide comments at national and regional meetings or via mail and the Internet. A report by the Institute of Medicine, National Academy of Sciences, provided several scientific models on which to support a set of indicators. Research using focus groups ensured the indicators are meaningful and motivating to the public.

Each of the 10 Leading Health Indicators has one or more objectives from Healthy People 2010 associated with it. As a group, the Leading Health Indicators reflect the major health concerns in the United States at the beginning of the 21st century. The Leading Health Indicators, selected based on the availability of data to measure progress, and their importance as public health issues, are listed below.

1. Physical Activity
2. Overweight and Obesity
3. Tobacco Use
4. Substance Abuse
5. Responsible Sexual Behavior
6. Mental Health
7. Injury and Violence
8. Environmental Quality
9. Immunization
10. Access to Health Care

Each LHI represents an important health issue by itself. Together, the set of indicators helps us understand that many factors influence the health of individuals, communities, and the nation. Each of the indicators depends to some extent on

- The information people have about their health status as well as information on how to make improvements in their health.
- Choices people make (behavioral factors).
- Where and how people live (environmental, economic, and social conditions).
- The type, amount, and quality of health care people receive (access to health care and characteristics of the healthcare system).

The Leading Health Indicators motivate citizens and communities to take actions to improve the health of individuals, families, communities, and the nation. The indicators can help us determine *what each one of us can do and where we can best focus our energies*—at home, and in our communities, worksites, businesses, or states—to live better and longer. Some possible actions are

- Adopt the 10 LHIs as personal and professional guides for choices about how to make health improvements.
- Encourage public health professionals and public officials to adopt the LHIs as the basis for public health priority-setting and decision-making.
- Urge our public and community health systems and our community leadership to use the LHIs as measures of local success for investments in health improvements.

Realizing improvements for the 10 Leading Health Indicators will require effective public and private sector programs that address multiple factors. Significant reductions in infant mortality, fewer teen pregnancies, and childhood vaccination rates at record highs are recent positive healthy trends. However, obesity is now epidemic in the United States. Diabetes rates among people ages 30 to 39 rose by 70% in the past decade. About 46.5 million adults in the United States smoke cigarettes, even though this single behavior will result in disability and premature death for half of them. More than 60% of American adults do not get enough physical activity, and more than 25% are not active at all (HealthierUS.gov, 2005). There is much work to be done!

The indicators can provide the foundation for new partnerships across health issues and new thinking about how to address the many health concerns we face as a nation. An example of this type of innovative thinking is collaboration among those who want to increase the amount of physical activity individuals do and promote weight loss to reach a healthy weight. In short, the Leading Health Indicators serve as a tool to develop comprehensive health activities that work simultaneously to improve many aspects of health. The following table identifies which indicators most closely relate to each of the 28 focus areas and suggests opportunities for collaboration across focus areas.

Table 2.2 *Leading Health Indicators*

Focus Area	Physical activity	Overweight and obesity	Tobacco Use	Substance Abuse	Responsible Sexual Behavior	Mental Health	Injury and Violence	Environmental Quality	Immunization	Access to Health Care
Access to Quality Health Services	•	•	•	•	•	•	•		•	•
Arthritis, Osteoporosis, and Chronic Back Conditions	•	•					•			
Cancer	•	•	•	•	•				•	•
Chronic Kidney Disease	•	•	•					•		
Diabetes	•	•	•						•	•
Disability and Secondary Conditions	•	•	•	•		•			•	•
Educational and Community-Based Programs	•	•	•	•	•	•	•	•	•	•
Environmental Health								•		
Family Planning					•	•				•
Food Safety								•		•
Health Communication	•	•	•	•	•	•	•	•	•	•
Heart Disease and Stroke	•	•	•					•		
HIV					•	•	•			•
Immunization and Infectious Diseases									•	•
Injury and Violence Prevention				•	•		•	•		
Maternal, Infant, and Child Health	•	•	•	•	•	•	•		•	•
Medical Product Safety						•				
Mental Health and Mental Disorders				•	•	•	•			•
Nutrition and Overweight	•	•	•			•				
Occupational Safety and Health				•				•	•	
Oral Health		•	•	•					•	•
Physical Activity and Fitness	•	•	•			•	•	•		
Public Health Infrastructure	•	•	•	•	•	•	•	•	•	•
Respiratory Diseases	•	•						•		
Sexually Transmitted Diseases					•	•				
Substance Abuse			•	•	•			•		•
Tobacco Use			•						•	•
Vision and Hearing										•

Source: Leading Health Indicators Touch Everyone, http://www.healthypeople.gov/LHI/Touch_fact.htm

Leading Health Indicators and Healthy People 2010 Objectives

The following descriptions provide a basic illustration of the concepts addressed by each of the Leading Health Indicators. Examples of some Healthy People 2010 objectives demonstrate the goals and identify benchmarks for measuring improvement. The complete set of 467 science-based objectives is available at www.healthypeople.gov. In most objectives, baseline data provide understanding of the current known measurements; the targets indicate the expected or desired improvement by 2010. For objectives that address health services and protection (for example, access to prenatal care, health insurance coverage, etc.) the targets have been set so that there is an improvement for all racial/ethnic segments of the population (that is, the targets are set to "better than the best" for the racial/ethnic subgroup shown for the objective). For objectives that can be influenced in the short term by policy decisions, lifestyle choices, and behaviors (for example, physical activity, diet, smoking, suicide, alcohol-related motor vehicle deaths, etc.), the target setting method is also "better than the best" group. For objectives that are unlikely to achieve an equal health outcome in the next decade, regardless of the level of investment (for example, occupational exposure and resultant lung cancer), the target represents an improvement for a substantial proportion of the population and is regarded as a minimum acceptable level. Implicit in setting targets for these objectives is the recognition that population groups with baseline rates already better than the identified target should continue to improve.

Most objectives are tracked by a single measure to assess progress made over the decade. For these objectives, progress is assessed by the change from the baseline measure toward the target. Some objectives seek to increase positive behaviors or outcomes while others are defined in terms of decreasing negative behaviors or outcomes. A number of objectives contain multiple measures. Progress will be assessed separately for each measure. For these objectives, therefore, the progress may be mixed if some measures are progressing toward the target and others are regressing. For some objectives, precise measures that match the objective are not available. In these cases, similar proxy measures may be used to track progress. The tracking data and methods for assessing progress will be reviewed during the midcourse review in 2005, and a determination will be made at that time whether any changes will be made.

Developmental objectives are those that currently do not have national baseline data established, therefore, they currently have no operational definitions. Some objectives that contain several measures may have parts that are developmental. Developmental objectives indicate areas that need to be placed on the national agenda for data collection. They address subjects of sufficient national importance that investments should be made over the next decade to measure their change.

Healthy People 2010 uses population estimates from the US Census Bureau to calculate morbidity and mortality rates for many of the objectives. Every 10 years, the Census Bureau conducts a full census of the resident population of the United States, Puerto Rico, and US territories and collects data on gender, race, age, and marital status; the estimates produced represent the US population as of April 1 of the census year. More detailed data on education, housing, occupation, income, and other information are also collected from a representative sample of the population (about 17% of the total population).

Midway through the decade, a Midcourse Review assesses the status of the national objectives determined by Healthy People 2010. The Midcourse Review process identifies significant trends and gaps in preventive health issues and assesses whether objectives are moving away or toward their target. The final Midcourse Review, released in 2006, is available at the Healthy People 2010 Web site at www.healthypeople.gov.

Physical Activity

I have never taken any exercise except sleeping and resting.
Mark Twain (1835–1910)

Millions of Americans suffer from illnesses prevented or improved through regular physical activity. Regular physical activity reduces people's risk for heart attack, colon cancer, diabetes, and high blood pressure and may reduce their risk for stroke. It also helps to control weight; contributes to healthy bones, muscles, and joints; reduces falls among older adults; helps to relieve the pain of arthritis; reduces symptoms of anxiety and depression; and is associated with fewer hospitalizations, physician visits, and medications. Moreover, physical activity need not be strenuous to be beneficial; people of all ages benefit from moderate-intensity physical activity, such as 30 minutes of brisk walking 5 or more times a week.

Despite the proven benefits of physical activity, more than 50% of US adults do not get enough physical activity to provide health benefits; 26% are not active at all in their leisure time. Activity decreases with age, and sufficient activity is less common among women than men and among those with lower incomes and less education. Insufficient physical activity is not limited to adults. More than a third of young people in grades 9 through 12 do not regularly engage in vigorous physical activity. Daily participation in high school physical education classes dropped from 42% in 1991 to 28% in 2003 (CDC, 2004).

The US Surgeon General estimates 13.5 million people have coronary heart disease and 1.5 million people suffer from a heart attack in a given year. Approximately 8 million people have adult-onset (non-insulin-dependent) diabetes and 250,000 people suffer from hip fractures each year. Over 60 million people (a third of the population) are overweight and 50 million people have high blood pressure. Millions of Americans suffer from illnesses that can be prevented or improved through regular physical activity (CDC, 2005).

Sample Healthy People 2010 Objectives for Physical Activity

22-2. **Increase the proportion of adults who engage regularly, preferably daily, in moderate physical activity for at least 30 minutes per day.**

Target: 30 percent.

Baseline: 15 percent of adults aged 18 years and older engaged in moderate physical activity for at least 30 minutes 5 or more days per week in 1997 (age adjusted to the year 2000 standard population).

22-7. **Increase the proportion of adolescents who engage in vigorous physical activity that promotes cardiorespiratory fitness 3 or more days per week for 20 or more minutes per occasion.**

Target: 85 percent.

Baseline: 65 percent of students in grades 9 through 12 engaged in vigorous physical activity 3 or more days per week for 20 or more minutes per occasion in 1999.

Overweight and Obesity:

Getting my lifelong weight struggle under control has come from a process of treating myself as well as I treat others in every way.
Oprah Winfrey (1954–), *O Magazine*, August 2004

During the past 20 years, obesity among adults has risen significantly in the United States. Results of the National Health and Nutrition Examination Survey for 1999–2002 indicate that an estimated 30 percent of US adults aged 20 years and older—over 60 million people—are obese, defined as having a body mass index (BMI) of 30 or higher. Approximately 65% of US adults aged 20 years and older are either overweight or obese, defined as having a

BMI of 25 or higher. This increase is not limited to adults. The percentage of young people who are overweight has more than tripled since 1980. Among children and teens aged 6–19 years, 16 percent, over 9 million young people, are overweight (CDC, 2005b).

These increasing rates raise concern because of their implications for Americans' health. Although one of the national health objectives for the year 2010 is to reduce the prevalence of obesity among adults to less than 15%, current data indicate that the situation is worsening rather than improving (see Figure 2.2). Obese individuals are at increased risk for heart disease, high blood pressure, diabetes, arthritis-related disabilities, and some cancers. The estimated annual cost of obesity in the United States in 2000 was about $117 billion. Promoting regular physical activity and healthy eating and creating an environment that supports these behaviors are essential to reducing this epidemic of obesity (CDC, 2005b).

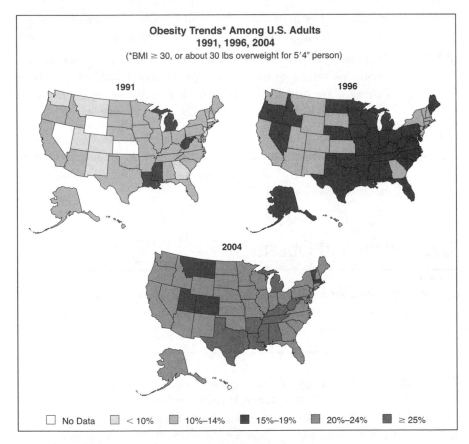

Figure 2.2   *Obesity Trends* Among U.S. Adults 1991, 1996, 2004*
Note: (*BMI ≥30, or about 30 lbs overweight for 5'4" person)
Source: Behavioral Risk Factor Surveillance System, CDC.

As a society, we can no longer afford to make poor health choices such as being physically inactive and eating an unhealthy diet; these choices have led to a tremendous obesity epidemic. As policy makers and health professionals, we must embrace small steps toward coordinated policy and environmental changes that will help Americans live longer, better, healthier lives.

—Vice Admiral Richard H. Carmona,
MD, MPH, FACS, US Surgeon General

Sample Healthy People 2010 Objectives for Overweight and Obesity

19-2. **Reduce the proportion of adults who are obese.**

Target: 15 percent.

Baseline: 23 percent of adults aged 20 years and older were identified as obese (defined as a BMI of 30 or more) in 1988–94 (age adjusted to the year 2000 standard population).

19-3. **Reduce the proportion of children and adolescents who are overweight or obese.**

Target and baseline:

Objective	Reduction in Overweight or Obese Children and Adolescents*	1988–94 Baseline	2010 Target
		Percent	
19-3a.	Children aged 6 to 11 years	11	5
19-3b.	Adolescents aged 12 to 19 years	11	5
19-3c.	Children and adolescents aged 6 to 19 years	11	5

*Defined as at or above the gender- and age-specific 95th percentile of BMI based on the revised CDC Growth Charts for the United States.

Tobacco Use

For thy sake, tobacco, I would do anything but die.
Charles Lamb, English Critic, Poet and Essayist (1775–1834)

Tobacco is the second major cause of death in the world. It is currently responsible for the death of one in ten adults worldwide, about 5 million deaths each year. If current smoking patterns continue, it will cause some 10 million deaths each year by 2020. Half the people that smoke today—that is about 650 million people—will eventually be killed by tobacco (WHO, 2005b). In spite of decades of Surgeon General warnings on every package of cigarettes, tobacco use remains the leading preventable cause of death in the United States, causing more than 400,000 deaths every year in this country. Each year, smoking kills more people than AIDS, alcohol, drug abuse, car crashes, murders, suicides, and fires—combined! Approximately 80% of adult smokers started smoking before the age of 18. Every day, nearly 3,000 young people under the age of 18 become regular smokers. More than 5 million children living today will die prematurely because of a decision they will make as adolescents—the decision to smoke cigarettes. Though 30% of Americans over age 12 still smoke, the trend with tobacco use continues to be good; rates keep coming down. The rate of lifetime cigarette use among youth ages 12 to 17 declined from 37% in 2001 to 33% in 2002. Since 1980, when girls' smoking caught up with boys', the two sexes have smoked at nearly the same rates. The rate of teen youth who smoke daily is going down, from 11% in 2001 to 8% in 2002 (SAMHSA, 2003). Cigarette smoke contains roughly 4,000 chemicals, including 200 known poisons of which 43 are carcinogenic (cancer causing). Smoking remains the leading cause of preventable death and has negative health impacts on people at all stages of life. It harms unborn babies, infants, children, adolescents, adults, and seniors.

Coronary heart disease and stroke—the primary types of cardiovascular disease caused by smoking—are the first and third leading causes of death in the United States. Smoking causes coronary heart disease, the leading cause of death in the United States. In 2003, an estimated 1.1 million Americans had a new or recurrent coronary attack. Cigarette smoking has been associated with sudden cardiac death of all types in both men and women (Surgeon General, 2004a).

Lung cancer is the leading cause of cancer death, and cigarette smoking causes most cases. Compared to nonsmokers, men who smoke are about 23 times more likely to develop lung cancer and women who smoke are about 13 times more likely. Smoking causes about 90% of lung cancer deaths in men and almost 80% in women. In 2003, an estimated 171,900 new cases of lung cancer occurred and approximately 157,200 people died from lung cancer. The 2004 Surgeon General's report adds more evidence to previous conclusions that smoking causes cancers of the oral cavity, pharynx, larynx, esophagus, lung, and bladder (Surgeon General, 2004a). Even environmental tobacco smoke (ETS) or secondhand smoke, has been designated a class-A carcinogen (a substance or agent producing cancer) by the US Environmental Protection Agency, comparable to asbestos (EPA, 1993).

In 2001, chronic obstructive pulmonary disease (COPD) was the fourth leading cause of death in the United States, resulting in more than 118,000 deaths. More than 90% of these deaths were attributed to smoking. According to the American Cancer Society's second Cancer Prevention Study, female smokers were nearly 13 times as likely to die from COPD as women who had never smoked. Male smokers were nearly 12 times as likely to die from COPD as men who had never smoked. Roughly, 10 million people in the United States have been diagnosed with COPD, which includes chronic bronchitis and emphysema. COPD is consistently among the top 10 most common chronic health conditions in women (Surgeon General, 2004a).

While regulations on smoking limit some exposure to Environmental Tobacco Smoke (ETS) in the United States, the problem continues around the globe. Smoking rates are still high in most European countries, exposing more than 50% of all children to ETS in some areas. Young children's exposure to ETS occurs mainly in the home, but also in other indoor environments (for example, vehicles, schools, and other public places). Rising smoking rates among children and teenagers in many countries and a decrease in the age of onset are additional reasons for concern. The World Health Organization issued a summary of the proven health effects of exposure to ETS, including respiratory problems; irritation of eyes, nose, and throat; and lung cancer. A person in a smoke-filled room for 8 hours a day smokes the equivalent of one cigarette each hour. The nonsmoking spouse of a smoker has a 30% greater risk of lung cancer compared to spouses of non-smokers. Exposure to ETS is a serious health threat to children. Compared to children of nonsmokers, children exposed to high levels of ETS have a much higher risk of upper respiratory infection, pneumonia, bronchitis, asthma, reduced hearing (middle-ear effusion), ear infections, and long-term lung damage. Children and adolescents who smoke are less physically fit and have more respiratory illnesses than their nonsmoking peers. In general, smokers' lung function declines faster than that of nonsmokers (WHO, 2005b).

Sample Healthy People 2010 Objectives for Tobacco:

27-1. **Reduce tobacco use by adults.**

Target and baseline:

Objective	Reduction in Tobacco Use by Adults Aged 18 Years and Older	1988 Baseline	2010 Target
		Percent	
27-1a.	Cigarette smoking	24	12
27-1b.	Spit tobacco	2.6	0.4
27-1c.	Cigars	2.5	1.2
27-1d.	Other products	Developmental	

*Age adjusted to the year 2000 standard population.

Substance Abuse

If we burn ourselves out with drugs or alcohol,
we won't have long to go in this business.
John Belushi (1949–1982), *Playboy* Interview, May 1977

John Belushi, one of the original comedians on *Saturday Night Live,* died
from a lethal combination of drugs and alcohol. His death is one of many
tragic losses due to substance abuse. Substance abuse problems, both those
of individuals and communities at large, impose a staggering burden on the
people and resources in our nation. Drug and alcohol abuse and dependence
affect individuals of all ages, from all geographic areas, and all ethnicities,
education, and employment levels. Alcohol or drug abuse occurs when individuals repeatedly drink or use drugs even though it causes significant problems in their lives. If the substance abuse continues, it can lead to dependence—a physical and emotional addiction to alcohol or drugs. In 2002, an
estimated 22 million Americans suffered from substance dependence or
abuse, according to the newest results of the Substance Abuse and Mental
Health Services Administration's (SAMHSA) 2002 National Survey on Drug
Use and Health, or NSDUH (formerly called the National Household Survey
on Drug Abuse). The primary source of statistics on substance abuse in the
United States, NSDUH is based on 68,126 interviews nationwide. Other new
NSDUH findings include the following:

- Abuse of pain relievers and stimulants otherwise used legitimately as
  medicine continues to be one of the few classes of drug abuse that is rising. Four times as many people have begun to abuse pain relievers in
  2001 (2.4 million) as did in 1990 (628,000).
- African-Americans and whites abuse substances at about the same rate
  (9.5 and 9.3%, respectively). Fourteen percent of Native Americans (the
  highest rate), 4 percent of Asian Americans (the lowest), and 10 percent
  of Hispanic Americans abuse substances.
- Of those youth whose parents "strongly" disapprove of marijuana use,
  only 5.5 percent had used it in the past month; of those whose parents
  disapproved somewhat or were indifferent, 30 percent were past month
  marijuana smokers.

Marijuana continues to be the most widely used illicit drug, though youth 12
to 17 who had *ever* tried it declined slightly (from 22% in 2001 to 21% in
2002). Unfortunately, in the college-to-young adult bracket (18 to 25) the rate
of those who have *ever* tried marijuana has been increasing for almost a decade.

In 2002, the rate (53.8%) reached its highest level since 1982 (54.4%). At the same time, only 6% of the population over 12 years of age were "current" marijuana smokers (used in the past month). A marked increase in use of hallucinogens from 1992 to 2002 (14% to 24%) among youth 18–25 appears driven by the popularity of ecstasy (MDMA). At the same time, new use of LSD, which like ecstasy is an extremely toxic hallucinogen, has dropped precipitously (33%) in only one year (2000 to 2001). Lifetime use of pain relievers non-medically by youth ages 12 to 17 increased from 9.6% in 2001, to 11.2% in 2002, a 10-fold increase in a little over a decade (from 1.2% in 1989).

An estimated 120 million Americans reported being current drinkers (drank in the past month). About 23% of Americans report binge-drink (5 or more drinks at a sitting) at least once in the 30 days prior to completing the NSDUH survey. Seven percent of Americans are classified as heavy drinkers (binge drinking on 5 different days in the past month). In the 12 to 20 age bracket, 29% are current drinkers and 19 percent binge drinkers. Current drinking rates increase exponentially as students get older: 20% at age 15, 29% at 16, and 36% at 17.

In 2002, nearly 8% of Americans 12 and over needed treatment for a serious alcohol problem, and 3% needed treatment for a diagnosable drug problem. Yet less than half with a drug problem got treatment, and less than one fifth with a drinking problem sought treatment (SAMHSA, 2003). Science has proven that the abuse of alcohol and alcohol dependency can adversely affect physical and mental health, both in the individual who drinks, and those around them.

- Accidents—Alcohol-related motor vehicle crashes kill someone every 30 minutes and injure someone every 2 minutes. Forty-one percent of all traffic-related deaths are alcohol related. In 2002, the National Highway Traffic Safety Administration reported arrests of about 1.5 million drivers for driving under the influence of alcohol or narcotics (NHTSA, 2004). That's slightly more than one percent of the 120 million self-reported episodes of alcohol–impaired driving among U.S. adults each year (Dellinger, et al., 1999) with 17,419 of those episodes resulting in death in 2002. Though there is significant progress to reduce drunk driving since the 1980s, the number of alcohol-related fatalities is again trending upward.

- Violence—Perpetrators of family violence are often using alcohol or drugs when they lash out at their victims.

- Increase in birth defects—Alcohol can have a number of harmful effects on a baby, including mental retardation, and learning and behavioral problems.

- Drinking-related medical conditions—Those who are alcohol dependent run a higher risk of liver disease, and various forms of cancer, including breast cancer. They are also more likely to be injured by falling.

Sample Healthy People 2010 Objectives for Substance Abuse

26-10. **Reduce past-month use of illicit substances.**

26-10a. Increase the proportion of adolescents not using alcohol or any illicit drugs during the past 30 days.

Target: 89 percent.

Baseline: 79 percent of adolescents aged 12 to 17 years reported no alcohol or illicit drug use in the past 30 days in 1998.

26-10b. Reduce the proportion of adolescents reporting use of marijuana during the past 30 days.

Target: 0.7 percent.

Baseline: 8.3 percent of adolescents aged 12 to 17 years reported marijuana use in the past 30 days in 1998.

26-10c. Reduce the proportion of adults using any illicit drug during the past 30 days.

Target: 2.0 percent.

Baseline: 5.8 percent of adults aged 18 years and older used any illicit drug during the past 30 days in 1998.

Responsible Sexual Behavior

In America sex is an obsession; in other parts of the world it is a fact.
Marlene Dietrich, Actor (1901–1992)

Sexual intercourse is the most powerful of human behaviors. In the same instant, intercourse can start a new life (pregnancy) and begin a deadly disease (HIV/AIDS). Five of the ten most commonly reported infectious diseases in the United States are sexually transmitted diseases. Nearly one-half of all pregnancies in the United States are unintended. Unintended pregnancy is not only medically costly, it is also socially costly in terms of out-of-wedlock births, reduced educational attainment and employment opportunity, increased welfare dependency, and later child abuse and neglect (Surgeon General, 2004b).

Teen pregnancy and birth rates have declined steadily in the United States in recent years. Despite these declines, the United States continues to have the highest teen birth rate among all industrialized nations and a higher teen birth rate than over 50 developing nations. Experts attribute the declining rates to a substantial increase in contraceptive use by sexually active teens and to a decrease in sexual activity among adolescents. Yet, millions of American youth are still engaging in behaviors that put them at risk for unintended pregnancy and sexually transmitted infections (STIs), including HIV. Each year in the United States, about 900,000 adolescent females become pregnant, 20,000 young people are newly infected with HIV, and nearly four million new STI infections occur among 15- to 19-year-olds (Advocates for Youth, 2005).

Sample Healthy People 2010 Objectives for Responsible Sexual Behavior

13-6.   **Increase the proportion of sexually active persons who use condoms.**

Target and baseline:

Objective	Increase in Sexually Active Persons Using Condoms	1995 Baseline	2010 Target
		Percent	
13-6a.	Females aged 18 to 44 years	23	50
13-6b.	Males aged 18 to 49 years	Developmental	

Target-setting method: Better than the best.

Data source: National Survey of Family Growth (NSFG), CDC, NCHS.

25-11.   **Increase the proportion of adolescents who abstain from sexual intercourse or use condoms if currently sexually active.**

Target: 95 percent.

Baseline: 85 percent of adolescents in grades 9 through 12 abstained from sexual intercourse or used condoms in 1999 (50 percent had never had intercourse; 14 percent had intercourse but not in the past 3 months; and 21 percent currently were sexually active and used a condom at last intercourse).

Mental Health

A crust eaten in peace is better than a banquet partaken in anxiety.
Aesop (620 BC–560 BC), *The Town Mouse and the Country Mouse*

Mental health influences the ways individuals look at themselves, their lives, and others in their lives. Like physical health, mental health is important at every stage of life. According to the World Health Organization, 450 million people worldwide are affected by mental, neurological, or behavioral problems at any time. About 873,000 people die by suicide every year. Mental illnesses are common to all countries and cause immense suffering. People with these disorders may be subject to social isolation, poor quality of life, and increased mortality. These disorders are the cause of staggering economic and social costs. Mental illnesses affect and are affected by chronic conditions such as cancer, heart and cardiovascular diseases, diabetes, and HIV/AIDS. Untreated, they bring about unhealthy behavior, noncompliance with prescribed medical regimens, diminished immune functioning, and poor prognosis. Cost-effective treatments exist for most disorders and, if correctly applied, could enable most of those affected to become functioning members of society. Barriers to effective treatment of mental illness include lack of recognition of the seriousness of mental illness and lack of understanding about the benefits of services. In addition, the stigma attached to mental illness, and to the people who have it, is a major obstacle to better care and to the improvement of the quality of their lives. Policy makers, insurance companies, health and labor policies, and the public at large all discriminate between physical and mental problems (WHO, 2005a).

The National Institute of Mental Health (NIMH) states "the burden of psychiatric conditions has been heavily underestimated." Mental illness, including suicide, accounts for over 15% of the burden of disease in established market economies, such as the United States. This is more than the disease burden caused by all cancers. This measure is called Disability Adjusted Life Years (DALYs). DALYs measure lost years of healthy life regardless of whether the years were lost to premature death or disability. The disability component of this measure is weighted for severity of the disability. For example, disability caused by major depression was found to be equivalent to blindness or paraplegia, whereas active psychosis seen in schizophrenia produces disability equal to quadriplegia. Using the DALYs measure, major depression ranked second only to ischemic heart disease in magnitude of disease burden in established market economies. Schizophrenia, bipolar disorder, obsessive-compulsive disorder, panic disorder, and post-traumatic stress disorder also contributed significantly to the total burden of illness attributable to mental disorders (NIMH, 2005). Mental illness clearly has a negative impact on quality of life.

Sample Healthy People 2010 Objective for Mental Health

18-9. **Increase the proportion of adults with mental disorders who receive treatment.**

Target and baseline:

Objective	Increase in Adults with Mental Disorders Receiving Treatment	1997 Baseline (unless noted)	2010 Target
		Percent	
18-9a.	Adults aged 18 to 54 years with serious mental illness	47 (1991)	55
18-9b.	Adults aged 18 years and older with recognized depression	23	50
18-9c.	Adults aged 18 years and older with schizophrenia	60 (1984)	75
18-9d.	Adults aged 18 years and older with generalized anxiety disorder	38	50

Injury and Violence

> *We live in a time when the words impossible and unsolvable are no longer part of the scientific community's vocabulary. Each day we move closer to trials that will not just minimize the symptoms of disease and injury but eliminate them.*
>
> Christopher Reeve, Actor (1952–2004),
> 1999 Testimony to US House of Representatives

Christopher Reeve, the actor perhaps best known for portraying Superman on the big screen, suffered permanent disability after a horseback riding injury. Injuries and violence can affect everyone, even "Superman." Some injuries, however, disproportionately affect different groups of individuals. The following is a look at how injuries affect different groups of Americans and what the CDC is doing to address them (NCIPC, 2002).

Males are at higher risk for motor vehicle crashes, falls, drowning, and homicide. Several factors may account for these differences. For instance, males are more likely than females to engage in behaviors that put them at risk, such as driving or boating after drinking alcohol, failing to wear seat belts, participating in potentially dangerous sports and leisure activities, and perpetrating violent acts.

The injury rate for African-Americans is higher than that for nearly all other racial and ethnic groups. This disparity may be due in part to the fact that a greater percentage of African-Americans have lower education levels and higher poverty levels. Such characteristics may increase risk for injury. They are clearly associated with higher pedestrian fatality rates and higher fatality rates from residential fires. These factors are also linked to an increase in violence-related injuries and deaths.

Overall, the injury rate for Hispanic Americans is lower than for non-Hispanics. However, for some injury problems, Hispanics are at a higher risk than other racial or ethnic groups. Among this group, pedestrian fatalities are nearly twice as high as for whites. One possible explanation is that Hispanics make 55% more walking trips than do non-Hispanics. This difference may be attributable to a lower vehicle ownership rate among Hispanics. Hispanic youth are at higher risk than whites for injuries resulting from violence. This disparity may be due in part to the fact that a greater percentage of Hispanic Americans have lower education levels and higher poverty levels. Such characteristics, along with family disruption and weak intergenerational ties in families and communities, may increase risk for violent behavior.

Native Americans and Alaska Natives are at higher risk for several types of injuries, both unintentional and violence-related. This group has a higher rate than many racial and ethnic groups for injuries resulting from fires in their homes. This disparity may be attributable to a higher percentage of Native Americans and Alaska Natives living in rural areas and in manufactured housing, a known risk for fire-related injuries and deaths. Teens and young adults among this racial group are at increased risk for suicide. This higher risk may be due to several factors, including limited availability of employment and educational opportunities, alcohol use among this population, and loss of traditional spiritual practices and indigenous languages.

Infants and young children are also at greater risk for many injuries. This increased risk may be attributable to many factors. Children are curious and like to explore their environment. This characteristic may lead children to sample the pills in the medicine cabinet, play with matches, or venture into the family pool. Young children have limited physical coordination and cognitive abilities, leading to a greater risk for falls from bicycles and playground equipment and may make it difficult for them to escape from a fire. Their small size and developing bones and muscles may make them more susceptible to injury in car crashes if they are not properly restrained.

Sample Healthy People 2010 Objective for Injury and Violence

15-15. Reduce deaths caused by motor vehicle crashes.
Target and baseline:

Objective	Reduction in Deaths Caused by Motor Vehicle Crashes	1998 Baseline	2010 Target
		Percent	
15-15a.	Deaths per 100,000 population	15.6*	9.2
15-15b.	Deaths per 100 million vehicle miles traveled	1.6	0.8

*Age adjusted to the year 2000 standard population.

Environmental Quality

The environment is everything that isn't me.
Albert Einstein

Einstein is right; the environment is everything that is not you. Your environment can contribute to health problems. The water you drink, the air you breathe, even the bugs in your home, can influence your health. For example, the quality of our air, whether indoors or outdoors, affects everyone. The National Center for Environmental Health at the Centers for Disease Control and Prevention strives to promote health and quality of life by preventing or controlling those diseases or deaths that result from interactions between people and their environment. The Air Pollution and Respiratory Health Program of the National Center for Environmental Health leads CDC's fight against environmental-related respiratory illnesses, including asthma, and studies indoor and outdoor air pollution. Research-based intervention conducted in partnership with international, national, and local partners is applied to CDC's work in preventing carbon monoxide poisoning, studying the health effects of exposure to forest fire smoke, battling chronic obstructive pulmonary disease, and investigating human health effects of mold exposure. One health-related outcome related to air quality is chronic obstructive pulmonary disease, or COPD, which refers to a group of diseases that cause airflow blockage and breathing-related problems. It includes emphysema, chronic bronchitis, and in some cases asthma. COPD is a leading cause of death, illness, and disability in the United States. In 2000, COPD was responsible for 119,000 deaths, 726,000 hospitalizations, and 1.5 million hospital emergency department visits.

An additional 8 million cases of hospital outpatient treatment or treatment by personal physicians were linked to COPD in 2000. In the United States, tobacco use is a key factor in the development and progression of COPD, but asthma, exposure to air pollutants in the home and workplace, genetic factors, and respiratory infections play a role. In the developing world, indoor air quality is thought to play a larger role in the development and progression of COPD than it does in the United States.

Sample Healthy People Objectives for Environmental Air Quality

8-1.   Reduce the proportion of persons exposed to air that does not meet the US Environmental Protection Agency's health-based standards for harmful air pollutants.

Target and baseline:

Objective	Reduction in Air Pollutants	1997 Baseline	2010 Target
		Percent	
8-1a.	Ozone*	43	0
8-1b.	Particulate matter*	12	0
8-1c.	Carbon monoxide	19	0
8-1d.	Nitrogen dioxide	5	0
8-1e.	Sulfur dioxide	2	0
8-1f.	Lead	<1	0
		Number	
8-1g.	Total number of people	119,803,000	0

*The targets of zero percent for ozone and particulate matter are set for 2012 and 2018, respectively.

27-10.   Reduce the proportion of nonsmokers exposed to environmental tobacco smoke.

Target: 45 percent.

Baseline: 65 percent of nonsmokers aged 4 years and older had a serum cotinine level above 0.10 ng/mL in 1988–94 (age adjusted to the year 2000 standard population).

Target-setting method: Better than the best.

Data source: National Health and Nutrition Examination Survey (NHANES), CDC, NCHS.

Immunization

Thanks to support from individuals like Bill Gates, researchers may one day find a vaccine for AIDS. While this is not yet available, there are many immunizations used to prevent life-threatening diseases across the lifespan. Vaccination (Latin: *vacca—cow*) is so named because the first vaccine was derived from a virus affecting cows—the cowpox virus—a relatively benign virus that, in its weakened form, provides a degree of immunity to smallpox, a contagious disease that is sometimes deadly to humans. "Vaccination" and "immunization" generally have the same meaning. The process of triggering immune response, in an effort to protect against infectious disease, works by "priming" the immune system with an "immunogen." Stimulating immune response, via use of an infectious agent, is known as *immunization*. Vaccinations involve the administration of one or more immunogens, in the form of live, but weakened, infectious agents. These agents normally are derived from either weaker, but closely related, species (as with smallpox and cowpox), or strains weakened by some process. In such cases, an immunogen is called a *vaccine*.

In recent years, the Centers for Disease Control and Prevention (CDC) announced that the nation's childhood immunization rates continue at record high levels, with about 81% of the nation's 19-to-35-month-old children receiving all the vaccinations in the recommended series. This is the first time that coverage for the baseline series of vaccines in children has exceeded 80%, which also represents the Healthy People 2010 goal. Vaccines are not just for kids. Far too many adults become ill, disabled, or die each year from diseases easily prevented by vaccines. Thus, everyone, from young adults to senior citizens, can benefit from immunizations.

Vaccine-preventable adult diseases:

- Diphtheria
- Haemophilus influenzae type b (Hib)
- Hepatitis A
- Hepatitis B
- Influenza (flu)

- Measles
- Mumps
- Pneumococcus
- Polio
- Rubella (German measles)
- Tetanus (lockjaw)
- Varicella* (chicken pox)

*You do *not* need the varicella vaccine if you have a reliable history of having had chicken pox.

Vaccines needed for teenagers and college students:

- Varicella (chicken pox) vaccine
- Hepatitis B vaccine
- Measles-Mumps-Rubella (MMR) vaccine
- Tetanus-Diphtheria vaccine
- Meningococcus vaccine

Children's vaccine-preventable diseases:

- Diphtheria
- Hepatitis A
- Hepatitis B
- Haemophilus influenzae type b (Hib)
- Influenza (flu)
- Measles
- Mumps
- Pertussis
- Pneumococcal
- Polio
- Rubella (German measles)
- Tetanus (lockjaw)
- Varicella (chicken pox)

Sample Healthy People 2010 Objectives for Immunization

14-24. Increase the proportion of young children and adolescents who receive all vaccines that have been recommended for universal administration for at least 5 years.

Target and baseline:

Objective	Increase in Coverage Levels of Universally Recommended Vaccines	1998 Baseline	2010 Target
		Percent	
14-24a.	Children aged 19 to 35 months who receive the recommended vaccines (4DTaP, 3 polio, 1 MMR, 3 Hib, 3 hep B)	73	80
14-24b.	Adolescents aged 13 to 15 years who receive the recommended vaccines	Developmental	

14-29. Increase the proportion of adults who are vaccinated annually against influenza and ever vaccinated against pneumococcal disease.

Target and baseline:

Objective	Increase in Adults Vaccinated	1998 Baseline* (unless noted)	2010 Target
		Percent	
	Noninstitutionalized adults aged 65 years and older		
14-29a.	Influenza vaccine	64	90
14-29b.	Pneumococcal vaccine	46	90
	Noninstitutionalized high-risk adults aged 18 to 64 years		
14-29c.	Influenza vaccine	26	60
14-29d.	Pneumococcal vaccine	13	60
	Institutionalized adults (persons in long-term care or nursing homes)†		
14-29e.	Influenza vaccine	59 (1997)	90
14-29f.	Pneumococcal vaccine	25 (1997)	90

*Age adjusted to the year 2000 standard population.
†National Nursing Home Survey estimates include a significant number of residents who have an unknown vaccination status. See *Tracking Healthy People 2010* for further discussion of the data issues.

Access to Health Care

The health care system is really designed to reward you
for being unhealthy. If you are a healthy person and
work hard to be healthy, there are no benefits.

Mike Huckabee, Governor of Arkansas

The debate about improving access to health care continues to rage on in conference rooms and living rooms across the nation. All the wonderful advances in primary, secondary, and tertiary prevention have little benefit to those individuals with no resources to access or pay for those services. The Census Bureau reported that 45 million Americans lacked health insurance in 2003, up by 1.4 million from 2002 and 5.2 million from 2000.

A combination of factors—including America's liability crisis and a decrease in employment-based health insurance coverage—has contributed to the increase in the number of uninsured. Medical liability is a legal practice to regulate and reduce medical malpractice, which is an act or omission by a healthcare provider which deviates from accepted standards of practice in the medical community, causing injury to the patient. The nation's medical liability crisis affects every patient and physician in some way. The cost of litigation per person in the United States is higher than any other major industrialized nation in the world. Skyrocketing medical liability premiums are forcing some physicians to limit services, retire early, or move to a state with reforms where premiums are more stable. The crisis is threatening access to care for patients in states without liability reforms. The cost of medical liability insurance for healthcare providers, then passed onto patients, escalates the cost for medical care, thus making health insurance more expensive. Higher insurance rates force some companies to stop offering or limit the health insurance benefits they provide for employees. In 2005, President Bush proposed a need for common-sense medical liability reform to make health care more affordable and accessible for all Americans, and to keep necessary services in communities that need them the most.

The percentage of people covered by government health insurance programs rose in 2003, from 25.7% to 26.6%, largely as the result of increases in Medicaid and Medicare coverage. Medicaid is the largest source of government funding for medical and health-related services for people with limited income. Medicare is publicly funded health insurance for the elderly and disabled only. Medicaid coverage rose 0.7 percentage points to 12.4% in 2003, and Medicare coverage increased 0.2 percentage points to 13.7%. The proportion of uninsured children did not change in 2003, remaining at 11.4%

of all children, or 8.4 million. Studies about access to care include the uninsured and those with low incomes as well as racial and ethnic minorities and people with chronic conditions.

Sample Healthy People 2010 Objectives for Access to Health Care

1-1.   **Increase the proportion of persons with health insurance.**

Target: 100 percent.

Baseline: 83% of persons under age 65 years were covered by health insurance in 1997 (age adjusted to the year 2000 standard population).

Target-setting method: Total coverage.

Data source: National Health Interview Survey (NHIS), CDC, NCHS.

1-4.   **Increase the proportion of persons who have a specific source of ongoing care.**

Target and baseline:

Objective	Increase in Specific Source of Ongoing Care	1998 Baseline*	2010 Target
		Percent	
1-4a.	All ages	87	96
1-4b.	Children and youth aged 17 years and under	93	97
1-4c.	Adults aged 18 years and older	85	96

*Age adjusted to the year 2000 standard population.

Target-setting method: Better than the best.

Data source: National Health Interview Survey (NHIS), CDC, NCHS.

16-6.   **Increase the proportion of pregnant women who receive early and adequate prenatal care.**

Target and baseline:

Objective	Increase in Maternal Prenatal Care	1998 Baseline	2010 Target
		Percent of Live Births	
16-6a.	Care beginning in first trimester of pregnancy	83	90
16-6b.	Early and adequate prenatal care	74	90

Target-setting method: Better than the best.

SUMMARY

The 20th century brought remarkable and unprecedented improvements in the lives of the people of the United States. In spite of the dramatic increase in life expectancy seen in the last century, all members of our society do not equally enjoy the benefits of modern medicine, both in the United States and around the world. The discrepancies in health status noted between genders, races, ethnic groups, and socioeconomic groups continue to separate citizens within this country. Developed with the best scientific knowledge available, Healthy People 2010 is a comprehensive set of disease-prevention and health-promotion objectives for America. It reflects the best in public health planning and provides a comprehensive picture of the nation's health at the beginning of the decade, establishes goals and targets to achieve, and monitors national progress over time. Healthy People 2010 challenges all of us— individuals, communities, and healthcare professionals—to take steps to enjoy good health and a long life.

ADDITIONAL RESOURCES

General

US Department of Health and Human Services
240-453-8280
http://odphp.osophs.dhhs.gov/

Physical Activity

President's Council on Physical Fitness and Sports
202-690-9000
http://www.fitness.gov

Centers for Disease Control and Prevention (CDC)
888-232-3228
http://www.cdc.gov/nccdphp/dnpa

Overweight and Obesity

Obesity Education Initiative, National Heart, Lung, and Blood Institute Information Center
301-592-8573
http://www.nhlbi.nih.gov/about/oei/index.htm

The Weight-Control Information Network
National Institutes of Health (NIH)
877-946-4627
http://www.niddk.nih.gov/health/nutrit/win.htm

Tobacco Use

Office on Smoking and Health, National Center for Chronic Disease Prevention and Health Promotion, CDC
800-CDC-1311
http://www.cdc.gov/tobacco

Cancer Information Service, NIH
800-4-CANCER
http://cis.nci.nih.gov

Substance Abuse

National Clearinghouse for Alcohol and Drug Information Substance Abuse and Mental Health Services Administration (SAMHSA)
800-729-6686; 800-487-4889 (TDD)
http://www.health.org

National Institute on Drug Abuse, NIH
301-443-1124
http://www.nida.nih.gov

National Institute on Alcohol Abuse and Alcoholism, NIH
301-443-3860
http://www.niaaa.nih.gov

Responsible Sexual Behavior

CDC National AIDS Hotline
800-342-AIDS (800-342-2437)
http://www.cdc.gov/hiv/hivinfo/nah.htm

CDC National Sexually Transmitted Diseases
(STD) Hotline
800-227-8922
http://www.cdc.gov/nchstp/dstd/dstdp.html

CDC National Prevention Information Network
800-458-5231
http://www.cdcnpin.org

Office of Population Affairs
301-654-6190
http://opa.osophs.dhhs.gov

Mental Health

Center for Mental Health Services, SAMHSA
http://www.mentalhealth.org/cmhs/index.htm

National Mental Health Information Center, SAMHSA
800-789-2647
http://www.mentalhealth.org

National Institute of Mental Health Information Line, NIH
800-421-4211
http://www.nimh.nih.gov/publicat/depressionmenu.cfm

Injury and Violence

National Center for Injury Prevention and Control, CDC
770-488-1506
http://www.cdc.gov/ncipc/ncipchm.htm

Office of Justice Programs, U.S. Department of Justice
202-307-0703
http://www.ojp.usdoj.gov/home.htm

National Highway Traffic Safety Administration
US Department of Transportation
Auto Safety Hotline 888-DASH-2-DOT (888-327-4236)
http://www.nhtsa.dot.gov/hotline

Environmental Quality

Indoor Air Quality Information Clearinghouse
US Environmental Protection Agency
800-438-4318 (IAQ hotline)
800-SALUD-12; (725-8312) Spanish
http://www.epa.gov/iaq/iaqinfo.html

Information Resources Center (IRC)
US Environmental Protection Agency
202-260-5922
http://www.epa.gov/natlibra/hqirc/about.htm

Agency for Toxic Substances and Disease Registry, CDC
888-442-8737
http://www.atsdr.cdc.gov

Immunization

National Immunization Program/CDC
800-232-2522 (English); 800-232-0233 (Spanish)
888-CDC-FAXX (Fax-back)
http://www.cdc.gov/nip

Access to Health Care

Agency for Healthcare Research and Quality
Office of Healthcare Information
301-594-1364
http://www.ahrq.gov/consumer/index.html#plans

"Insure Kids Now" Initiative
Health Resources and Services Administration
877-KIDS NOW (877-543-7669)
http://www.insurekidsnow.gov

Maternal and Child Health Bureau
Health Resources and Services Administration
1-888-ASK-HRSA (HRSA Information Center)
http://www.mchb.hrsa.gov

Office of Beneficiary Relations
Centers for Medicare & Medicaid Services
800-444-4606 (customer service center)
800-MED-ICARE (Info Line)
http://www.Medicare.gov

OTHER RESOURCES

For more health promotion and disease prevention information:
Search online for thousands of free federal health documents using healthfinder® at http://www.healthfinder.gov/

For health promotion and disease prevention information in Spanish:
Visit http://www.healthfinder.gov/espanol/

REFERENCES

Advocates for Youth. (2005). Adolescent sexual behavior and contraceptive use. Retrieved August 15, 2005, from http://www.advocatesforyouth.org/arsh.htm.

Agency for Healthcare Research and Quality (AHRQ). (2002, March). *AHRQ focus on research: Disparities in health care.* AHRQ Publication No. 02-M027, March 2002. Agency for Healthcare Research and Quality, Rockville, MD. Retrieved June 24, 2005, from http://www.ahrq.gov/news/focus/disparhc.htm.

Centers for Disease Control and Prevention (CDC). (2004, September). Participation in high school physical education—United States, 1991–2003, 2004. *Mortality and Morbidity Weekly Report (MMWR), 53*(36), 844–847.

Centers for Disease Control and Prevention (CDC). (2005a). Health burdens that could be reduced through physical activity: Report from the U.S. Surgeon General. Retrieved December 7, 2005, from http://www.cdc.gov/nccdphp/sgr/mm.htm.

Centers for Disease Control and Prevention (CDC). (2005b). Overweight and obesity. Retrieved August 12, 2005, from http://www.cdc.gov/nccdphp/dnpa/obesity/.

Centers for Medicare and Medicaid Services (CMS). (2003). National Health Expenditures, 2003. Retrieved August 31, 2005, from http://www.cms.hhs.gov/National-HealthExpendData/02_NationalHealthAccountsHistorical.asp.

Dellinger, A. M., Bolen, J., & Sacks, J. J. (1999). A comparison of driver- and passenger-based estimates of alcohol-impaired driving. *American Journal of Preventive Medicine, 16*(4), 283–288.

Environmental Protection Agency (EPA). (1993). EPA designates passive smoking a "Class A" or known human carcinogen. Retrieved August 11, 2005, from http://www.epa.gov/history/topics/smoke/01.htm.

HealthierUS.gov. (2005). Retrieved November 4, 2006.

National Center for Injury Prevention and Control (NCIPC). (2002). Injury fact book 2001–2002. Centers for Disease Control and Prevention, National Center for Injury Prevention and Control. Retrieved August 14, 2005, from http://www.cdc.gov/ncipc/fact_book/factbook.htm.

National Highway Traffic Safety Administration (NHTSA). (2004). Traffic safety facts 2003: Alcohol. Retrieved December 12, 2005, from www-nrd.nhtsa.dot.gov/pdf/nrd-30/NCSA/TSF2003/809761.pdf.

National Institute of Mental Health (NIMH). (2005). The impact of mental illness on society. National Institute of Mental Health. Retrieved August 15, 2005, from http://www.nimh.nih.gov/publicat/burden.cfm.

Substance Abuse and Mental Health Services Administration (SAMHSA). (2003). 2002 National survey on drug use and health. Retrieved August 16, 2005, from http://www.samhsa.gov.

UC Atlas of Global Inequality (UC Atlas). (2005). Health expenditures. Retrieved July 15, 2005, from http://ucatlas.ucsc.edu/health/expenditure.html.

US Surgeon General's Office (Surgeon General). (2004a). *The health consequences of smoking: A report of the Surgeon General.* U.S. Department of Health and Human Services, Centers for Disease Control and Prevention, National Center for Chronic Disease Prevention and Health Promotion, Office on Smoking and Health. Washington, DC: Government Printing Office.

US Surgeon General's Office (Surgeon General). (2004b). The surgeon general's call to action to promote sexual health and responsible sexual behavior, 2004. Retrieved on August 15, 2005, from http://www.surgeongeneral.gov/library/sexual health/glancelist.htm.

World Health Organization (WHO). (2005a). Mental health. Retrieved August 10, 2005, from http://www.who.int/mental_health/en/.

World Health Organization (WHO). (2005b). Tobacco free initiatives. Retrieved August 15, 2005, from http://www.who.int/tobacco/en/.

Chapter 3

Paying for Health Care

Stephanie Chisolm

OBJECTIVES

After studying this chapter, the student should be able to

1. Explain the role of health insurance in the healthcare system.
2. Describe the historical evolution of health insurance in the United States.
3. Identify different kinds of government and non-government health insurance.
4. Explain the difference in eligibility and coverage between Medicare and Medicaid programs.

INTRODUCTION

> *Medical professionals, not insurance company bureaucrats,*
> *should be making health care decisions.*
> US Senator Barbara Boxer, California

Senator Boxer and others are committed to making quality health care more accessible and affordable for Americans. Presidential candidates have health care availability at the forefront of every campaign. The United States has some of the finest health care in the world, yet not all citizens can afford the high cost of healing. The best way to provide health care to all is an ongoing debate in political arenas and living rooms across the nation. As you read about the significant training, education, and advances in treatment and diagnostic technology in the professional chapters of this text, you may begin to understand why health care is the 1.7 trillion dollar business it is. As an example, Blue Cross/Blue Shield estimates a couple having their first baby in a hospital is facing a medical bill ranging from $6,800–$9,800 for prenatal care and the delivery at a hospital (BCBS, 2006). That estimate is for a normal, healthy, vaginal birth without complications. A cesarean birth with the surgery, anesthesiology, and extended hospital stay can easily cost double that. Considering that many pregnancies in this country are unintended, it may be safe to assume that often couples do not have the funds to pay for this in their pockets. Could you save that much money in nine months?

Your Money for Your Life

Because of advances in medicine and medical technology, medical treatment is more expensive. People in developed countries are living longer, thus the population of those countries is aging. A larger group of senior citizens requires more medical care than a young healthier population. Some other factors that cause an increase in health insurance prices are health related: insufficient exercise; unhealthy food choices; a shortage of doctors in impoverished or rural areas; excessive use of alcohol or street drugs, smoking, and obesity among some parts of the population; and the modern sedentary lifestyle of the middle classes.

Fortunately, many individuals have some type of health insurance to cover the cost of receiving health care. According to the United States Census Bureau figures, roughly 85% of Americans have health insurance. Approximately 60% obtain health insurance through their place of employment or as individuals, and various government agencies provide health insurance to 25% of Americans. Unfortunately, many individuals do not have a means to help pay for expensive medical treatments. If you recall from Chapter 2, the Census Bureau reported that 45 million Americans lacked health insurance in 2003, an increase of 1.4 million from 2002 (DeNavas-Walt et al., 2005). The high cost of health care ultimately reaches into all of our pockets. For example, manufacturers may charge more for their products to recover the expense of providing insurance to their employees. Federal government and state taxes pay for services like Medicare and Medicaid and health insurance for children. Both the federal government and states support mental health programs, health departments, community hospitals, and other healthcare programs. All feel the social costs of limited access to health care. To improve the quality and quantity of life and reduce disparities between populations, goals of Healthy People 2010 is expensive business.

Health Insurance

Illness or non-work-related injury can be financially devastating, especially when considering the rising cost of health care over the past 20 years. Health insurance can help protect against large out-of-pocket healthcare expenses that can accumulate during an acute or chronic illness. Health insurance is a prepayment plan providing services or medical care needed in times of illness or disability. Health insurance includes voluntary plans, either commercial or nonprofit, or compulsory national insurance plans, usually connected with a Social Security program. Understanding the options, benefits, and limitations of health insurance is important for both personal and professional reasons. Eventually, students will graduate and join the work force, or at least that is what their parents hope! Employees often have to select health insurance from their employer's options. Many students in the health professions will rely on health insurance to pay their salaries in their future careers. A basic understanding will benefit both perspectives, as it is wise to be informed consumers when health is the product.

As with other forms of insurance, for your car and your home, health insurance helps relieve the burden of unexpected events: a little money is put away regularly in case expensive medical care is needed later. Every year, the cost of health care increases dramatically. Simple same-day surgeries, required tests, and emergency attention can add up to thousands of dollars or more. Having health insurance provides many benefits. Individuals are less likely to avoid seeking care because it costs too much. This may improve health, extend life expectancy, and add to quality of life. A health insurance policy is a contract between an insurer and an individual or group, in which the insurer agrees to provide specified health insurance at an agreed-upon price (the premium). Depending on the type of policy, the premium may be payable either in a lump sum or in installments. Health insurance usually provides either direct payment or reimbursement for expenses associated with illnesses and injuries.

Health insurance is one of the most controversial forms of insurance because of the perceived conflict between the need for the insurance company to remain solvent versus the need of its customers to remain healthy, which many view as a basic human right. Critics of private health insurance claim that this conflict of interest is why state and federal regulation of health insurance companies is necessary. Some say that this conflict exists in a liberal healthcare system because of the unpredictability of how patients respond to medical treatment. Proponents of regulation argue that too many health insurance companies put their desire for profits above the welfare of the consumer or patient.

Why Do You Need Health Insurance?

Let's face it—health insurance is a necessity in today's world. Even if you are healthy today and have never had any major problems in the past, you simply cannot predict the future. The costs of medical care and treatment have soared to new heights in recent years. There are enormous medical costs for individuals with a major injury or suddenly stricken with a life-threatening illness. In addition to medical emergencies, routine conditions requiring visits to a physician happen all the time. This is especially true for children. Ear infections, rashes, and high fevers are commonplace with infants and children; numerous trips to the doctor can be expensive without health insurance. Uninsured people live with such risk every day of their lives. Health insurance protects against that risk.

Historical Perspective on Health Insurance in the United States

While perpetually a topic of heated conversation in the political arena, paying for health care is not a new issue. In the past, health insurance in the United States took the form of voluntary programs. Such programs date from about 1850, when cooperative mutual benefit and fraternal beneficiary associations provided health insurance. Commercial companies introduced limited coverage, and subsequently established many plans offered by industries and labor unions.

Advocacy of government health insurance in the United States began in the early 1900s. Theodore Roosevelt made national health insurance one of the major planks of the Progressive Party during the 1912 presidential campaign, and in 1915 a model bill for health insurance was presented, but defeated, in numerous state legislatures. After 1920, opposition to government-sponsored plans led by the American Medical Association (AMA), was said to be motivated by the fear that government participation in medical care might lead to socialized medicine, a government-regulated system for providing health care for all by means of subsidies derived from taxation. Even today, the AMA opposes socialized medicine because these programs seek to impose predetermined clinical practice guidelines on patients without consideration of the best interests of those patients based on the advice of their physicians (*Columbia Encyclopedia*, 2006).

Over the years in the United States, societies of practicing physicians set up many health insurance plans, but the largest enrollment has been in Blue Cross and Blue Shield plans. These were set up as community-sponsored, nonprofit service plans based on contracts with hospitals and with subscribers or health-care consumers. Most general voluntary plans accept subscribers, in groups or as individuals. These plans extend coverage to dependents and exclude accidents and diseases covered by workers' compensation laws. Although valuable in cushioning the financial distress caused by illness or injury, voluntary health insurance not only limits benefits in order to avoid prohibitive premium rates but also excludes many people, particularly the poor, who cannot afford it, and senior citizens, for whom the cost is often prohibitive. By the mid-1990s, many of the Blue Cross companies, which had been suffering financially, were reorganizing, and by 2002 more than 20% of Blue Cross members were covered by plans that had converted to for-profit status (*Columbia Encyclopedia*, 2006).

During the middle of the 20th century, it became apparent that legislation was necessary to provide medical care for the elderly. In 1965, during President Lyndon B. Johnson's administration, federal legislation in the form of Medicare for the aged and Medicaid for the indigent was enacted. Since 1966, both public and private health insurance has played a key role in financing healthcare costs in the United States (*Columbia Encyclopedia*, 2006).

Government programs and insurance now cover the bulk of all medical bills. While the number of people covered by some form of health insurance increased over the past decades, those individuals have seen significant cost increases. As premiums increased, many businesses increased the amount of money employees contribute toward their health insurance. This situation has led to continuing political pressure for restructuring of the national healthcare insurance system.

Congress debated many bills for a national health insurance plan in the 1960s and 1970s, and in 1973 it passed the Health Maintenance Organization (HMO) Act, which provided grants to employers who set up HMOs. Unlike insurers, HMOs provide care directly to patients; hence, they are viewed as low-cost alternatives to hospitals and private doctors (*Columbia Encyclopedia*, 2006).

Managed care is a concept in US health care that rose to dominance during the presidency of Ronald Reagan as a means to control Medicare payouts. Managed care is based on an effort to control escalating healthcare costs by the health insurance industry, which supposedly defines a reasonable maximum fee which healthcare providers may charge for any given service. Providers are ostensibly bound to accept these maximum fees if they wish to be listed in directories of specific insurance companies, which are provided to their policy holders as referral directories of "approved" physicians.

The rise of managed care was credited by the health insurance industry for the lessened rate of medical inflation seen in much of the 1990s in the United States; in some years of that decade the rate of increase in the price of medical goods and services was little more than the overall rate of general inflation.

However, this effect now seems to largely have ended, and US medical inflation is once again two or three times the rate of overall inflation, as it was during much of the 1980s (*Columbia Encyclopedia*, 2006).

In 1993, President Clinton, elected on a promise of healthcare reform, proposed a national health insurance program that ultimately would have provided coverage for most citizens. Opposition by insurance, medical, small business, and other groups killed it. In 1999, Clinton and Congress battled over developing a "patient's bill of rights," to protect people from denial of service and other HMO limitations. Many individual states have developed their own health insurance alternatives by

- Using managed healthcare systems that monitor the type of services offered and have set fees for each service.
- Expanding Medicaid to help serve formerly ineligible patients.
- Establishing statewide or small-business health insurance alliances that pool people into a large group that has more buying power.

While we cannot ignore the millions that have no health insurance, it is helpful to understand the wide variety of programs available to the individuals who do have coverage. According to the National Center for Health Statistics of the CDC, there are private plans, government plans, state-specific plans, and even insurance plans offered by the Indian Health Service. Private health insurance is coverage by a health plan provided through an employer or union or purchased by an individual from a private health insurance company. These may be offered by an employer or a union. Employment-based health insurance is coverage offered through one's own employment or a relative's. Direct-purchase health insurance is coverage though a plan purchased by an individual from a private company (NCHS, 2006). The different types of coverage will be discussed in detail later in this chapter.

Government health insurance includes plans funded at the federal, state, or local level. The major categories of government health insurance are Medicare, Medicaid, the State Children's Health Insurance Program (SCHIP), military health care, state plans, and the Indian Health Service. Medicare is the federal program that helps pay healthcare costs for people 65 and older and certain people under 65 with long-term disabilities. Medicaid is a program administered at the state level that provides medical assistance to the needy. Families with dependent children, the aged, blind, and disabled who are in financial need are eligible for Medicaid. The State Children's Health Insurance Program is a program administered at the state level, providing health care to low-income children whose parents do not qualify for Medicaid. SCHIP may be known by different names in different states.

Military health care includes TRICARE/CHAMPUS (Civilian Health and Medical Program of the Uniformed Services) and CHAMPVA (Civilian

Health and Medical Program of the Department of Veterans Affairs), as well as care provided by the Department of Veterans Affairs (VA).

Some states have their own health insurance programs for low-income uninsured individuals. These health plans, known by different names in different states, vary in coverage and eligibility. Indian Health Service (IHS) is a healthcare program through which the Department of Health and Human Services provides medical assistance to eligible Native Americans at IHS facilities. In addition, the IHS helps pay the cost of selected healthcare services provided at non-IHS facilities (NCHS, 2006).

What Kinds of Non-government Health Insurance are There?

According to the Insurance Information Institute, there are essentially two kinds of health insurance: Fee-for-Service and Managed Care. Although these plans differ, they both cover an array of medical, surgical, and hospital expenses. Most plans cover prescription drugs and some also offer dental coverage (III, 2006b). A brief description of each type follows.

- **Fee-for-Service**

  These plans generally assume that the medical professional is paid a fee for each service provided to the patient. Patients are seen by a doctor of their choice and the insurance claim is filed by either the medical provider or the patient.

- **Managed Care**

  More than half of all Americans have some kind of managed-care plan for their health insurance. Various plans work differently and can include health maintenance organizations (HMOs), preferred provider organizations (PPOs), and point-of-service (POS) plans. These plans provide comprehensive health services to their members and offer financial incentives to patients who use the providers in the plan.

Traditional Fee-for-Service Insurance (Indemnity Policies)

Most indemnity policies allow individuals to choose any doctor and hospital that they wish when seeking healthcare services. Indemnity in this case means protection, as by insurance, from liabilities or penalties incurred by one's actions. The hallmark of traditional fee-for-service insurance is choice—the choice of what provider to visit when seeking covered medical services with few if any geographic limitations. When purchasing an indemnity policy there is often a deductible, the amount required to pay before policy benefits are provided. There may be options regarding the amount of the deductible. If individual healthcare charges are covered, or eligible for payment under the policy, any applicable deductible will apply. Once the deductible has been paid, the remaining charges are reimbursed to the individual at a specified percentage according to the policy contract. A *co-payment* is the difference between eligible charges and the percentage paid, and is normally the participant's responsibility. The policy or an employee benefit booklet (if the indemnity policy is group coverage) will spell out the terms and conditions of what is covered and what is not covered (III, 2006b).

Health Maintenance Organizations

A health maintenance organization (HMO) is a type of managed healthcare system. HMOs and preferred provider organizations (PPOs) share the goal of reducing healthcare costs by focusing on preventative care and implementing utilization management controls. Unlike many traditional insurers, HMOs do not merely provide financing for medical care. The HMO actually delivers the treatment as well. Doctors, hospitals, and insurers all participate in the business arrangement known as an HMO. In practice, an HMO is an insurance plan under which an insurance company controls all aspects of the health care of the insured. In the design of the plan, each member is assigned a "gatekeeper," a primary care physician (PCP), who is responsible for the overall care of members assigned to him/her. Specialty services require a specific referral from the PCP to the specialist. Non-emergency hospital admissions also require specific pre-authorization by the PCP. Typically, services are not covered if performed by a provider who is not an employee of, or specifically approved by, the HMO, unless it is an emergency situation as defined by the HMO. Instead of deductibles, most HMO's have nominal co-payments. In return for this fee, most HMOs provide a wide variety of medical services, from office visits to hospitalization and surgery. With a few exceptions, HMO members must receive their medical treatment from physicians and facilities within the HMO network. The size of this network varies depending on the individual HMO.

The focus of many HMOs is on wellness and preventative care. By reducing out-of-pocket costs and paperwork, HMOs encourage members to seek medical treatment early, before health problems become severe. In addition, many HMOs offer health education classes and discounted health club memberships. Unlike most health insurance plans, HMOs generally do not place a limit on your lifetime benefits. The HMO will continue to cover your treatment as long as you are a member (III, 2006b).

Preferred Provider Organizations

Like an HMO, a preferred provider organization (PPO) is a managed healthcare system. However, there are several important differences between HMOs and PPOs. A PPO is actually a group of doctors and/or hospitals that provides medical service only to a specific group or association. The PPO may be sponsored by a particular insurance company, by one or more employers, or by some other type of organization. PPO physicians provide medical services to the policyholders, employees, or members of the sponsor(s) at discounted rates and may set up utilization-control programs to help reduce the cost of medical care. In return, the sponsor(s) attempts to increase patient volume by creating an incentive for employees or policyholders to use the physicians and facilities within the PPO network.

Rather than prepaying for medical care, PPO members pay for services as rendered. The PPO sponsor (employer or insurance company) generally reimburses the member for the cost of the treatment, less any co-payment percentage. In some cases, the physician may submit the bill directly to the insurance company for payment. The insurer then pays the covered amount directly to the healthcare provider, and the member pays his or her co-payment amount. The healthcare providers and the PPO sponsor negotiate the price for each type of service in advance. PPO members are not required to seek care from PPO physicians. However, there is generally strong financial incentive to do so. Reimbursement for PPO physicians is often greater than for non-network physicians. For example, members may receive 90% reimbursement for care obtained from network physicians but only 60% for treatment provided by non-network physicians.

Healthcare costs paid out of your own pocket (for example, deductibles and co-payments) are limited with most PPOs. Typically, out-of-pocket costs for network care are limited to $1,200 for individuals and $2,100 for families. Out-of-pocket costs for non-network treatment are typically capped at $2,000 for individuals and $3,500 for families (III, 2006).

Point of Service Plans

A Point of Service (POS) plan is a type of managed healthcare system that combines characteristics of the HMO and the PPO. Like an HMO, members pay no deductible and usually only a minimal co-payment when they use a healthcare provider within the PPO network. Members also must choose a primary care physician who is responsible for all referrals within the POS network. If they choose to go outside the network for health care, POS coverage functions more like a PPO. Members will likely be subject to a deductible (around $300 for an individual or $600 for a family), and the co-payment required will be a substantial percentage of the physician's charges (usually 30–40%).

POS coverage allows you to maximize your freedom of choice. As with a PPO, you can mix the types of care you receive. For example, your child could continue to see his pediatrician who is not in the network, while you receive the rest of your health care from network providers. This freedom of choice encourages members to use network providers but does not require it, as with HMO coverage. As with HMO coverage, members pay only a nominal amount for network care. Usually, their co-payment is around $10 per treatment or office visit. Unlike HMO coverage, however, they always retain the right to seek care outside the network at a lower level of coverage. When choosing to use network providers, there is generally no deductible, as long as members stay within the POS network of physicians. If members choose to go outside the POS network for treatment, they are free to see any doctor or specialist they choose without first consulting a primary care physician (PCP). Of course, they will pay substantially more out-of-pocket charges for non-network care. Healthcare costs paid out of the member's own pocket (that is, deductibles and co-payments) are typically limited. The average yearly limit for individuals is around $2,400. For families, the average yearly limit is approximately $4,000. In a catastrophic illness, these limits help reduce the financial burden to the members.

As in a PPO, there is generally strong financial incentive to use POS network physicians. For example, the co-payment may be only $10 for care obtained from network physicians, but members could be responsible for up to 40% of the cost of treatment provided by non-network doctors. In most cases, individuals must reach a specified deductible before coverage begins on out-of-network care. On average, individual deductibles are around $300 per year, and the average annual family deductible is about $600. This deductible amount is *in addition* to the higher co-payment for out-of-network care. As in an HMO, members must choose a primary care physician (PCP) who provides general medical care and must be consulted before seeking care from another doctor or specialist within the network. This screening process helps to reduce costs both for the POS and for POS members, but it can also lead to complications if a PCP does not provide the referral needed (III, 2006).

Other Types of Health-Related Insurance

Vision care insurance is insurance that provides coverage for services relating to the care and treatment of the eyes. It typically covers services delivered by an optometrist or opthamologist. Some vision plans may provide more extensive coverage (such as certain eye surgeries), while others may limit coverage to "reasonable and customary" charges incurred during routine eye exams. Reasonable and customary charges generally don't include the cost of glasses and contact lenses. With some employer-sponsored vision plans, coverage may be even more narrowly limited to the medical treatment of certain eye conditions. This is rare, however.

Dental insurance may provide direct payment to the dentist for the dental care and treatment you receive. Or you may be required to cover the applicable charges out-of-pocket at the time of service, and then file a claim for reimbursement. It depends on the specific plan. Dental insurance has become more common in recent years. Of the roughly 55% of Americans who have dental insurance, most receive their coverage through their employer. Employer-sponsored dental insurance may take the form of a health insurance plan that includes dental coverage, a separate dental plan, or a benefit choice within a cafeteria plan (III, 2006b).

Picking a Non-government Health Plan: Considerations

With so many health insurance options, how do you choose? There are some important differences between indemnity plans, HMOs, PPOs, and POS plans worthy of understanding. As a future (or current) consumer, you should make every effort to understand your own health insurance policy, and become familiar with common health insurance provisions, including limitations, exclusions, and riders. It is important to know what your policy covers, and what you will have to pay in out-of-pocket expenses. When comparing health insurance policies, you should strive to balance coverage against cost. While price is an important consideration, other factors also may influence your decision when the time comes to choose a health insurance plan.

A good health insurance policy contains several types of coverage. Basic insurance includes hospital, surgical, and physicians' expense coverage. In addition, major medical coverage is necessary in case of a catastrophic accident or illness. These may be purchased separately, but you will generally get more complete coverage if they are combined in a single policy. Your policy should discuss the cost of each type of coverage and describe exactly what each pays for. A health insurance policy also contains important information regarding out-of-pocket costs, namely deductibles and co-payments. The family coverage provisions will be important as well, if a spouse or dependents are covered by the policy. Information about out-of-pocket maximums and benefit ceilings should also be included.

The Insurance Information Institute suggests employees ask the following questions when deciding on health insurance options. It is crucial to understand health insurance choices and pick the insurance that is best for you and your family (III, 2006a).

How affordable is the cost of care?

- What is the monthly premium I will have to pay?
- Should I try to insure most of my medical expenses or just the large ones?
- What deductibles will I have to pay out-of-pocket before insurance starts to reimburse me?
- After I've met my deductible, what percentage of my medical expenses are reimbursed?
- How much less am I reimbursed if I use doctors outside the insurance company's network?

Does the insurance plan cover the services I am likely to use?

- Are the doctors, hospitals, laboratories, and other medical providers that I use in the insurance company's network?
- If I want to use a doctor outside the network, will the plan permit it?
- How easily can I change primary care physicians if I want to?
- Do I need to get permission before I see a medical specialist?
- What are the procedures for getting care and being reimbursed in an emergency situation, both at home and out of town?
- If I have a preexisting medical condition, will the plan cover it?
- If I have a chronic condition such as asthma, cancer, AIDS, or alcoholism, how will the plan treat it?

- Are the prescription medicines that I use covered by the plan?
- Does the plan reimburse alternative medical therapies such as acupuncture or chiropractic treatment?
- Does the plan cover the costs of delivering a baby?

What is the quality of the insurance plan I'm looking at?

- How have independent government and non-government organizations rated the plan? For example, the National Committee for Quality Assurance (NCQA) (http://www.ncqa.org) issues a Consumer Assessment of Health Plans (CAHPS) report for every medical plan and facility.
- What kind of accreditation has the plan received from groups such as NCQA or the Joint Commission on Accreditation of Healthcare Organizations (JCAHO) (http://www.jcaho.org)?
- How many patient complaints were filed against the plan last year and how many were upheld by state regulatory agencies like the state insurance commission or the state medical licensing board?
- How many members drop out of the plan each year? State insurance departments keep track of "dis-enrollment rates."
- Do the doctors, pharmacies, and other services in the plans offer convenient times and locations?
- Does the plan pay for preventive health care such as diet and exercise advice, immunizations, and health screenings?
- What do my friends and colleagues say about their experiences with the plan?
- What does my doctor say about his or her experience with the plan?

If you do not have health insurance right now, you should seriously consider purchasing it as soon as possible. No one can predict the future—you do not know when you might suffer an accident or become seriously ill. Health insurance can help to protect you against financial ruin.

Government-Sponsored Health Insurance Programs

Some people would like to see some form of national health insurance to pay for medical care for everyone. Others would keep the system as it currently exists. Congress, the President, state legislatures, doctors, insurance companies, and private citizens are talking about rising health costs and proposing ways to deal with this issue. Government-sponsored programs such as Medicare and Medicaid do not provide care directly, but rather contract with healthcare professionals, hospitals, and HMOs to deliver services to their beneficiaries.

On July 30, 1965, President Lyndon Johnson signed legislation that created the Medicaid program. Medicaid has grown from its origins as a health coverage program for welfare recipients into a public health insurance program for the nation's low-income population as well as the predominant long-term care program for the elderly and individuals with disabilities. The combined federal, state, and local governments' role in financing healthcare services has evolved from a relatively minor one, to one of major importance for the healthcare services provided to millions of people in the United States. However, like many "40-somethings," a mid-life crisis is in the making for Medicaid. Will its programs be able to support the health care needs of the surge of citizens over 65?

Overview of Medicaid

Title XIX of the Social Security Act is a federal/state entitlement program that pays for medical assistance for certain individuals and families with low incomes and resources. This program, known as Medicaid, became law in 1965 as a cooperative venture jointly funded by the federal and state governments (including the District of Columbia and the Territories) to assist states in furnishing medical assistance to eligible needy persons. It was created as a joint federal-state program to provide medical assistance to aged, disabled, or blind individuals (or to needy, dependent children) who could not otherwise afford the necessary medical care. Medicaid is the largest source of funding for medical and health-related services for some of America's poorest people (DeParle, 2000).

Within broad national guidelines established by federal statutes, regulations, and policies, each state (1) establishes its own eligibility standards; (2) determines the type, amount, duration, and scope of services; (3) sets the rate of payment for services; and (4) administers its own program. Medicaid policies for eligibility, services, and payment are complex and vary considerably, even among states of similar size or geographic proximity. Thus, a person who is eligible for Medicaid in one state may not be eligible in another state, and the services provided by one state may differ considerably in amount, duration, or scope from services provided in a similar or neighboring state. In addition, state legislatures may change Medicaid eligibility, services, and/or reimbursement during the year.

Medicaid pays for a number of medical costs, including hospital bills, physician services, home health care, and long-term nursing home care. States may elect to provide other services for which federal matching funds are available.

Some of the most frequently covered optional services are clinic services, medical transportation, services for the mentally retarded in intermediate care facilities, prescribed drugs, optometrist services and eyeglasses, occupational therapy, prosthetic devices, and speech therapy.

Who Is Eligible for Medicaid?

Medicaid does not provide medical assistance for *all* poor persons. Under the broadest provisions of the federal statute, Medicaid does not provide health-care services even for very poor persons unless they are in a "categorically needy" eligibility group. Low income is only one test for Medicaid eligibility; individuals' resources also are tested against threshold levels determined by each state within federal guidelines.

The poverty thresholds are the original version of the federal poverty measure. They are updated each year by the Census Bureau. The thresholds are used mainly for statistical purposes—for instance, preparing estimates of the number of Americans in poverty each year. (In other words, all official poverty population figures are calculated using the poverty thresholds, not the guidelines.) The poverty guidelines issued by the Department of Health and Human Services (DHHS) are the other version of the federal poverty measure. The guidelines are a simplification of the poverty thresholds for use for administrative purposes—for instance, determining financial eligibility for federal programs such as Medicaid. The poverty guidelines are sometimes loosely referred to as the "federal poverty level" (FPL).

States generally have broad discretion in determining which groups their Medicaid programs will cover and the financial criteria for Medicaid eligibility. To be eligible for federal funds, however, states are required to provide Medicaid coverage for certain individuals who receive federally assisted income-maintenance payments, as well as for related groups not receiving cash payments. In addition to their Medicaid programs, most states have additional "state-only" programs to provide medical assistance for specified poor persons who do not qualify for Medicaid. Federal funds do not support state-only programs. The following enumerates the mandatory Medicaid "categorically needy" eligibility groups for which federal matching funds are provided (CMS, 2005):

- Most individuals who meet the requirements for the Aid to Families with Dependent Children (AFDC) program that were in effect in their state on July 16, 1996.
- Children under age 6 whose family income is at or below 133% of the federal poverty level (FPL).

- Pregnant women whose family income is below 133% of the FPL (services to these women are limited to those related to pregnancy, complications of pregnancy, delivery, and postpartum care).
- Supplemental Security Income (SSI) recipients in most states (some states use more restrictive Medicaid eligibility requirements that pre-date SSI).
- Recipients of adoption or foster care assistance under Title IV of the Social Security Act.
- Special protected groups (typically individuals who lose their cash assistance due to earnings from work or from increased Social Security benefits, but who may keep Medicaid for a period of time).
- All children born after September 30, 1983 who are under age 19, in families with incomes at or below the FPL.
- Certain Medicare beneficiaries.

States also have the option of providing Medicaid coverage for other "categorically related" groups. These optional groups share characteristics of the mandatory groups (that is, they fall within defined categories), but the eligibility criteria are somewhat more liberally defined.

The Balanced Budget Act (BBA) of 1997 amended federal Medicaid law in the areas of eligibility, benefits, premiums and cost sharing, provider reimbursement and participation, managed care, and federal financial assistance. In addition to making Medicaid changes, the BBA also created the State

Table 3.1 *2006 HHS Poverty Guidelines*

Persons in Family or Household	48 Contiguous States and D.C.	Alaska	Hawaii
1	$ 9,800	$12,250	$11,270
2	13,200	16,500	15,180
3	16,600	20,750	19,090
4	20,000	25,000	23,000
5	23,400	29,250	26,910
6	26,800	33,500	30,820
7	30,200	37,750	34,730
8	33,600	42,000	38,640
For each additional person, add 3,400	4,250	3,910

Source: Federal Register, 2006.

Children's Health Insurance Program (SCHIP), or Title XXI of the Social Security Act. SCHIP allows states to expand their Medicaid programs to cover additional uninsured children, or to create non-Medicaid insurance programs to accomplish the same goal (CMS, 2005).

Welfare reform also repealed the open-ended federal entitlement program known as Aid to Families with Dependent Children (AFDC) and replaced it with Temporary Assistance for Needy Families (TANF), which provides states with grants to be spent on time-limited cash assistance. TANF generally limits a family's lifetime cash welfare benefits to a maximum of 5 years and permits states to impose a wide range of other requirements as well—in particular, those related to employment. However, the impact on Medicaid eligibility is not expected to be significant. Under welfare reform, persons who would have been eligible for AFDC under the AFDC requirements in effect on July 16, 1996 generally will still be eligible for Medicaid. Although most persons covered by TANF will receive Medicaid, it is not required by law (CMS, 2005).

Scope of Medicaid Services

Title XIX of the Social Security Act allows considerable flexibility within the states' Medicaid plans. However, some federal requirements are mandatory if federal matching funds are to be received. A state's Medicaid program must offer medical assistance for certain basic services to most categorically needy populations (CMS, 2005). These services generally include the following:

- Inpatient hospital services
- Outpatient hospital services
- Prenatal care
- Vaccines for children
- Physician services
- Nursing facility services for persons aged 21 or older
- Family planning services and supplies
- Rural health clinic services
- Home health care for persons eligible for skilled-nursing services
- Laboratory and x-ray services
- Pediatric and family nurse practitioner services
- Nurse-midwife services
- Federally qualified health-center (FQHC) services, and ambulatory services of an FQHC that would be available in other settings

- Early and periodic screening and diagnostic and treatment (EPSDT) services for children under age 21

States may also receive federal matching funds to provide certain optional services. Following are the most common of the 34 currently approved optional Medicaid services:

- Diagnostic services
- Clinic services
- Intermediate care facilities for the mentally retarded (ICFs/MR)
- Prescribed drugs and prosthetic devices
- Optometrist services and eyeglasses
- Nursing facility services for children under age 21
- Transportation services
- Rehabilitation and physical therapy services
- Home and community-based care to certain persons with chronic impairments

The BBA included a state option known as Programs of All-inclusive Care for the Elderly (PACE). PACE provides an alternative to institutional care for persons aged 55 or older who require a nursing facility level of care. The PACE team offers and manages all health, medical, and social services and mobilizes other services as needed to provide preventative, rehabilitative, curative, and supportive care. This care, provided in day health centers, homes, hospitals, and nursing homes, helps the person maintain independence, dignity, and quality of life. PACE functions within the Medicare program as well.

Amount and Duration of Medicaid Services

The Centers for Medicare & Medicaid Services (CMS) is a federal agency within the US Department of Health and Human Services. The CMS administers the Medicare program and works in partnership with the states to administer Medicaid and State Children's Health Insurance Programs. Within broad federal guidelines and certain limitations, states determine the amount and duration of services offered under their Medicaid programs. States may limit, for example, the number of days of hospital care or the number of physician visits covered. Two restrictions apply: (1) limits must result in a sufficient level of services to reasonably achieve the purpose of the benefits; and (2) limits on benefits may not discriminate among beneficiaries based on medical diagnosis or condition (CMS, 2005).

In general, states are required to provide comparable amounts, duration, and scope of services to all categorically needy and categorically related eligible persons. There are two important exceptions: (1) medically necessary healthcare services that are identified under the Early Periodic Screening, Diagnosis, and Treatment (EPSDT) program for eligible children, and that are within the scope of mandatory or optional services under federal law, must be covered even if those services are not included as part of the covered services in that state's plan; and (2) states may request "waivers" to pay for otherwise uncovered home and community-based services (HCBS) for Medicaid-eligible persons who might otherwise be institutionalized. As long as the services are cost effective, states have few limitations on the services that may be covered under these waivers (except that, other than as a part of respite care, states may not provide room and board for the beneficiaries). With certain exceptions, a state's Medicaid program must allow beneficiaries to have some informed choices among participating providers of health care and to receive quality care that is appropriate and timely (CMS, 2005).

Payment for Medicaid Services

Medicaid operates as a vendor payment program. States may pay healthcare providers directly on a fee-for-service basis, or states may pay for Medicaid services through various prepayment arrangements, such as health maintenance organizations (HMOs). Within federally imposed upper limits and specific restrictions, each state for the most part has broad discretion in determining the payment methodology and payment rate for services. Generally, payment rates must be sufficient to enlist enough providers so that covered services are available at least to the extent that comparable care and services are available to the general population within that geographic area. Providers participating in Medicaid must accept Medicaid payment rates as payment in full. States must make additional payments to qualified hospitals that provide inpatient services to a disproportionate number of Medicaid beneficiaries and/or to other low-income or uninsured persons under what is known as the "disproportionate share hospital" (DSH) adjustment. States may impose nominal deductibles, coinsurance, or co-payments on some Medicaid beneficiaries, for certain services.

Medicaid, initially formulated as a medical care extension of federally funded programs, provided cash income assistance for the poor with an emphasis on dependent children and their mothers, the disabled, and the elderly. Legislative changes over the years resulted in incremental expansion of Medicaid focusing on increased access, better quality of care, specific benefits, enhanced outreach programs, and fewer limits on services.

As with all health insurance programs, most Medicaid beneficiaries incur relatively small average expenditures per person each year, and a relatively small proportion incurs very large costs. Moreover, the average cost varies substantially by type of beneficiary. National data for 2001, for example, indicate that Medicaid payments for services for 23.3 million children, who constitute 50% of all Medicaid beneficiaries, average about $1,305 per child (a relatively small average expenditure per person). Similarly, for 11.6 million adults, who comprise 25% of beneficiaries, payments average about $1,725 per person. However, certain other specific groups have much larger per-person expenditures. Medicaid payments for services for 4.4 million aged, constituting 9% of all Medicaid beneficiaries, average about $10,965 per person; for 7.7 million disabled, who comprise 16% of beneficiaries, payments average about $10,455 per person. When expenditures for these high- and lower-cost beneficiaries are combined, the 2001 payments to healthcare vendors for 47.0 million Medicaid beneficiaries average $3,965 per person (CMS, 2005).

Long-term care is an important provision of Medicaid that will be increasingly utilized as our nation's population ages. The Medicaid program paid for over 41% of the total cost of care for persons using nursing facility or home health services in 2001. National data for 2001 show that Medicaid payments for nursing facility services totaled $37.2 billion for more than 1.7 million beneficiaries of these services—an average expenditure of $21,890 per nursing home beneficiary. The national data also show that Medicaid payments for home health services totaled $3.5 billion for more than 1.0 million beneficiaries—an average expenditure of $3,475 per home healthcare beneficiary. With the percentage of our population who are elderly or disabled increasing faster than that of the younger groups, the need for long-term care is expected to increase (CMS, 2005).

Another significant development in Medicaid is the growth in managed care as an alternative service delivery concept different from the traditional fee-for-service system. Under managed care systems, HMOs, prepaid health plans (PHPs), or comparable entities agree to provide a specific set of services to Medicaid enrollees, usually in return for a predetermined periodic payment per enrollee. Managed care programs seek to enhance access to quality care in a cost-effective manner. Waivers may provide the states with greater flexibility in the design and implementation of their Medicaid managed care programs to develop innovative healthcare delivery or reimbursement systems. The number of Medicaid beneficiaries enrolled in some form of managed care program is growing rapidly, from 14% of enrollees in 1993 to 59% in 2003 (CMS, 2005).

More than 46.0 million persons received healthcare services through the Medicaid program in 2001. In 2003, total outlays for the Medicaid program (federal and state) were $278.3 billion, including direct payment to providers of $197.3 billion, payments for various premiums (for HMOs, Medicare, etc.) of $52.1 billion, payments to disproportionate share hospitals of $12.9 billion, and administrative costs of $16.0 billion. Outlays under the SCHIP program in 2003 were $6.1 billion. With no changes to either program, expenditures under Medicaid and SCHIP are projected to reach $445 billion and $7.5 billion, respectively, by 2009 (CMS, 2005).

The Centers for Medicare & Medicaid Services (CMS) estimates that Medicaid currently provides some level of supplemental health coverage for about 6.5 million Medicare beneficiaries. Starting January 2006, the new Medicare prescription drug benefit provides drug coverage for Medicare beneficiaries, including those who also receive coverage from Medicaid. In addition, individuals eligible for both Medicare and Medicaid also receive the low-income subsidy for both the Medicare drug plan premium and assistance with cost sharing for prescriptions. Medicaid will no longer provide drug benefits for Medicare beneficiaries.

Medicare

Medicare is a federal program that provides health insurance to retired individuals, regardless of their medical condition. Most people become eligible for Medicare upon reaching age 65 and becoming eligible for Social Security retirement benefits. In addition, individuals may be eligible if they are disabled or have end-stage renal disease. Any individual who is receiving Social Security benefits is automatically enrolled in Medicare at age 65 when he or she becomes eligible. However, those who delay retirement until after age 65 must remember to enroll in Medicare at age 65 anyway, because enrollment won't be automatic. Medicare coverage consists of two parts—Medicare Part A (hospital insurance) and Medicare Part B (medical insurance). A third part, Medicare Part C (Medicare+Choice), is a program that allows you to choose from several types of healthcare plans. Everyone with Medicare, regardless of income, health status, or prescription drug usage, will have access to prescription drug coverage as of January 1, 2006 under Medicare Part D. Medicare Part D prescription drug coverage is insurance that covers both brand-name and generic prescription drugs at participating pharmacies in your area. Medicare prescription drug coverage provides protection for people who have very high drug costs (CMS, 2005). Each category of Medicare coverage is described in the following sections.

- **Medicare Part A (hospital insurance):** Generally known as hospital insurance, Part A covers services associated with inpatient hospital care (that is, the costs associated with an overnight stay in a hospital, skilled nursing facility, or psychiatric hospital, such as charges for the hospital room, meals, and nursing services). Part A also covers hospice care and home health care.

- **Medicare Part B (medical insurance):** Generally known as medical insurance, Part B covers other medical care. Physician care—whether it was received while you were an inpatient at a hospital, at a doctor's office, or as an outpatient at a hospital or other healthcare facility—is covered under Part B. Also covered are laboratory tests, physical therapy or rehabilitation services, and ambulance service.

- **Medicare Part C (Medicare+Choice):** The 1997 Balanced Budget Act expanded the kinds of private healthcare plans that may offer Medicare benefits to include managed care plans, medical savings accounts, and private fee-for-service plans. The new Medicare Part C programs are in addition to the fee-for-service options available under Medicare Parts A and B.

- **Medicare Part D prescription drug coverage**: This insurance covers both brand-name and generic prescription drugs at participating pharmacies in your area. Medicare prescription drug coverage provides protection for people who have very high drug costs. Everyone with Medicare is eligible for this coverage, regardless of income and resources, health status, or current prescription expenses.

Who Administers the Medicare Program?

The Centers for Medicare and Medicaid Services (CMMS), a division of the US Department of Health and Human Services, has overall responsibility for administering the Medicare program. Although the Social Security Administration processes Medicare applications and claims, the CMMS sets standards and policies. However, beneficiaries deal mostly with the private insurance companies that actually handle the claims on the local level for individuals receiving Medicare coverage. Insurance companies handling Medicare Part A claims are called Medicare intermediaries, and insurance companies handling Part B claims are called Medicare carriers. Managed care plans handle Part C claims. Although the same private insurance company may handle both Part A and Part B claims, Part A and Part B are very different regarding administration (for example, different deductibles and co-payment requirements). There is virtually no overlap; it is as if participants have two separate health insurance policies.

Medicare beneficiaries who have low incomes and limited resources may also receive help from the Medicaid program. For such persons who are eligible for full Medicaid coverage, the Medicare healthcare coverage is supplemented by services that are available under their state's Medicaid program, according to eligibility category. These additional services may include, for example, nursing facility care beyond the 100-day limit covered by Medicare, prescription drugs, eyeglasses, and hearing aids. For persons enrolled in both programs, any services that are covered by Medicare are paid for by the Medicare program before any payments are made by the Medicaid program, since Medicaid is always the "payer of last resort."

Medicaid and Long-Term Nursing Home Care

Over 60% of all nursing home residents receive Medicaid benefits that help pay for their care. An aging population and the increased cost of long-term care have made Medicaid planning an important topic. In years past, attorneys and financial planners devised strategies for the middle class and people of means to qualify for Medicaid by transferring funds to family members and by establishing trusts. Consequently, Congress tightened the Medicaid rules regarding the transfer of assets. The Omnibus Reconciliation Act of 1993 makes qualifying for Medicaid more difficult for those people who transfer their assets away without receiving fair value in return. If individuals transfer assets away for less than fair consideration within 36 months of their application for Medicaid, the law creates a waiting period before they can collect Medicaid benefits. Transfers into certain trusts within 60 months of a Medicaid application also will also cause a period of ineligibility.

Health Insurance Covering our Smallest Citizens: State Children's Health Insurance

Although Medicaid has made great strides in enrolling low-income children, significant numbers of children remain uninsured. From 1988 to 1998, the proportion of children insured through Medicaid increased from 15.6% to 19.8%. At the same time, however, the percentage of children without health insurance increased from 13.1% to 15.4%. The increase in uninsured children is mostly the result of fewer children being covered by employer-sponsored health insurance. Title XXI of the Social Security Act, known as the State Children's Health Insurance Program (SCHIP), is a program initiated by the Balanced Budget Act. In addition to allowing states to craft or expand an existing state insurance program, SCHIP provides more federal funds for states to expand Medicaid eligibility to include a greater number of children who are currently uninsured. With certain exceptions, these are low-income children who would not qualify for Medicaid based on the plan that was in effect on April 15, 1997. Funds from SCHIP also may be used to provide medical assistance to children during a presumptive eligibility period for Medicaid. As part of the Balanced Budget Act of 1997, SCHIP was designed as a federal/state partnership, similar to Medicaid, with the goal of expanding health insurance to children whose families earn too much money to be eligible for Medicaid, but not enough money to purchase private insurance. SCHIP is the single largest expansion of health insurance coverage for children since the initiation of Medicaid in the mid-1960s (CMS, 2005).

SCHIP is designed to provide coverage to "targeted low-income children." A "targeted low-income child" is one who resides in a family with income below 200% of the Federal Poverty Level (FPL) or whose family has an income 50% higher than the state's Medicaid eligibility threshold. Some states have expanded SCHIP eligibility beyond the 200% FPL limit, and others are covering entire families and not just children. As of September 30, 1999, each of the states and territories had an approved SCHIP plan in place. SCHIP offers states three options when designing a program. The state can either

- use SCHIP funds to expand Medicaid eligibility to children who previously did not qualify for the program;
- design a separate children's health insurance program entirely separate from Medicaid; or,
- combine both the Medicaid and separate program options.

Children's health insurance programs are not welfare programs. Everyone has a stake in making sure America's children are healthy. These programs support working families and low-income families alike in providing health insurance to their children. *Insure Kids Now!* is a national campaign to link the nation's 10 million uninsured children—from birth to age 18—to free and low-cost health insurance. Many families simply do not know their children are eligible. The states have different eligibility rules, but in most states, uninsured children 18 years old and younger whose families earn up to $34,100 a year (for a family of four) are eligible (CMS, 2005).

Nationalized Health Care

Many countries have made the societal choice to avoid this important conflict by nationalizing the health industry so that doctors, nurses, and other medical workers become state employees, all funded by taxes; or setting up a national health insurance plan that all citizens pay into with tax or quasi-tax payments and which pays private doctors for health care. These national healthcare systems also have their problems. Some of these countries have citizen groups which protest bureaucracy and cost-cutting measures that unduly delay medical treatment. Similar issues exist with private health management insurances (HMO) in countries with privately funded medicine.

Future Challenges

With the advent of DNA testing, previously unknown risk factors involving genetic makeup will become known and this is expected to lead to greater pressure on the private health insurance industry as they try to limit their exposure to high-risk individuals. As larger groups of these individuals are identified and charged higher premiums (if they can get coverage at all) the pressure on privacy laws to limit the flow of personal medical data will only increase. HIPAA is the acronym for the Health Insurance Portability and Accountability Act of 1996. The Centers for Medicare & Medicaid Services (CMS) are responsible for implementing various unrelated provisions of HIPAA, therefore HIPAA may mean different things to different people. This legislation is important to healthcare providers as well as a protection of the healthcare consumer. Chapter 4 addresses HIPAA and the implications for healthcare professionals.

SUMMARY

In April 2006, the state of Massachusetts became the first to propose universal health care for all its citizens, requiring all state residents to have health insurance through an individual mandate on the purchase of health insurance, with government subsidies to ensure affordability. This innovative bipartisan bill is an attempt to cover 95% of the state's uninsured population within 3 years (Kaiser, 2006). Those with access to health insurance are often asked to pay increasing premiums and co-payments for their health coverage.

Employers, in efforts to curb costs of providing insurance to their workers, raise deductibles to reduce their premium rates. Quality health care is expensive! The economic impact of the current epidemic of obesity alone, and the subsequent health problems related to obesity and lack of physical activity in this country, will be staggering. To achieve Healthy People 2010 objectives of improving the quality and quantity of life and reduce disparities within populations, access to health care is critical. Someone has to pay for that care. As a nation, we will likely see many innovative proposals to expand coverage to keep more individuals healthy.

ADDITIONAL RESOURCES

Consumer information on the various health insurance plans that exist today is available from the following leading insurance trade associations. They are:

America's Health Insurance Plans

601 Pennsylvania Avenue, NW
South Building
Suite 500
Washington, DC 20004
http://www.ahip.org

Insurance Information Institute
110 William Street
New York, NY 10038
212-346-5500
http://www.iii.org/

Life and Health Foundation for Education

2175 K Street, NW—Suite 250
Washington, DC 20037
http://www.life-line.org

Medicare and Medicaid and SCHIP

Centers for Medicare & Medicaid Services
7500 Security Boulevard
Baltimore, MD 21244-1850
1-800-MEDICARE
http://www.cms.hhs.gov/

REFERENCES

Blue Cross Blue Shield (BCBS). (2006). Healthcare cost estimator, inpatient hospital admissions, pregnancy, and childbirth: Average cost by condition. Retrieved September 15, 2006, from http://www.bcbsnc.com/apps/costestimator/report.do?type=inpatient&sub=14.

Centers for Medicare & Medicaid Services (CMS). (2005, December). Technical summary. Retrieved August 1, 2006, from http://www.cms.hhs.gov/MedicaidGen-Info/03_TechnicalSummary.asp.

The Columbia Encyclopedia (6th ed). (2006). Health insurance in the United States. New York: Columbia University Press. Retrieved March 30, 2006, from www.bartleby.com/65/.

DeNavas-Walt, C., Proctor, B., & Lee, C. (2005). *Income, poverty, and health insurance coverage in the United States: 2004.* U.S. Census Bureau, Current Population Reports. Washington, DC: Government Printing Office.

DeParle, N. (2000, Fall). Celebrating 35 years of Medicaid and Medicare. *Health Care Financing Review, 22*(1).

Federal Register. (2006, January 24). The HHS federal poverty guidelines. Retrieved April 8, 2006, from http://aspe.hhs.gov/poverty/06poverty.shtml.

Insurance Information Institute (III). (2006a). How do I pick a health plan? Retrieved March 30, 2006, from http://www.iii.org/individuals/health/health/howdoi/.

Insurance Information Institute (III). (2006b). What kinds of health insurance are there? Retrieved March 30, 2006, from http://www.iii.org/individuals/health/health/whatkinds/.

Kaiser Commission on Key Facts (Kaiser). (2006). Massachusetts health care reform plan. Washington, DC: The Henry J. Kaiser Foundation.

National Center for Health Statistics (NCHS). (2006). Health insurance coverage, NCHS definitions. Retrieved September 12, 2006, from http://www.cdc.gov/nchs/datawh/nchsdefs/healthinsurancecov.htm.

Chapter 4

Understanding HIPAA: The Health Insurance Portability and Accountability Act

Jennifer McCabe

OBJECTIVES

After studying this chapter, the student should be able to

1. Explain the historical development process of HIPAA.
2. Describe the goals and function of HIPAA.
3. Recognize the impact of disclosure of private health information without patient consent.
4. Differentiate between reportable patient private health information and non-reportable information.

INTRODUCTION

Most of us feel that our health information is private and should be protected. Healthcare providers, insurance companies, and the general public are moving away from paper records toward the convenience and cost savings of electronic information. The Health Insurance Portability and Accountability Act (HIPAA) sets national standards for electronic healthcare transactions. This federal law sets limits on who can look at and receive your health information. It addresses the security and privacy of health data. Adopting these standards improves the efficiency and effectiveness of the nation's healthcare system by encouraging the widespread use of electronic data interchange in health care. To ensure your health information does not interfere with your health care, your information can be used

- For your treatment and care coordination.
- To pay doctors and hospitals for your health care and help run their businesses (or your business in the future).
- With your family, relatives, friends, or others you identify who are involved with your health care or your healthcare bills, unless you object.
- To make sure doctors give good care and nursing homes are clean and safe.
- To protect the public's health, such as reporting when the flu is in your area.
- To make required reports to the police, such as reporting gunshot wounds.

Your health information cannot be used or shared without your written permission unless this law allows it. Without patient authorization, a healthcare provider generally cannot:

- Provide health information to an individual's employer.
- Use or share personal information for marketing or advertising purposes.
- Share private notes about a patient's mental health counseling sessions.

The first-ever federal privacy standards to protect patients' medical records and other health information provided to health plans, doctors, hospitals, and other healthcare providers took effect on April 14, 2003. Developed by the Department of Health and Human Services (HHS), these new standards provide patients with access to their medical records and more control over how their personal health information is used and disclosed. They represent a uniform, federal floor of privacy protections for consumers across the country. State laws providing additional protections to consumers are not affected by this new rule.

> *It is the purpose... to improve the Medicare program under Title XVIII of the Social Security Act, the Medicaid program under Title XIX of such Act, and the efficiency and effectiveness of the health care system, by encouraging the development of a health information system through the establishment of standards and requirements for the electronic transmission of certain health information (Public Law 104-191, 1996).*

[This chapter is not legal advice. It is provided for informational use only to help understand HIPAA and how it came to be law. All facilities and personnel must comply with state and federal laws and should consult their legal counsel and risk management personnel.]

HIPAA

The Health Insurance Portability and Accountability Act of 1996, known as HIPAA, includes important new—but limited—protections for millions of working Americans and their families. HIPAA may

1. Increase individuals' ability to get health coverage for themselves and their dependents if they start a new job;
2. Lower the chance of losing existing healthcare coverage, whether individuals have that coverage through a job, or through individual health insurance;
3. Help maintain continuous health coverage for themselves and their dependents when they change jobs; and
4. Help them buy health insurance coverage on their own if they lose coverage under an employer's group health plan and have no other health coverage available.

Among its specific protections, HIPAA

1. Limits the use of pre-existing condition exclusions;
2. Prohibits group health plans from discriminating by denying coverage or charging people extra for coverage based on their individual or family member's past or present poor health;
3. Guarantees certain small employers, and certain individuals who lose job-related coverage, the right to purchase health insurance; and
4. Guarantees, in most cases, that employers or individuals who purchase health insurance can renew the coverage regardless of any health conditions of individuals covered under the insurance policy.

In short, HIPAA may lower the chance of losing existing coverage, ease the ability to switch health plans, and/or help individuals buy coverage on their own if they lose their employer's plan and have no other coverage available. The federal HIPAA law presents the single largest change in the healthcare business environment since the advent of Medicare and Medicaid in 1965. HIPAA is not a state or federal program, but an industry-wide effort to enhance consumer control of insurance coverage, create healthcare industry standards to improve administration, and protect and secure personal health information.

To understand the HIPAA law as it applies to communication among healthcare providers (or to students studying to be healthcare providers in the future), it is important to understand how HIPAA defines "covered entity," "healthcare provider," and "health care" as they are described here.

HIPAA applies only to "covered entities." Covered entities include individuals who are, or are employed by, a health plan, a healthcare clearinghouse, or a healthcare provider who transmits any health information electronically. Individuals are "healthcare providers" if they provide (or will in the future) health services, or they are "any other person or organization who furnishes, bills, or is paid for health care in the normal course of business" (Centers for Medicare and Medicaid Services, 2005a). For HIPAA purposes, "health care" refers to the care, services, or supplies related to the health of an individual. This includes preventive, diagnostic, therapeutic, rehabilitative, mainte-nance, or palliative care, and counseling, services, assessment, or procedures with respect to the physical or mental condition, or functional status, of an individual, or that affects the structure or function of the body (CMS, 2005a). In short, if you are (or are employed by) a covered entity, HIPAA's Privacy Rule applies to you—even as a student who may report on information obtained from contact with a patient or that patient's medical records.

Most of us feel that our health and medical information is private and should remain so. HIPAA laws give patients rights over their own health information and set rules and limits regarding who can have access to that information. The focus of this chapter will be the privacy aspect of HIPAA, and the applicability to healthcare providers.

How HIPAA Began

It could be said that the journey to HIPAA began with the advent of managed care. This is the point in the history of health care in America when payers began to seek ways of making health care more efficient. Doctors historically have been primarily concerned with care of the ill, not with running businesses. But thanks to hundreds of years of scientific advances, as well as the recognition that health-care services take place in many settings, not just private doctor's offices, it became necessary to examine the traditional model of delivering health care and ask some difficult questions. Could health care be modified to make it affordable for everyone? How could the most recent advances in the science of medicine be integrated into practices? And, perhaps most difficult of all, who should ulti-mately decide what kind of care patients receive: doctors or insurance compa-nies? As the government became more involved in paying doctors to treat those who could not pay for their own health care, managed care was born. Managed care (discussed in Chapter 3) involves many complicated laws and regulations, and the application of business models to the delivery of healthcare services.

As managed care began to catch on as a way to administer health care, those involved began to ask if there were ways to make health care more effi-cient, thus lowering the cost of providing it. In 1991, Louis Sullivan, Secre-tary of Health & Human Services, convened a working group to study what effect moving to more economical electronic transmission of information would have on health care. This can be considered the genesis of HIPAA, though it was not signed into law until 1996 (Hartley & Jones, 2004).

HIPAA changed the way that healthcare facilities operate in a number of important ways. Most notable perhaps is the fact that all healthcare professionals need to be familiar with the law so that they handle information responsibly and legally. The Privacy and Security rules of the HIPAA law came out in April of 2003, and these were the rules that all covered entities, healthcare providers and administrators alike, must follow. The Final Rule adopting HIPAA standards for the security of electronic health information, published in the Federal Register on February 20, 2003, specifies a series of administrative, technical, and physical security procedures to assure the confidentiality of electronic protected health information (CMS, 2005b).

HIPAA was just one part of President Clinton's healthcare reform plan. The original intent of HIPAA was to assure that health insurance was portable, so that people could keep their insurance when they changed jobs. The accountability part of the law refers to the efficient and cost-effective management of healthcare services. In any healthcare facility, money is spent on administration as well as supplies, services, and the salaries of clinicians. If facilities can operate efficiently, the cost of providing health care will go down. The government wants the cost of health care to be affordable: for people who pay for their own and for people who are covered by government-sponsored programs like Medicare and Medicaid. HIPAA is a very complex piece of legislation, but parts of it are essential for anyone working in a healthcare environment.

Title II Subtitle F of HIPAA contains the Administrative Simplification provisions of the Act. It is also the part of the law intended to make the business of providing health care more efficient. There are four main areas of impact of Title II: privacy of records, standards for transmitting information electronically, security measures to protect the patient's privacy, and the establishment of national identifiers (like Social Security numbers) for healthcare providers and facilities (Beaver & Herold, 2004).

Covered Entities

The sections of HIPAA that healthcare providers need to understand were written to provide guidance and regulations for handling information for all covered entities. Covered entities are essentially any organization that deals with health information and therefore must abide by HIPAA rules. As organizations, they must create and enforce policies and practices that ensure that all employees comply with, or obey, HIPAA. These covered entities include persons, businesses, and agencies that furnish, bill, or receive payment for healthcare services in the normal course of business. Public and private clinics, pharmacies, home health agencies, nursing homes, college health centers, providers of mental health services, etc. are also subject to regulations established by HIPAA.

The actual healthcare providers covered by HIPAA rules include professionals, such as physicians, nurses, physician assistants, occupational therapists, counselors, and some social workers. Students who do clinical rotations are also considered covered entities, even though they may only be in a specific facility for a short time. Essentially, anyone who uses or sees confidential patient information, including students, is considered a covered entity. Health plans like HMOs and insurance plans that pay for health care are also covered entities, because they have full access to medical records. Healthcare clearinghouses are organizations that assist clinics with billing, coding, and other aspects of the business of providing and being reimbursed for medical care. A busy private practice may contract their coding and billing to a clearinghouse, to help them operate more efficiently, making the clearinghouse a covered entity. Finally, business associates of providers are covered under HIPAA. These would be lawyers, accountants, data processors, and any other organization that does work for the provider.

Some agencies that aren't exclusively healthcare providers are also considered covered entities by HIPAA. These include city, county, and state social service agencies, mail order pharmacies, retirement centers, outpatient treatment centers, and correctional facilities. Employees in these facilities must also understand and operate under the HIPAA guidelines. It is possible to encounter protected health information (PHI) even when working in a non-healthcare facility. Agency supervisors should have clear policies in place for handling confidential health information before anyone gets access to it. Anyone who enters a fieldwork placement or permanent position in health care is wise to remember that treating patients is a privilege. All patients must share very private details of their lives with clinicians if they are to receive and participate in their care. It is morally and legally important to treat this information with the care and discretion it deserves.

HIPAA and Privacy

We must protect our citizens' privacy—the bulwark of personal liberty, the safeguard of individual creativity.
Bill Clinton, 42nd President of the United States (1946–)

Here are some real cases of private health information falling into the wrong hands.

- A doctor's laptop, stolen at a medical conference, contained the names and medical histories of his patients in North Carolina (Santana, 2000).

- A hacker downloaded medical records, health information, and Social Security numbers of more than 5,000 patients at the University of Washington Medical Center. The hacker claimed to be motivated by a desire to expose the vulnerability of electronic medical records (O'Harrow, 2000).

- The 13-year-old daughter of a hospital employee took a list of patients' names and phone numbers from the hospital when visiting her mother at work. As a joke, she contacted patients and told them they had been diagnosed with HIV ("Hospital Clerk's Child," 1995).

- A banker who also served on his county's health board cross-referenced customer accounts with patient information. He then called due the mortgages of anyone suffering from cancer (Lavelle, 1994).

- An Orlando woman had her doctor perform some routine tests and received a letter weeks later from a drug company touting a treatment for her high cholesterol ("Many Can Hear," 1997).

The privacy rules of HIPAA protect health information from intentional or unintentional abuse. Protected health information (PHI) is any information about an individual and their current, past, or future physical or mental health. It includes treatment or diagnostic tests, current conditions, and even predictors of future health conditions. For example, if a person has a genetic condition that increases the likelihood of their developing an illness or disability in the future, the presence of that condition now, even though they may have no symptoms, is protected health information. Likewise, any past medical procedures and any current diagnoses, therapy, or prescriptions are all Protected Health Information.

Transmitted or stored information in a healthcare setting can be verbal, written, or electronic. Therefore, all three ways of transmitting information require measures to protect the privacy of patients. To appreciate the privacy rules, it is helpful to reflect on the nature of privacy. Most people can probably think of personal information that they do not want widely known. There is some information that they are willing to share with some individuals, but not others. In the context of HIPAA, privacy is really about controlling access to information, and assuring that patients are informed about how personal information may be used.

Some people try to protect their privacy by omitting or lying about information. If a patient is worried that something in their lifestyle will prevent them from being eligible for health insurance, they are likely to try and hide that information. For example, a patient who regularly smokes marijuana may not disclose this to their doctor out of concern about who else the doctor may tell. Yet this omission may delay diagnosis and treatment of a serious condition.

Clearly, a lack of trust hinders the delivery of the best possible care because important pieces of information may be missing. Patients must trust their caregivers if they are to receive quality care and participate in their own care.

Under HIPAA, patients may see their records, and must be informed of who else may have access to them. Patients may also grant permission to specific people to see their records, like a spouse or other family member. Patients may also request changes to their records, although those requests are not always granted. The point to remember is that patients do have some control of the content and sharing of their private health records.

Since April 2003, visitors to doctors' offices, pharmacies, clinics, or even eye glasses shops have been asked to read and sign a notice of privacy practices. This notice is a HIPAA-required document that explains what the facility will do with PHI. The notice of privacy practices spells out, in plain English, what kinds of information is collected, and who may have access to it. It also advises patients how to view and request changes to their record. HIPAA requires that all covered entities inform their patients of their privacy practices. The federal government, through the Health Resources and Services Administration (HRSA), provides guidance on preparing privacy notices. All notices require the following elements: header with specific language; uses and disclosure; a separate statement for certain uses and disclosure; individual rights; covered entity's duties; complaints; and contact information for further explanation (Health Research & Services Administration, n.d.).

Access to Health Information

Many people consider clinicians to be the frontline providers of healthcare services. Clinicians come from a variety of backgrounds and have a wide variety of levels of education. Licensed Practical Nurses (LPNs) and even nurse's aides have access to extremely private information about their patients. Sometimes this information is recorded, and other times it is simply observed. Likewise, physicians and surgeons have access to the most personal information about their patients. Therapists, nurses of all levels, case managers, pharmacists, physician assistants, counselors, and even emergency medical technicians are all required to protect the privacy of those they treat. Anyone who, in the course of their employment, has access to PHI is covered by HIPAA privacy rules.

Administrators may not encounter PHI on a regular basis, as they tend to deal with a larger picture of the care provided. However, administrators and their non-clinical support staff need access to the various databases and storage facilities where patient data is typically stored. New patient records systems are sometimes compared to existing systems. When billing systems are upgraded, vast amounts of data are migrated from one system to another. When analyzing billing data for epidemiological or other reasons, individual information is scaled up to the macro level, and vice versa. All of these scenarios represent opportunities for administrators to legitimately need access to PHI. It is important that they, too, understand the privacy rules and abide by them. Just because their access to PHI is not firsthand, does not mean that they are exempt from the rules.

Most important, administrators must assure that policies and procedures are in place to apprise all employees of the basic tenets of HIPAA. Administrators also must assure that staff follow proper policies and procedures for the disposal of records containing PHI. Record-retention policies must be HIPAA compliant, and disposal procedures must include safeguards against theft of PHI.

Many larger healthcare facilities contract with third parties to provide billing and other data-management tasks. This often requires combining patient records with the appropriate codes corresponding to their diagnoses and treatments. Maintaining good-quality data is an important part of the healthcare picture, as it improves the efficiency of reimbursement, and helps to form an accurate picture of the health of a community. Employers may want to know what the most frequent musculoskeletal injuries are among their employees in order to improve the safety of the workplace. They may find that through simple changes, like improved lighting and safety training, they are able to decrease the numbers of repetitive stress injuries and doctors' visits, and improve their employees' productivity and satisfaction. Insurance companies do complicated analyses of healthcare diagnoses and treatments in order to study the real costs associated with specific diagnoses. This is done to bring down the cost of providing health care. Obviously, accessing PHI enables companies to mine the existing data for clues to improving health. As with administrators, third parties must be aware of the privacy rule and operate under it.

Information technology professionals are the people who maintain the systems on which PHI is stored. They are also the people who control the amount of information to which each employee has access. When a new employee begins, the information technology staff creates an electronic profile for the person that includes the kinds of information they will need to do their jobs. If the new employee is a pharmacy technician, he or she may need access to the pharmaceutical inventory system, but may not need patients' home addresses. If the new employee is a geriatric nurse practitioner, he or she will need access to all of the information about his or her patients, but not those patients in the pediatric ward.

Information technology managers also have the responsibility for maintaining a network that has sufficient security in place. Security measures can be firewalls, to prevent outside information from entering the internal system, password-changing policies, to prevent hackers from guessing them and gaining access, and even encryption, to scramble electronic communication so that no one can intercept messages that may contain PHI. Maintaining up-to-date virus protection is another important part of providing security for PHI, as viruses often allow for remote, unauthorized users to access protected information. It is very important for information technology staff to understand the privacy and security rules of HIPAA in order to incorporate them into the information infrastructure.

Many healthcare facilities are businesses. They deal with companies selling everything from drugs, to office and clinic supplies, to educational materials. As such, vendors working for suppliers often visit their customers, to help them place their orders and apprise them of new products. And these visits usually include access to spaces where PHI may be stored or displayed. If vendors enter patient care areas of healthcare facilities, they can access as much PHI as clinicians through simple observation. However, most vendors do not have the kind of HIPAA training that healthcare facilities provide their own employees. Therefore it is incumbent on the facility to have and follow procedures for protecting PHI from vendors and others who may not have HIPAA training.

De-identification and Disclosure

Certain elements of PHI may associate a specific person with the record of their health. These must be removed from a record in order for it to be de-identified. Even students who make presentations or write papers about patients seen on clinical rotations must de-identify or strip the PHI descriptions of individual cases. Most faculty will stop reading as soon as they realize that PHI has been included in a description. For instance, you cannot say "Joe is a 28-year-old plumber from Elkton who was admitted to Memorial Hospital on July 4 after a fireworks accident." But you can de-identify the case by saying "Joe is a 28-year-old who was hospitalized this summer after a fireworks accident."

Elements of PHI That Must Be Removed

The following is a list of PHI elements that must be removed.

1. Name
2. Address
3. City

4. County

5. Zip code

6. Telephone #

7. Fax #

8. E-mail

9. Social Security #

10. Medical record #

11. Health plan #

12. Account #

13. All dates pertaining to care

14. Birth date

15. Certificate or license #

16. Vehicle identification

17. URLs

18. IP addresses

19. Biometric identifiers

20. Full face photographs

21. Unique numbers or characteristics

Obviously, disclosing PHI is necessary in order to carry out patient care. Routine disclosure occurs during the normal course of treatment and operations, and this is permitted under HIPAA. Anyone involved in the treatment of patients may, and should, have access to their medical record. Likewise, anyone involved in collecting payment for the services rendered, and in maintaining records for the facility, must have access to PHI. The people who have access to protected information should receive training in protecting patient confidentiality.

Non-routine disclosure occurs when PHI is given out for reasons other than providing or billing for care. There are a number of other reasons PHI is sometimes disclosed without the patient's consent. Certain diseases and conditions are considered "reportable," meaning that states keep track of how many people have them. Reportable diseases include highly infectious diseases like cholera and hepatitis, those that may indicate bioterrorism like tularemia or small pox, and sexually transmitted diseases. Many states also keep track of cancers in cancer registries, considered non-routine disclosure. Likewise if any member of the care team suspects neglect or abuse of a patient, PHI may be disclosed to the proper authorities. From time to time, records containing PHI may be subpoenaed for court cases, or requested by law enforcement for use in an investigation or in cases of on-site crimes. These non-routine disclosures of protected health information are all allowable under HIPAA.

To provide guidance on how much PHI should be disclosed in specific circumstances, a "Minimum Necessary" rule applies to the routine and non-routine disclosure of information. Essentially it means that information should be released on a "need to know" basis. For example, if a non-routine disclosure is being made to report suspected child abuse, releasing the PHI that pertains to the abuse, but not the entire medical record of the patient, is permissible. A history of broken limbs and burns may reveal a pattern of abuse, but a prescription for antibiotics is not germane to the case. In a routine disclosure, the facility uses the minimum necessary rule to create policies regarding which classes of employees need access to which elements of PHI. As a rule, employees have access to the information they need to perform their jobs, and no more. Understanding the minimum necessary rule requires a good degree of professional judgment and experience. All healthcare facilities should have policies and procedures in place to handle non-routine situations.

HIPAA and Security

Another major area of impact of HIPAA is security. Security refers to the steps an organization takes to assure that information remains in their control at all times. Organizations need to record, index, and store information for it to retain its value. It may be recorded as a note written on a piece of paper and stored in a metal filing cabinet; it may be recorded in an e-mail communication and stored in a database; or it may be a series of codes entered into an electronic patient record. Regardless of format, it must be secured to maintain the integrity of the data and protect the patients to whom it pertains.

Organizations are responsible for creating security policies and practices. They limit access to information in databases by assigning passwords that include varying degrees of permissions. Information management personnel are also responsible for installing and maintaining anti-virus software and other security software on their networks. Individual clinicians and others with access to PHI are responsible for following policies to safeguard personal information. These responsibilities include not sharing passwords, protecting paper records, and any other security measures.

Security measures are important not only to protect patients' privacy, but also to protect their credit. To a thief looking to establish fraudulent bank accounts and credit card accounts, healthcare records often contain just the right information to allow them to "steal" someone's identity.

As mentioned earlier, PHI is transmitted in one of three ways: spoken, written, and electronically. Each of these means of transmission can be made secure by following some guidelines. PHI always contains private details of patients' lives. When entering a patient's room while others are in it, knock first, and ask the patient's permission before revealing anything. Sometimes patients will want their guests to participate in the conversation; healthcare providers should not assume this. Providers across all healthcare professions should never speak about a patient or a case in a public place, like an elevator or cafeteria. If a conversation must take place in a common area like a waiting room, using a low tone of voice and moving out of the earshot of others reduces the risk of sharing PHI with unauthorized persons. Even students often need to discuss work with fellow students and faculty members. Keep confidentiality of information in mind during these conversations, and do not disclose PHI inappropriately. While it may seem a little unnatural at first, it is better to err on the side of caution when protecting PHI.

Many healthcare facilities are still using paper for part of their record keeping. Because paper can be lost or stolen easily, it presents special security concerns. Never leave charts, files, billing information, and other tangible PHI out in the open or in unsecured areas. Healthcare facilities utilizing shared printers and fax machines bear special consideration. Call before faxing information out, to confirm the correct number and alert the recipient that it is coming. Collect faxes or printouts immediately and file in the appropriate, secure location. Facilities should all have procedures in place for destroying documents they no longer need.

When accessing PHI through a networked computer, remember that most computer activity is recorded and may be monitored. Once a password is used to access information, records can be kept of every key stroke made. This safeguard is in place to make it easier to investigate breaches of security. Local and institutional policies usually forbid sharing passwords, since that makes it more difficult to establish exactly who was using a computer or program at a given time. Always terminate a session with a database by logging out when finished, thus preventing someone else from using your session to retrieve information. Keeping virus software updated is standard practice, and helps protect individual machines and networks from hackers and other security risks. Finally, if policy allows you to use a portable computer like a laptop or PDA to store PHI, remember to pass-word-protect these files.

Students should never have any PHI on *personal* laptops or home com-puters. If you use information from a healthcare agency for an assignment, all information should be de-identified. Be especially mindful when using computers in the public labs on campus—these machines often make tem-porary backup files that are not secure. Agency work that involves PHI *must* be done on agency computers, where the responsibility to keep soft-ware password-protected and virus detection programs updated rests with the agency.

Even casual communications like instant messaging and e-mail are con-sidered electronic transmissions. Students must never include any PHI in these messages.

HIPAA Violations and Ramifications

Much of what is in this chapter may seem like common sense, and it is. With the exception of some of the details, most people probably know it is impor-tant to protect patient privacy. But with the passage of HIPAA these regula-tions now contain the force of law, meaning that *severe penalties* exist for fail-ure to comply. Not only should facilities have their own procedures and penalties for breaches of privacy, but there are legal ramifications for these infractions as well. Figure 4.1 outlines the range of penalties imposed if HIPAA privacy and security rules are breached.

These fines and sentences apply to both the organization as a whole, and the individual or individuals involved in the violations. While the organiza-tion has an obligation to create policies, the ultimate responsibility rests with the individual. Individuals who breach HIPAA regulations for privacy or security may receive penalties in addition to those of the organization. HIPAA has set up ways for violations to be reported. You should know these are available, but seek advice before using them.

HIPAA Training

The kind of training each person involved in health care receives will vary according to the kinds of PHI their jobs require them to access. Human Resources departments typically conduct training programs, with input

- **Wrongful disclosure**—up to $50,000 fine and/or up to 1 year in prison.
- **Gaining access by false pretense**—up to $100,000 fine and/or up to 5 years in prison.
- **Intentional misuse**—up to $250,000 fine and/or up to 10 years in prison.

Figure 4.1 *Penalties for HIPAA Breaches*

provided by the attorneys who provide legal advice. HIPAA does not regulate the format of the training; agencies may choose to use live trainers, video tapes, discussion groups, assigned readings, or a combination of these techniques. They are required to assess their training in some way, to ensure that the message is registering with the participants. It is always a good precautionary measure to build in some repetition over time. Employees must not feel that HIPAA is a one-day event to endure; they must understand that it is a "way of life" in today's healthcare environment.

Organizations are also required to keep track of the training program, and assure that it reflects the current state of the law. As mentioned earlier, rules may change, and it is important to stay up to date. Record keeping on the training program is not only a requirement of HIPAA, it is also good business practice.

SUMMARY

This chapter has only introduced the various applicable provisions of the Health Insurance Portability and Accountability Act that future health professionals should know. Each healthcare facility should have policies and procedures in place for communicating with their clients, training their employees, and securing the information they collect.

HIPAA ought not to be seen as an obstacle, but rather a way to instill a sense of trust between patients and their healthcare providers. Only when patients feel secure in sharing the most private details of their lives will they be able to participate in and receive the highest quality health care. Clinicians should view the HIPAA rules as an agreement they have with their patients, a covenant to honor their privacy and include them in the most important conversations that they may ever have.

REFERENCES

Beaver, K. & Herold, R. (2004). *The practical guide to HIPAA privacy and security compliance*. New York: Auerbach Publications.

Centers for Medicare and Medicaid Services (CMS). (2005a). Covered entity decision tools. Retrieved September 23, 2005, from http://www.cms.hhs.gov/hipaa/hipaa2/support/tools/decisionsupport/default.asp.

Centers for Medicare and Medicaid Services (CMS). (2005b). HIPAA administrative simplification—Security. Retrieved September 23, 2005, from http://www.cms.hhs.gov/hipaa/hipaa2/regulations/security/default.asp.

Hartley, C. P. & Jones, E. D. (2004). *HIPAA plain and simple: A compliance guide for health care professionals*. Chicago: AMA Press.

Health Resources & Services Administration. (n.d.). *Plain language principles and thesaurus for making HIPAA privacy notices more readable*. Retrieved September 21, 2005, from http://www.hrsa.gov/language.htm.

Hospital clerk's child allegedly told patients that they had AIDS. (1995, March 1). *The Washington Post*, A17.

Krager, D. & Krager, C. (2005). *HIPAA for medical office personnel*. Clifton Park, NY: Thomson/Delmar Learning.

Lavelle, M. (1994, May 30). Health plan debate turning to privacy: Some call for safeguards on medical disclosure. Is a federal law necessary? *The National Law Journal*, A1.

Many can hear what you tell your doctors: Records of patients are not kept private. (1997, November). *Orlando Sentinel*, A1.

O'Harrow, R. (2000, December 9). Hacker accesses patients' records. *The Washington Post*, E1.

Public Law 104-191. (1996). Health Insurance Portability and Accountability Act of 1996. Retrieved September 23, 2005, from http://aspe.hhs.gov/admnsimp/pl104191.htm#261.

Chapter 5

E-health Resources

Stephanie Chisolm

OBJECTIVES

After studying this chapter, the student should be able to

1. Describe different types of Internet health information resources.
2. Identify questions consumers can utilize to ascertain the reliability of Internet information.
3. Describe the Federal Trade Commission efforts to combat Internet health fraud.
4. Identify reliable resources for health information on the World Wide Web.

INTRODUCTION

Health care has been evolving away from a "disease-centered model" and toward a "patient-centered model." In the older, disease-centered model, physicians make almost all treatment decisions based largely on clinical experience and data from various medical tests. In a patient-centered model, patients become active participants in their own care and receive services designed to focus on their individual needs and preferences, in addition to advice and counsel from health professionals. The patient-centered model relies on individuals becoming informed consumers of healthcare services. Think about a time, perhaps when you are preparing to study for a test, when you have felt overwhelmed by all the information you are required to know to earn a good grade. Now imagine you have a chronic or life-threatening health condition or disease. Thanks to the World Wide Web and other resources, patients have more information today about their diseases and treatment options than ever before. While this information is valuable, it may feel a bit like trying to get a drink of water from an open fire hydrant. There is so much information available so quickly, it can be overwhelming, even for a healthy student, let alone a sick patient!

Finding Health Information on the World Wide Web

When I took office, only high energy physicists had
ever heard of what is called the Worldwide Web....
Now even my cat has its own page.
Bill Clinton, 42nd President of the United States (1946–),
announcement of Next Generation Internet initiative, 1996

As the US healthcare system continues to evolve, patients and their families must take a more active role in the care they and their loved ones receive. Today, it is more important than ever that individuals take more responsibility for understanding health care and communicating with healthcare providers. With constant innovations in treatment and prevention, patients must become savvy consumers of health information from a plethora of resources to ensure they receive the best care available.

The Internet is one source of health information that, when used cautiously, can aid informed health decision making. Anyone with computer access can find information on primary, secondary, and tertiary prevention for health issues from A to Z. Using any available Internet search engine to look up a health condition can provide a sometimes overwhelming volume of resources. However, as both a consumer of health information and a future health professional, you should be aware that anyone with computer skills can set up a slick, professional-appearing Web site and sell anything from information to medications directly to unsuspecting individuals searching for guidance in an ever-changing healthcare landscape.

The fact that it is easy to publish health and medical information and reach vast audiences without having the information verified by other sources presents potential issues for the Food and Drug Administration (FDA) and other government agencies. Product information on the Internet is unlike traditional forms of advertising and labeling. Current regulations on prescription drug advertising differ between print and broadcast media. The anonymity of cyberspace presents additional challenges.

While regulatory agencies try to devise ways of ensuring that accurate and well-balanced health and medical information is presented on the Internet, consumers should use a lot more discretion in evaluating what they see. A Web page, either changed quickly or quickly obsolete, is easy to put up and easy to take down. There is no guarantee that what you see one day will be there the next (FDA, 1996). When it comes to health information, the term "caveat emptor," let the buyer beware, may mean the difference between life and death.

By far, the most consumer-friendly part of the Internet is the World Wide Web, which has the ability to display colorful graphics and utilize multimedia (sound, video, virtual reality). Many legitimate providers of reliable health and medical information, including the medical professional associations, the FDA, and other government agencies, are taking advantage of the Web's popularity by offering brochures and in-depth information on specific topics on their Web sites designed for consumers as well as healthcare industry and medical professionals. Even students can find valuable resources on the Web. Although there is a wealth of reliable sources of information on the Web, it is important to be aware that what is available there is only as good as the quality and integrity of the original information. Exercise caution before believing information or products found on the Web are scientific truth. Checking both information and products against other sources can prevent costly or even painful mistakes.

Exchanging Information On-line

In Internet "newsgroups," such as Usenet groups, people post questions and read messages much as they would on regular bulletin boards. Through "mailing lists," participants exchange messages by e-mail, and all subscribers, perhaps located anywhere in the world, may receive messages. We have come a long way from the old cork and thumbtack bulletin boards! In "chat" areas on some services and on the Internet's IRC (Internet Relay Chat) users can communicate with each other, "live." Assessing the value and validity of health and medical information in news and chat groups demands at least the same—and maybe more—discrimination as that required for Web sites, because the information is more ephemeral and you often can't identify the source. Although these groups can provide reliable information about specific diseases and disorders, they can also perpetuate misinformation. It is always a good idea to check the source of the information and when it was last updated to help determine credibility. As with any medical decision, obtaining a second opinion before acting on information exchanged in this way is a good idea.

Other information services are commercial on-line services, fee-charging companies that provide vast amounts of proprietary information. They often include health and medical databases, electronic versions of popular newspapers and magazines, and their own chats and newsgroups, as well as Internet access. The fact that a commercial service may screen information does not necessarily make it more reliable than other sources. Most services do not verify information posted in their newsgroups, nor do they control what is "said" in chat rooms. Healthcare providers should corroborate health and medical material obtained through on-line information resources and services. Most professional associations in the healthcare field have their own Web sites that offer members access to timely information regarding treatments, certifications, or continuing education, as well as bulletin boards and chat rooms for professional issues. Some organizations also provide electronic access to professional journals and other sources of information specific to their scope of practice.

Is This Site Reliable?

FDA staff and others familiar with Internet medical offerings suggest asking the following questions to help determine the reliability of a Web site (FDA, 1996):

- *Who maintains the site?*

  Government or university-run sites are among the best sources for scientifically sound health and medical information. Private practitioners or lay organizations may have marketing, social, or political agendas that can influence the type of material they offer on-site and which sites they link to.

- *Is there an editorial board or another listing of the names and credentials of those responsible for preparing and reviewing the site's contents?*

  Can the organization or individual be contacted if visitors to the site have questions or want additional information?

- *Does the site link to other sources of medical information?*

  A reputable organization will not position itself as the sole source of information on a particular health topic. On the other hand, links alone are not a guarantee of reliability. Since anyone with a Web page can create links to any other site on the Internet—and the owner of the site that is "linked to" has no say over who links to it—then a person offering suspect medical advice could conceivably try to make his or her advice appear legitimate by, say, creating a link to the FDA's Web site. What's more, health information produced by the FDA or other government agencies is not copyrighted; therefore, someone can quote FDA information at a site and be perfectly within his or her rights. By citing a source such as the FDA, experienced marketers using careful wording can make it appear as though the FDA endorses their products.

- *When was the site last updated?*

  Generally, the more current the site, the more likely it is to provide timely material. Ideally, health and medical sites should be updated weekly or monthly.

- *Are informative graphics and multimedia files such as video or audio clips available?*

  Such features can assist in clarifying medical conditions and procedures. Bear in mind, however, that multimedia should help explain medical information, not make up for the lack of it. Some sites provide dazzling "bells and whistles," lending an aura of authenticity, but little scientifically sound information.

- *Does the site charge an access fee?*

  Many reputable sites with health and medical information, including FDA and other government sites, offer access and materials for free. If a site does charge a fee, be sure that it offers value for the money. Use a search engine to see whether you can get the same information without paying additional fees. If you find something of interest at a site—say, a new drug touted to relieve disease symptoms with fewer side effects—look for information to determine whether legitimate research sources, such as journal articles or proceedings from a scientific meeting support the information.

In addition, before taking medications or herbal remedies found on the Internet, patients should consult their healthcare provider. The healthcare provider can determine if the drug is appropriate for the individual's situation, even if the information comes from a source that is reputed to be reliable. Specific situations (such as taking other drugs or having other health conditions) may make the therapy an inadvisable choice; the drug may not be suitable for the individual; or there may be alternative treatments that are more appropriate.

Search Programs

Because the Internet contains no central indexing system, getting the information wanted quickly can be a major challenge. Internet search engines can be useful, powerful tools to help narrow the field if you have a specific topic to pursue, or the name of a specific organization, but no address for its site. Input a few key words relating to the desired topic, and the search engine returns a list of sites related to the query. Be aware, however, that although a search engine can point the way, it does not evaluate the information it identifies. For example, a search on the words "breast cancer" is just as likely to point to a page advertising a reconstructive surgeon or a health food store's article on the purported benefits of phytochemicals as it is to the National Cancer Institute. It is up to the visitor to evaluate the information the site contains. Here are a few of the many search engines:

- Alta Vista: http://www.altavista.com
- Dogpile: http://www.dogpile.com
- Excite: http://www.excite.com/
- Google: http://www.google.com/
- Lycos: http://www.lycos.com/
- Webcrawler: http://www.webcrawler.com/
- Yahoo: http://www.yahoo.com/Health/Medicine/

Credibility and the Public Interest

The Internet Healthcare Coalition (www.ihealthcoalition.org) is the first and only nonpartisan organization of its kind, representing constituents from every sector of the Internet health space. Since 1999, the Coalition has been actively involved in developing guidelines for the ethical use of the Internet in health care. The Internet Healthcare Coalition (IHCC) began as a grass-roots response to issues raised initially by the Food and Drug Administration. The IHCC is an independent and non-industry-aligned group, incorporated as a nonprofit organization dedicated to

- Educating healthcare consumers, professionals, educators, marketers, and both health care and mainstream media, as well as public policy-makers on the full range of uses of the Internet—current and potential—to deliver high-quality healthcare information and services.
- Furnishing clear models, not only of good and bad sources of online healthcare information and services, but of the potentially disparate methods of evaluating disparate sources of information—from product- or disease-information sites developed by regulated manufacturers to peer-reviewed electronic publications and patient support groups.
- Publicizing and promoting the use of currently available resources and developing new resources that exemplify ethical, innovative, and high-quality uses of the Internet to deliver healthcare information and services.
- Acting as a representative of their constituencies in areas of mutual concern before public policymakers and with the media.

Since the beginning, the Coalition has been a leader in helping to improve the quality of health information on the Internet. It has developed the eHealth Code of Ethics and has an active, ongoing educational program, which includes the Annual Quality Healthcare Information on the Net Conference, eHealth Ethics Workshops, books, and speakers' bureaus. The IHCC is developing materials to help consumers evaluate online health resources and information. The Internet Healthcare Coalition works to provide clear guidance for evaluating on-line sources of health information—from product- or disease-related sites developed by regulated manufacturers, to peer-reviewed electronic publications, to patient support and discussion groups. The Coalition's goal is to develop well-informed Internet healthcare consumers, professionals, educators, marketers, and media. The Internet Healthcare Coalition offers the following advice in their publication *Tips for Healthy Surfing Online, Finding Quality Health Information on the Internet* (iHealth, 2005).

1. Choosing an online health information resource is like choosing your doctor. You would not go to just any doctor and you may get opinions from several doctors. Therefore, you should not rely on just any one Internet site for all your health needs. A good rule of thumb is to find a Web site that has a person, institution, or organization in which you already have confidence. If possible, you should seek information from several sources and not rely on a single source of information.

2. Trust what you see or read on the Internet only if you can validate the source of the information. Authors and contributors should always be identified, along with their affiliations and financial interests, if any, in the content. Phone numbers, e-mail addresses, or other contact information should also be provided.

3. Question Web sites that credit themselves as the sole source of information on a topic, as well as sites that disrespect other sources of knowledge.

4. Do not be fooled by a comprehensive list of links. Any Web site can link to another and this in no way implies endorsement from either site.

5. Find out if the site is professionally managed and reviewed by an editorial board of experts to ensure that the material is both credible and reliable. Sources used to create the content should be clearly referenced and acknowledged.

6. Medical knowledge is continually evolving. Make sure that all clinical content includes the date of publication or modification.

7. All sponsorship, advertising, underwriting, commercial funding arrangements, or potential conflicts should be clearly stated and separated from the editorial content. A good question to ask is: Does the author or authors have anything to gain from proposing one particular point of view over another?

8. Avoid any on-line physician who proposes to diagnose or treat you without a proper physical examination and consultation regarding your medical history.

9. Read the Web site's privacy statement and make certain that any personal medical or other information you supply will be kept absolutely confidential.

10. Most important, use your common sense! Shop around, always get more than one opinion, be suspicious of miracle cures, and always read the fine print.

Sources of Internet Health Information

There are literally thousands of health-related Internet resources maintained by government agencies, universities, and nonprofit and commercial organizations in the United States and around the globe. The National Library of Medicine's MEDLINE, the Centers for Disease Control and Prevention, and even Merck Pharmaceutical Company are examples of organizations offering healthcare information for patients and professionals. The appendix for this chapter contains a list of reputable World Wide Web sites that is by no means complete; it is offered as a jumping-off point to illustrate the regulated resources available to consumers, students, and health professionals. Many of these sites have information available in English and Spanish; some offer translations into other languages as well.

Fraudulent Claims for Online Health Products

If a man defrauds you one time, he is a rascal;
if he does it twice, you are a fool.
Author Unknown

Online marketers—legitimate as well as fraudulent—market their products through Web sites, spam, and chat rooms. The cost is reasonable. Whether made on- or off-line, fraudulent health claims typically deal with serious diseases, such as AIDS, cancer, heart disease, multiple sclerosis, diabetes, and arthritis, as well as chronic medical conditions like headaches and back pain. Often, exaggerated claims are used to promote products such as DHEA (a hormone supplement), Cat's claw (an herbal product), and colloidal silver, as well as diagnostic tests and devices, such as electrical "zappers." In recent years, the Federal Trade Commission (FTC) and other law enforcement agencies have stepped up efforts to prevent the proliferation of fraudulent health claims on the Internet. They are using the latest technology to track down fraudulent marketers quickly and efficiently and bring about enforcement actions when appropriate (FDA, 2005).

The Internet provides unscrupulous health product hucksters low-cost access to a huge market of potential consumers. The World Wide Web is a medium that is hard to police. It may be difficult to discern who might actually be running a Web site or where they are located, and a few clicks of a mouse anywhere in the world can change that information in an instant. Internet health scams are common, so the FTC is also educating consumers on how to shop safely on-line for health products and encouraging them to talk to their doctor or other healthcare provider about the safe use of supplements and other alternative health products. They encourage the public to report suspicious health claims to government fraud fighters.

Why the concern about health fraud? Like other fraud, it cheats consumers out of their money and harms legitimate marketers striving to compete fairly. Health fraud can be deadly. Health fraud often targets the very sick and even desperate consumers, luring them away from treatments that have proven benefits. It can mislead people who use an advertised "cure-all" product into thinking they are disease-free. As a result, they may not seek or continue medical care, receive the drugs or legitimate treatment that could keep them healthier longer, or take precautions to prevent the spread of their disease. Some products can interact with other legitimate or fraudulent medicines, causing serious side effects or reducing a medicine's ability to work as it should. Some products may contain harmful substances. Consumers may spend billions of dollars a year on unproven, fraudulently marketed, often-useless, health-related products, devices, and treatments. Trading on false hope, health fraud promises quick cures and easy solutions to a variety of problems, from obesity to cancer and AIDS. Consumers who fall for fraudulent "cure-all" products do not find help or better health. Instead, they find themselves cheated out of their money, their time, and maybe even their lives (FDA, 2005).

To combat health fraud on the Internet, the FTC launched "Operation Cure-All" in 1999. It is an ongoing federal and state law enforcement and consumer education campaign. The FTC takes law enforcement action against Internet marketers for unsubstantiated health claims. One case resulted in a $1 million settlement with the maker of a shark cartilage product promoted as a cure for cancer. Two other settlements stopped companies from claiming that St. John's Wort was a safe and effective treatment for HIV/AIDS and required warnings about the serious drug interaction risks associated with St. John's Wort. Another settlement required consumer refunds for electronic devices and herbal remedies sold as cures for cancer, AIDS, Gulf War Syndrome, and many other diseases. All were required to remove their bogus claims from the

Web. In addition, the FTC estimates that more than 100 other Web sites have taken down their sites or removed their claims after the FTC contacted them. The FTC—through www.OperationCureAll.com—offers information for consumers on how to recognize health fraud. Guidance for businesses on how to market health products and services truthfully, as well as information about the FTC's initiatives, are available.

Education efforts—also key in fighting fraud—target consumers, as well as law enforcement. Last year, the FTC launched a program to teach state, local, and foreign law enforcers how to investigate Internet-related fraud. Education for consumers aims to help them learn how to determine the legitimacy of health claims. Two Web sites can help: the FTC's Virtual Health Treatments Web site (www.ftc.gov/cureall) and the FDA's Buying Medicines and Medical Products Online Web site (www.fda.gov/oc/buyonline/default.htm). The sites give tips on how to spot health fraud and where to report suspicious claims.

While the FTC works for the consumer to prevent fraudulent, deceptive, and unfair business practices in the marketplace, it also provides information to enable consumers to spot, stop, and avoid them. To file a complaint, or to get free information on any of 150 consumer topics, call toll-free, 1-877-FTC-HELP (1-877-382-4357), or use the complaint form at www.ftc.gov. The FTC enters Internet, telemarketing, identity theft, and other fraud-related complaints into Consumer Sentinel, a secure, online database available to hundreds of civil and criminal law enforcement agencies in the United States and abroad.

Food and Drug Administration Regulation of Health Claims

Federal law allows certain claims in the labeling of food and supplements. These include claims approved by the Food and Drug Administration (FDA) that show a strong link, based on scientific evidence, between a food substance and a disease or health condition. These approved claims can state only that a food substance *reduces the risk* of certain health problems—not that it can *treat or cure* a disease. Two examples of *approved* claims are: "The vitamin folic acid may reduce the risk of neural tube defect-affected pregnancies," and "Calcium may reduce the risk of the bone disease osteoporosis" (Claims That Can Be Made for Conventional Foods and Dietary Supplements, 2003).

Dietary supplements also may carry claims in their labeling that describe the effect of a substance in maintaining the body's normal structure or function, as long as the claims don't imply the product treats or cures a disease. The FDA does not review or authorize these claims. An example of such a claim is, "Product B promotes healthy joints and bones." When a company promotes a dietary supplement with a claim like this, the claim must be accompanied with the disclaimer, "This statement has not been evaluated by the Food and Drug Administration. This product is not intended to diagnose, treat, cure, or prevent disease."

When evaluating health-related claims, be skeptical. If something sounds too good to be true, it usually is. Here are some signs of a fraudulent claim (CFSAN, 2003):

- Statements that the product is a quick and effective cure-all or diagnostic tool for a wide variety of ailments. For example: "Extremely beneficial in the treatment of rheumatism, arthritis, infections, prostate problems, ulcers, cancer, heart trouble, hardening of the arteries, and more."
- Statements that suggest the product can treat or cure diseases. For example: "shrinks tumors" or "cures impotency."
- Promotions that use words like "scientific breakthrough," "miraculous cure," "exclusive product," "secret ingredient," or "ancient remedy." For example: "A revolutionary innovation formulated by using proven principles of natural health-based medical science."
- Text that uses impressive-sounding terms like these for a weight-loss product: "hunger stimulation point" and "thermogenesis."
- Undocumented case histories or personal testimonials by consumers or doctors claiming amazing results. For example: "My husband has Alzheimer['s disease]. He began eating a teaspoonful of this product each day. And now in just 22 days he mowed the grass, cleaned out the garage, weeded the flowerbeds, and we take our morning walk again."
- Limited availability and advance payment requirements. For example: "Hurry. This offer will not last. Send us a check now to reserve your supply."
- Promises of no-risk "money-back guarantees." For example: "If after 30 days you have not lost at least 4 pounds each week, your check will be returned to you."

It is easy to see why some people are taken in by promoters' promises, especially when successful treatments through legitimate healthcare providers have been elusive. Patients should be encouraged to resist pressure to decide "on the spot" about trying an untested product or treatment. Ask for more information and consult a knowledgeable doctor, pharmacist, or other healthcare professional. Promoters of legitimate healthcare products do not object to your seeking additional information (FDA, 2005).

To learn whether the FDA or the FTC has taken action against the promoter of a product you may be considering, visit www.fda.gov/oc/enforcement.html. Visit www.cfsan.fda.gov/~dms/ds-warn.html for a list of the dietary supplement ingredients for which the FDA has issued warnings. In addition, if individuals are considering a clinic that requires a person to travel and stay far from home for treatment, they should check it out with their doctor. Although some clinics offer effective treatments, others prescribe untested, unapproved, ineffective, and possibly dangerous "cures." The healthcare providers who work in these clinics may be unlicensed or lack other appropriate credentials. When dealing with online healthcare information and products it is better to err on the side of caution. There are wonderful resources available from the comfort of your own computer desk, but be careful, do not believe everything you read on the Internet. To stay safe, follow this simple rule, "When in doubt, check it out!"

SUMMARY: "CAVEAT EMPTOR!"

The Latin phrase above means "Let the buyer beware!" referring predominantly to real estate purchases. However, the application of "caveat emptor" to healthcare information and products is critical. While there may not be exchange of money for healthcare information, it could "cost" someone their life if they follow faulty advice! Efforts to improve health information access with the expansion of Internet resources, even to remote communities, put more responsibility on patients to sort the reliable and legitimate from the shady and questionable. Healthcare providers will see many patients enter their office armed with pages of information printed from the Internet. The Web is a valuable resource for patients and providers alike. All consumers of Internet information should carefully consider and evaluate the source before buying or believing the concepts or products promoted on glitzy Web sites.

ADDITIONAL RESOURCE:

Internet Healthcare Coalition
PO Box 286
Newtown, PA 18940
215-504-4164
215-504-5739 FAX
http://www.ihealthcoalition.org/

REFERENCES

Center for Food Safety and Applied Nutrition (CFSAN). (2003, September). Claims that can be made for conventional foods and dietary supplements, 2003. CFSAN/Office of Nutritional Products, Labeling, and Dietary Supplements. Retrieved September 16, 2005, from http://www.cfsan.fda.gov/~dms/hclaims.html.

Federal Food and Drug Administration (FDA). (1996, June). FDA: Health information online. *FDA Consumer, 30*(5).

Federal Trade Commission and the Food and Drug Administration (FDA). (2005). 'Miracle' health claims: Add a dose of skepticism. Retrieved September 16, 2005, from http://ftc.gov/bcp/conline/pubs/health/frdheal.htm.

Internet Healthcare Coalition (iHealth). (2005). Tips for healthy surfing online: Finding quality health information on the Internet. Retrieved February 4, 2005, from http://www.ihealthcoalition.org/content/tips.html.

APPENDIX: USEFUL WORLD WIDE WEB SITES

- Ask NOAH: http://www.noah-health.org/

  New York Online Access to Health, or NOAH, began in 1994 when four New York City library organizations joined forces to establish a single Web site to provide end-users a place on the World Wide Web to reach reliable consumer health information. The four organizations were: the City University of New York Office of Library Services (CUNY); the Metropolitan New York Library Council (METRO); the New York Academy of Medicine Library (NYAM); and the New York Public Library (NYPL). They were later joined by the Queens Borough Public Library and the Brooklyn Public Library. The initial goal, the development of a Web site which would provide healthcare information easily accessible and understandable to the layperson, resulted in NOAH. The NOAH-health.org site allows visitors to view a health topic listing by body area or disease category in English or Spanish. NOAH provides access to high-quality, full-text consumer health information that is accurate, timely, relevant, and unbiased.

- American Cancer Society: http://www.cancer.org/

  The American Cancer Society (ACS) site offers information for patients, family, and friends to learn about cancer, treatment options, and coping. A special section links cancer survivors to networks and support programs. Individuals seeking information can find statistics on cancer, prevention and early detection help, and a link to the ACS bookstore to purchase cancer-related literature. Professionals can find cancer facts and figures, publications, media information, and research programs related to many different types of cancer. Information is available in English, Spanish, and several Asian languages.

- American Heart Association: http://www.americanheart.org/

  Visitors to the American Heart Association Web site will find resources to identify warning signs of heart disease, as well as detailed information about various heart diseases and conditions, including strokes. There is also a section devoted to children's health concerns. CPR and Emergency Cardiovascular Care (ECC) are described and tools are available to find classes in local communities. Much of the information on this site is available in Spanish as well as English. The American Heart Association is committed to providing sound scientific information for healthcare professionals, from scientific statements to online versions of heart disease journals. The American Heart Association also works with government agencies to derive annual statistics for cardiovascular diseases, including coronary heart disease, stroke, high blood pressure, and others. This site also includes data on risk factors, nutrition, quality of care, medical procedures, and economic cost.

- Cancer Trials Help: http://www.CancerTrialsHelp.org

  If you are one of the 1.3 million people diagnosed with cancer each year, or involved in their health care, Cancer Trials provides information on the best available treatment and the opportunity to receive new, potentially more effective therapy. CancerTrialsHelp.org gives patients and caregivers in-depth content about cancer clinical trials, including information about insurance issues, and questions to ask a physician. The ABCs of cancer clinical trials utilizes an interactive guide to get the details about how researchers conduct clinical trials. As of 2005, this information was available in English only.

- Centers for Disease Control and Prevention: http://www.cdc.gov/

  The Centers for Disease Control and Prevention (CDC) is the principal agency in the United States government for protecting the health and safety of all Americans and for providing essential human services, especially for those people who are least able to help themselves. The CDC is globally recognized for conducting research and investigations and for its action-oriented approach. CDC applies research and findings to improve people's daily lives and responds to health emergencies—something that distinguishes CDC from its peer agencies. This Web site offers timely and thorough information about thousands of health topics in English and Spanish. Up-to-date national and state health statistics, programs, and healthcare initiatives, and links to other valuable resources are available on this site.

- Clinical Trials: http://ClinicalTrials.gov

  This site, created by the National Institutes of Health (NIH) and the National Library of Medicine (NLM), provides patients and the public easy access to information about the location of clinical trials, their design and purpose, criteria for participation, and additional disease and treatment information. ClinicalTrials.gov provides regularly updated information about federally and privately supported clinical research in human volunteers. ClinicalTrials.gov gives information about a trial's purpose, who may participate, locations, and phone numbers for more details. The information provided on ClinicalTrials.gov should be used in conjunction with advice from healthcare professionals. Visitors to the ClinicalTrials.gov Web site can search for information by disease, location, treatment, or sponsor of a clinical trial. As of 2005, this information was available only in English.

- Department of Health and Human Services: http://www.hhs.gov/
  The Department of Health and Human Services (HHS) is the US government's principal agency for protecting the health of all Americans and providing essential human services, especially for those who are least able to help themselves. HHS includes more than 300 programs, covering a wide spectrum of activities. Some highlights include:

  - Health and social science research
  - Preventing disease, including immunization services
  - Assuring food and drug safety
  - Medicare (health insurance for elderly and disabled Americans) and Medicaid (health insurance for low-income people)
  - Health information technology
  - Financial assistance and services for low-income families
  - Improving maternal and infant health
  - Head Start (preschool education and services)
  - Faith-based and community initiatives
  - Preventing child abuse and domestic violence
  - Substance abuse treatment and prevention
  - Services for older Americans, including home-delivered meals
  - Comprehensive health services for Native Americans
  - Medical preparedness for emergencies, including potential terrorism

  The Web site for the Department of Health and Human Services has extensive links to a wide range of resource topics, including Reference Collections, Grants & Funding, Disasters & Emergencies, Drug & Food Information, Safety & Wellness, Diseases & Conditions, Families & Children, Aging, Specific Populations, Resource Locators, and Policies & Regulations. Most of the information is available in English and Spanish.

- Healthfinder: http://www.healthfinder.gov/

  A Service of the National Health Information Center, US Department of Health & Human Services, Healthfinder is the US government's directory of authoritative health information, including links to online journals, medical dictionaries, and prevention and self-care information. Healthfinder has a *health library* with health information from A to Z, in English and Spanish, addressing prevention and wellness, diseases and conditions, and alternative medicine. The site also has medical dictionaries, an encyclopedia, journals, and more. Links to online health checkups, health news, and other health organizations are also available on Healthfinder.com. The *"Just for You"* section provides selected health topics organized by gender; by age, from kids to seniors; by race and ethnicity; and for parents, caregivers, health professionals, and others.

- Lab Tests Online: http://www.labtestsonline.org

  Like many areas in medicine, clinical lab testing often provides few simple answers to commonly asked questions. The issues—on topics like insurance reimbursement and reference ranges—can be very complex. Lab Tests Online is a peer-reviewed, non-commercial, patient-centered information resource on clinical lab testing from the American Association for Clinical Chemistry. This site breaks down a range of diagnostic laboratory tests in a way that will help patients to understand the issues, and perhaps, to ask the appropriate questions of healthcare providers. Lab Tests Online helps the patient better understand that many clinical lab tests are part of routine care, as well as diagnosis and treatment of conditions and diseases. Collaborating partners and sponsors are clearly identified on this Web site. As of 2005, the information was available in English.

- MayoClinic.com: http://www.mayoclinic.com/index.cfm

  The Mayo Clinic Web site contains easy-to-understand information on health and medical topics, reviewed for accuracy by Mayo Clinic experts. Content includes English language interactive resources and tools, information on specific diseases and disorders, management of particular chronic conditions, suggestions for healthy lifestyles, consumer drug information, first aid, specialists' answers to frequently asked questions about diseases, and health decision-making guides. This site is a service of Mayo Foundation for Medical Education and Research.

- Medline Plus: http://medlineplus.gov/

  MedlinePlus brings together authoritative information from the National Library of Medicine, the National Institutes of Health (NIH), and other government agencies and health-related organizations. Health professionals and consumers alike can depend on it for information that is authoritative and updated daily. MedlinePlus has extensive information from the National Institutes of Health and other trusted sources on over 700 diseases and conditions. There are also lists of hospitals and physicians, a medical encyclopedia and a medical dictionary, health information in Spanish, extensive information on prescription and nonprescription drugs, health information from the media, and links to thousands of clinical trials. There is no advertising on this site, nor does MedlinePlus endorse any company or product.

- MEDLINE/PubMed: http://www.ncbi.nlm.nih.gov/entrez/query.fcgi

  MEDLINE/PubMed is the National Library of Medicine's database of references to more than 14 million articles published in 4800 biomedical journals. When you search MEDLINE/PubMed:

  - You will find information about articles on your topic (the author, title of the article, name of the journal, date published, page numbers).
  - Many of the listings also have short summaries of the article (abstracts).
  - Sometimes you will find a link to the full article.

  Most of the articles listed in MEDLINE/PubMed are for health professionals. The articles are for educational use only and are not intended to replace advice from a health professional.

- Merck & Company/Merck Manual: http://www.merck.com/mmhe/index.html

  Merck & Co., Inc. is a global, research-driven pharmaceutical company dedicated to putting patients first. Established in 1891, Merck discovers, develops, manufactures, and markets vaccines and medicines in over 20 therapeutic categories. Merck also publishes unbiased health information as a not-for-profit service. The Merck Manual Web site contains anatomical drawings, multimedia health resources, pronunciations for medical terms, weights and measures, common medical tests, drug information, and other resources. The Merck Manual online also has over 25 different sections dedicated to providing health information on numerous topics. For example, the section devoted to common medical tests provides the normal test result ranges for blood tests as well as a chart of diagnostic procedures, body area tested, and descriptions. It describes disorders, who is likely to get them, their symptoms, diagnosis, prevention, and treatment; it also provides information about prognosis. It is based on the world's most widely used textbook of medicine—*The Merck Manual*—but written in everyday language by 300 contributors. Other manuals available through this site include the *Merck Manual of Diagnosis and Therapy, the Merck Manual of Health &*

Aging, the Merck Manual of Geriatrics, the Merck Index (a one-volume encyclopedia of chemicals, drugs, and biologicals) and *The Merck Veterinary Manual.*

- National Cancer Institute: http://www.nci.nih.gov/ or http://www.cancer.gov

  The National Cancer Institute (NCI) is a component of the National Institutes of Health (NIH), established under the National Cancer Act of 1937. It is the Federal Government's principal agency for cancer research and training. Visitors to the NCI Web site find valuable cancer-related health information. There are links to find out more about the work conducted by NCI-supported scientists throughout the country. For the general public and health professionals, www.cancer.gov provides consumer-oriented information on a wide range of topics as well as comprehensive descriptions of NCI research programs available in English and Spanish. Scientists will find detailed information on specific areas of research and funding opportunities.

- National Institutes of Health, Health Information: http://health.nih.gov/

  The National Institutes of Health (NIH), a part of the US Department of Health and Human Services, is the primary federal agency for conducting and supporting medical research. The NIH is the nation's medical research agency—making important medical discoveries that improve health and save lives. NIH scientists investigate ways to prevent disease as well as the causes, treatments, and even cures, for common and rare diseases. This site contains a mostly English language comprehensive file of health topics from A to Z. It includes links to national health databases, telephone hotlines, and other federal agencies.

Chapter 6

Government and Voluntary Health Agencies

Stephanie Chisolm

OBJECTIVES

After studying this chapter, the student should be able to

1. Explain the role of the governmental and voluntary health agencies in the United States today.
2. Identify major government and voluntary health agencies working to improve the health of Americans.
3. Identify career opportunities at these agencies.

INTRODUCTION

> *The ingredients of health and long life, are great temperance, open air, easy labor, and little care.*
>
> Sir Philip Sidney, English Statesman (1554–1586)

It is no easy task to increase the quality and quantity of life for all Americans while working to reduce disparities between different populations. Goals and objectives of Healthy People 2010, and the preceding objectives for the nation, would not be achievable with only brick-and-mortar healthcare facilities. This chapter introduces the many Public Health *government agencies* whose missions include improving the health care, health resources, or health information for our nations' citizens. Many of these organizations employ healthcare professionals from the US Public Health

Service as well as others. This chapter will provide details about some of the major government health agencies, and highlight some of the voluntary health agencies that serve as respected leaders for research, resources, and advocates for patients and professionals. The profiles of these agencies enable you to find the highest quality resources for health information as students and professionals. Understanding the role and mission of these organizations may identify new career opportunities for you, as many professionals in all aspects of healthcare find rewarding careers in government and voluntary health agencies.

What Is a Voluntary Health Agency?

Voluntary health agencies or *associations* often begin with the concerns expressed by a citizen, a mandate from officials, or with grass roots activism that result in an attempt to organize and support research to understand or cure a health condition. Some of these agencies are disease specific. The Lupus Foundation (http://lupus.org/) and the Hepatitis Foundation International (http://www.hepfi.org/) are examples of disease-specific agencies. Others such as the American Red Cross provide services across many areas. Some of these agencies deal directly with patients or victims; others provide national, regional, or state support for research. Advocacy, research, education, and support are common to most agencies or associations. Many voluntary health agencies have their national headquarters in or near Washington, DC or other large metropolitan areas to support advocacy. Some hire lobbyists to conduct activities aimed at influencing public officials and especially members of a legislative body on legislation specific to the health organization.

The Origin of Government Sponsored/Funded Health Agencies

Health agencies sponsored by the federal government generally fall under the umbrella of the Department of Health and Human Services. The Department of Health and Human Services (HHS) is the US government's principal agency for protecting the health of all Americans and providing essential human services, especially for those who are least able to help themselves. The roots of the Department of Health and Human Services go back to the earliest days of the nation. In 1709, the passage of an act which established a federal network of hospitals for the care of merchant seamen became a forerunner of today's US Public Health Service. In the last 100 years, significant legislation shaped the current role of the Department of Health and Human Services. The following milestones highlight the evolution of the public health infrastructure in this country, particularly as it pertains to the development of government health agencies.

- **1906**–Congress passed the Pure Food and Drugs Act, authorizing the government to monitor the purity of foods and the safety of medicines, now a responsibility of the FDA.
- **1912**–President Theodore Roosevelt's first White House Conference urged creation of the Children's Bureau, now known as the Maternal Child Health Bureau, to combat exploitation of children.
- **1921**–The Bureau of Indian Affairs Health Division was created, the forerunner to the Indian Health Service.
- **1930**–Creation of the National Institute of Health, out of the Public Health Service's Hygenic Laboratory.
- **1938**–Passage of the Federal Food, Drug, and Cosmetic Act.
- **1946**–The Communicable Disease Center was established, forerunner of the Centers for Disease Control and Prevention.
- **1953**–The Cabinet-level Department of Health, Education, and Welfare (HEW) was created under President Eisenhower, officially coming into existence in 1953. In 1979, the Department of Education Organization Act was signed into law, providing for a separate Department of Education. HEW officially became the Department of Health and Human Services in 1980.
- **1964**–Release of the first Surgeon General's Report on Smoking and Health.
- **1965**–Creation of the Medicare and Medicaid programs, making comprehensive health care available to millions of Americans.
- **1970**–Creation of the National Health Service Corps.
- **1977**–Creation of the Health Care Financing Administration to manage Medicare and Medicaid separately from the Social Security Administration.
- **1989**–Creation of the Agency for Health Care Policy and Research (now the Agency for Healthcare Research and Quality).
- **1996**–Enactment of the Health Insurance Portability and Accountability Act (HIPAA).
- **1997**–Creation of the State Children's Health Insurance Program (SCHIP), enabling states to extend health coverage to more uninsured children.
- **2001**–The Centers for Medicare & Medicaid is created, replacing the Health Care Financing Administration. HHS responds to the nation's first bioterrorism attack—the delivery of anthrax through the mail.

- **2002**–The Office of Public Health Emergency Preparedness created to coordinate efforts against bioterrorism and other emergency health threats.
- **2003**–Enactment of the Medicare Prescription Drug Improvement and Modernization Act of 2003, the most significant expansion of Medicare since its enactment, including a prescription drug benefit.

The Department of Health and Human Services represents almost a quarter of all federal outlays, an estimated $581 billion in 2005. It administers more grant dollars than all other federal agencies combined. HHS' Medicare program is the nation's largest health insurer, handling more than 1 billion claims per year. Medicare and Medicaid together provide healthcare insurance for 1 in 4 Americans (see Chapter 3 for additional information).

Most of the HHS departments are located in or around Washington, DC. The headquarters building of the US Department of Health and Human Services is the Hubert H. Humphrey Building, located at the foot of Capitol Hill. The largest Washington-area HHS facility is the campus of the National Institutes of Health in Bethesda, Maryland, where more than 17,000 employees, working in 40 buildings, are engaged in conducting the world's foremost biomedical research program. In addition, the campus of the Centers for Disease Control and Prevention and the offices of the Agency for Toxic Substances and Disease Registry are located in Atlanta, Georgia.

The Department of Health and Human Services works closely with state and local governments, with many HHS-funded services provided at the local level by state or county agencies as well as through private sector grantees. Eleven operating divisions administer the Department's more than 300 programs. These include eight agencies in the US Public Health Service and three human services agencies. In addition to the services they deliver, the HHS programs provide for equitable treatment of beneficiaries nationwide, and they enable the collection of national health and other data.

Major HHS-funded programs and their associated agencies are described in the sections which follow.

The National Institutes of Health – Web site: http://www.nih.gov

Established in 1887 as the Hygienic Laboratory in Staten Island, New York, the National Institutes of Health is the world's premier medical research organization, supporting over 38,000 research projects nationwide on a range of diseases, including cancer, Alzheimer's, diabetes, arthritis, heart ailments, and AIDS. The NIH, employing over 17,000 professionals, includes 27 separate health institutes and centers. Today, the headquarters are located in Bethesda, Maryland. Simply described, the goal of NIH research is to acquire new knowledge to help prevent, detect, diagnose, and treat disease and disability, from the rarest genetic disorder to the common cold. The NIH mission is to uncover new knowledge that will lead to better health for everyone. With a budget of $28.6 billion in 2005, NIH works toward that mission by conducting research in its own laboratories; supporting the research of non-Federal scientists in universities, medical schools, hospitals, and research institutions throughout the country and abroad; helping in the training of research investigators; and fostering the communication of medical and health sciences information.

Food and Drug Administration – Web site: http://www.fda.gov

The Food and Drug Administration (FDA) assures the safety of foods and cosmetics, and the safety and efficacy of pharmaceuticals, biological products, and medical devices—products which represent almost 25 cents out of every dollar in U.S. consumer spending. Established in1906, when the Pure Food and Drugs Act gave regulatory authority to the Bureau of Chemistry, the FDA has a budget of $1.8 billion and a team of over 10,000 public health employees that includes physicians, nurses, dietitians, consumer safety officers, lawyers, and scientists, with specialties ranging from biomaterials engineering to pharmacology. Decisions made by the FDA affect every American every day. In 2000, consumers spent $1 trillion—more than 20 percent of their income—on hundreds of thousands of products whose safety and effectiveness is the FDA responsibility. The public trusts the FDA to ensure that:

1. Foods are safe, wholesome, and truthfully labeled.
2. Drugs for both humans and animals, and vaccines for humans are safe and effective.
3. Blood used for transfusions is safe and in adequate supply.
4. Medical devices, from scalpels to CT scanners, are safe and effective.
5. Transplanted tissues are safe and effective.
6. Equipment that uses radiant energy, such as x-ray machines and microwave ovens, is safe.
7. Cosmetics are safe and properly labeled.

The FDA has identified the following four strategic priorities. Each reinforces the importance of *prevention* as the agency's primary response to the nation's health and safety concerns.

- *Assuring a Safe Food Supply*: The FDA is responsible for assuring the safety of 80% of the US food supply and annually monitors 4 million food import entries into the United States. That includes half of all seafood and more than 20% of the fresh fruits and vegetables consumed by Americans. The FDA is working with partners to significantly reduce food-borne illnesses and deaths. Prevention strategies based on strong scientific research and risk assessment are implemented through a nationwide inspection program in partnership with the states.

- *Assuring Medical Product Safety*: The FDA continues to ensure that drugs, vaccines, and medical devices are safe by conducting more than 15,000 inspections each year to make certain that these products are properly manufactured and distributed, and by monitoring their safe performance and use.

- *Managing Emerging Hazards*: The FDA is vigilant in assessing and then quickly and effectively reducing risks associated with unexpected health and safety threats to Americans such as bioterrorism, AIDS, and Bovine Spongiform Encephalopathy (BSE) known as "mad cow disease." The FDA's approach has been to counter these hazards through a regulatory framework and the agency's scientific expertise.

- *Bringing New Technologies to Market*: The FDA ensures that the products of new technologies are available to US consumers. Because of the agency's timely, science-based decisions, millions of Americans can get the medicines, biologics, and medical devices they need and be assured of their safety and effectiveness.

Centers for Disease Control and Prevention – Web site: http://www.cdc.gov

Established in 1946 as the Communicable Disease Center, the mission of the CDC today is to promote health and quality of life by preventing and controlling disease, injury, and disability. The CDC seeks to accomplish its mission by working with partners throughout the nation and the world to

- monitor health,
- detect and investigate health problems,
- conduct research to enhance prevention,
- develop and advocate sound public health policies,
- implement prevention strategies,
- promote healthy behaviors,
- foster safe and healthful environments, and
- provide leadership and training.

These functions are the backbone of the CDC's mission. Each of the CDC's component organizations undertakes these activities in conducting its specific programs. The steps needed to accomplish this mission, based on scientific excellence, require over 8,000 well-trained public health practitioners and leaders dedicated to high standards of quality and ethical practice. The CDC, as the sentinel for the health of people in the United States and throughout the world, strives to protect people's health and safety, provide reliable health information, and improve health through strong partnerships.

Working with states and other partners, the CDC provides a system of health surveillance to monitor and prevent disease outbreaks (including bioterrorism), implement disease-prevention strategies, and maintain national health statistics. The CDC provides for immunization services, workplace safety, and environmental disease prevention. The CDC also guards against international disease transmission, with personnel stationed in more than 25 foreign countries. The CDC director is also administrator of the Agency for Toxic Substances and Disease Registry (ATSDR), which helps prevent exposure and adverse human health effects and diminished quality of life associated with exposure to hazardous substances from waste sites, unplanned releases, and other sources of pollution present in the environment.

The CDC, with a budget for fiscal year 2005 of $8 billion, is committed to achieving true improvements in people's health. To do this, the agency is defining specific health impact goals to prioritize and focus its work and investments and measure progress. The following health impact goals and objectives drive the efforts to have healthy citizens at all ages, to have healthy environments, deal with emerging health threats, provide support, and encourage global health (CDC, 2005).

Healthy People in Every Stage of Life. All people, and especially those at greater risk of health disparities, will achieve their optimal lifespan with the best possible quality of health in every stage of life. To achieve this goal, individuals should follow the recommendations below:

- *Start Strong*: Increase the number of infants and toddlers that have a strong start for healthy and safe lives (Infants and Toddlers, ages 0-3 years).
- *Grow Safe and Strong*: Increase the number of children who grow up healthy, safe, and ready to learn (Children, ages 4-11 years).
- *Achieve Healthy Independence*: Increase the number of adolescents who are prepared to be healthy, safe, independent, and productive members of society (Adolescents, ages 12-19 years).
- *Live a Healthy, Productive, and Satisfying Life*: Increase the number of adults who are healthy and able to participate fully in life activities and enter their later years with optimum health (Adults, ages 20-64 years).

- *Live Better, Longer*: Increase the number of older adults who live longer, high-quality, productive, and independent lives (Older Adults, ages 65 and over).

Healthy People in Healthy Places. The places where people live, work, learn, and play will protect and promote their health and safety, especially those at greater risk of health disparities. To achieve this goal, the following recommendations should be implemented in the areas listed.

- *Healthy Communities*: Increase the number of communities that protect and promote health and safety and prevent illness and injury in all their members.
- *Healthy Homes*: Protect and promote health through safe and healthy home environments.
- *Healthy Schools*: Increase the number of schools that protect and promote the development, health, and safety of all students and staff.
- *Healthy Workplaces*: Promote and protect the health and safety of people who work by preventing workplace-related fatalities, illnesses, injuries, and personal health risks.
- *Healthy Healthcare Settings*: Increase the number of healthcare settings that provide safe, effective, and satisfying patient care.
- *Healthy Institutions*: Increase the number of institutions that provide safe, healthy, and equitable environments for their residents, clients, or inmates.
- *Healthy Travel and Recreation*: Ensure that environments enhance health and prevent illness and injury during travel and recreation.

People Prepared for Emerging Health Threats. People in all communities will be protected from infectious, occupational, environmental, and terrorist threats. Preparedness goals are under development to address scenarios that include natural and intentional threats. The first round of these goals include influenza, anthrax, plague, emerging infections, toxic chemical exposure, and radiation exposure. To meet this goal, the following areas must be addressed:

- *Prevention:* Increase the use and development of interventions known to prevent human illness from chemical, biological, and radiological agents, and naturally occurring health threats.
- *Detection and Reporting:* Decrease the time needed to classify health events as terrorism or naturally occurring in partnership with other agencies. This includes decreasing the time needed to detect and report chemical, biological, or radiological agents in tissue, food, or environmental samples that cause threats to the public's health.

Efforts also should be made to improve the timeliness and accuracy of communications regarding threats to the public's health.

- *Investigation:* Decrease the time to identify causes, risk factors, and appropriate interventions for those affected by threats to the public's health.

- *Control:* Decrease the time needed to provide countermeasures and health guidance to those affected by threats to the public's health.

- *Recover:* Decrease the time needed to restore health services and environmental safety to pre-event levels. Improve the long-term follow-up provided to those affected by threats to the public's health.

- *Improve:* Decrease the time needed to implement recommendations from after-action reports following threats to the public's health.

Healthy People in a Healthy World. People around the world will live safer, healthier, and longer lives through health promotion, health protection, and health diplomacy. This goal involves meeting sub-goals in the following areas:

- *Health Promotion*: Global health will improve by sharing knowledge, tools, and other resources with people and partners around the world.

- *Health Protection*: Americans at home and abroad will be protected from health threats through a transnational prevention, detection, and response network.

- *Health Diplomacy*: The CDC and the US Government will be a trusted and effective resource for health development and health protection around the globe.

Indian Health Service – Web site: http://www.ihs.gov

Established in 1921, the foundation of the IHS is to uphold the federal government's obligation to promote healthy American Indian and Alaska Native people, communities, and cultures and to honor and protect the sovereign rights of tribes. Their goal is to ensure that comprehensive, culturally acceptable personal and public health services are available and accessible to all American Indian and Alaska Native people. The IHS mission, in partnership with American Indian and Alaska Native people, is to raise their physical, mental, social, and spiritual health to the highest level.

Working with tribes, the over 16,000 health professionals of the IHS provide health services to 1.6 million American Indians and Alaska Natives of more than 560 federally recognized tribes. The IHS clinical staff consists of approximately 2,700 nurses, 900 physicians, 350 engineers, 450 pharmacists, 300 dentists, 150 sanitarians, and 83 physician assistants. The IHS also employs various allied health professionals, such as nutritionists, health administrators, engineers, and medical records administrators. The 2005 budget of $3.8 billion supports 49 hospitals, 247 health centers, 348 health stations, satellite clinics, residential substance abuse treatment centers, Alaska Native village clinics, and 34 urban Indian health programs. Headquartered in Rockville, Maryland, the IHS functions around the country to serve the members of federally recognized Indian tribes and their descendants who are eligible for services. The IHS is the agency within the Department of Health and Human Services that operates a comprehensive health service delivery system for more than half of the nation's estimated 2.6 million American Indians and Alaska Natives. The IHS strives for maximum tribal involvement in meeting the needs of its service population. In order to carry out its mission, uphold its foundation, and attain its goal, the IHS

1. Assists Indian tribes in developing their health programs through activities such as health management training, technical assistance, and human resource development;
2. Facilitates and assists Indian tribes in coordinating health planning, in obtaining and using health resources available through federal, state, and local programs, and in operating comprehensive health-care services and health programs.
3. Provides comprehensive healthcare services, including hospital and ambulatory medical care, preventive and rehabilitative services, and development of community sanitation facilities.
4. Serves as the principal federal advocate in the health field for Indians to ensure comprehensive health services for American Indian and Alaska Native people.

Preventive measures involving environmental, educational, and outreach activities are combined with therapeutic measures into a single national health system. Within these broad categories are special initiatives in traditional medicine, elder care, women's health, children and adolescent health, injury prevention, domestic violence and child abuse, healthcare financing, state health care, sanitation facilities, and oral health.

Health Resources and Services Administration – Web site: http://www.hrsa.gov

Established in 1982, the Health Resources and Services Administration (HRSA) envisions optimal health for all. It provides national leadership, program resources and services, and supports a healthcare system that assures access to comprehensive, culturally competent, quality care. As the nation's

Access Agency, HRSA focuses on uninsured, underserved, and special needs populations in its goals and program activities:

- Improve Access to Health Care.
- Improve Health Outcomes.
- Improve the Quality of Health Care.
- Eliminate Health Disparities.
- Improve the Public Health and Healthcare Systems.
- Enhance the Ability of the Healthcare System to Respond to Public Health Emergencies.
- Achieve Excellence in Management Practices.

While headquartered in Rockville, Maryland, HRSA employs about 2,000 individuals in the nation's capital and 10 regional offices. HRSA provides access to essential healthcare services for people who are low-income, uninsured, or who live in rural areas or urban neighborhoods where health care is scarce. Operating with a budget of approximately $6.8 billion, HRSA-funded health centers provided medical care to almost 14 million patients at more than 3,700 sites nationwide in 2005.

The agency helps prepare the nation's healthcare system and providers to respond to bioterrorism and other public health emergencies, maintains the National Health Service Corps, and helps build the healthcare workforce through training and education programs. HRSA administers a variety of programs to improve the health of mothers and children and serves people living with HIV/AIDS through the Ryan White CARE Act programs. HRSA also oversees the nation's organ transplantation system.

Substance Abuse and Mental Health Services Administration – Web site: http://www.samhsa.gov

The Substance Abuse and Mental Health Services Administration (SAMHSA), an agency of the US Department of Health and Human Services (HHS), was established by an act of Congress in 1992 under Public Law 102-321. The agency, separate and distinct from the National Institutes of Health or any other agency within the HHS, was created to focus attention, programs, and funding on improving the lives of people with or at risk for mental and substance abuse disorders. SAMHSA works to improve the quality and availability of substance abuse prevention, addiction treatment, and mental health services. The agency provides funding through block grants to states to support substance abuse and mental health services, including treatment for more than 650,000 Americans with serious substance abuse problems or mental health problems. SAMHSA's mission and vision have been more sharply focused and aligned with HHS goals and President Bush's administration priorities. It is a vision consistent with the President's New Freedom Initiative that promotes a life in the community for everyone. Moreover, SAMHSA is achieving that vision through a mission that is both action-oriented and measurable: to build resilience and facilitate recovery for people with or at risk for substance abuse and mental illness. In collaboration with the states, national and local community-based and faith-based organizations, and public and private sector providers, SAMHSA is working to ensure that people with or at risk for a mental or addictive disorder have the opportunity for a fulfilling life that includes a job, a home, and meaningful relationships with family and friends. The agency helps improve substance abuse prevention and treatment services through the identification and dissemination of best practices. SAMHSA monitors prevalence and incidence of substance abuse. Headquartered in Rockville, Maryland, SAMHSA employed 558 health professionals with a budget of $3.4 billion in 2005.

Agency for Healthcare Research and Quality (AHRQ) – Web site: http://www.ahrq.gov

Established in 1989 and located in Rockville, Maryland, AHRQ supports research designed to improve the outcomes and quality of health care, reduce its costs, address patient safety and medical errors, and broaden access to effective services. AHRQ sponsors and conducts research that provides evidence-based information on healthcare outcomes and quality, as well as cost, use, and access. The information helps healthcare decision makers—patients and clinicians, health system leaders, purchasers, and policymakers—make more informed decisions and improve the quality of healthcare services.

The World Health Organization – Web site http://www.who.int

On a global perspective, the World Health Organization, mentioned earlier in this text, is the United Nations' specialized agency for health. Established in 1948, WHO's objective, as set out in its constitution, is the attainment by all peoples of the highest possible level of health. Health is defined in WHO's constitution as a state of complete physical, mental, and social well-being and not merely the absence of disease or infirmity. WHO is governed by 192 Member States through the World Health Assembly. The Health Assembly is composed of representatives from WHO's Member States. The main tasks of the World Health Assembly are to approve the WHO program and the budget for the following biennium and to decide major policy questions.

Voluntary Health Agencies

Most voluntary health agencies fall within the nonprofit organization category. A "nonprofit" is an organization whose primary objective is to support an issue or matter of private interest or public concern for non-commercial purposes. Nonprofits may be involved in an innumerable range of health issues. Although nonprofits do not operate to generate profit, they still need to generate revenue in order to finance their activities. Most nonprofits receive funding by donations from the private or public sector. Many of the organizations identified in this chapter have a proportionately small paid staff to keep the organization or agency on task and operational. However, for most, the heart, soul, and hands to help come from volunteers that contribute time, talent, and treasures to benefit others or find a cure for a debilitating health condition. Voluntary health agencies may be disease specific or focus their efforts on general health concerns.

One key action of a nonprofit voluntary health agency is to work to advocate for those afflicted with their health conditions. Many have headquarters near Washington, DC or near other large metropolitan cities to have access to lawmakers and major healthcare providers. Most have local chapters and divisions to be of most help in the communities they serve. The voluntary health agencies are an excellent place for students interested in health careers to volunteer and gain valuable experience before going on to professional training. Some voluntary health agencies may also provide some direct care to individuals with respect to their health conditions, or provide support to patients or their caregivers. Local volunteer rescue squads are good examples of those providing direct service to their communities. Voluntary health organizations also support research into primary, secondary, or tertiary prevention of certain health problems. They also provide education and information to patients and the public to increase awareness and access to the best care possible. The voluntary health organizations profiled in this chapter are only a small sample of those working throughout this country and the world to find cures, advocate for legislation, and educate individuals to prevent, detect, and make informed decisions concerning treatment of diseases.

American Red Cross – Web site: http://www.redcross.org

The minute you think you've got it made, disaster is just around the corner.
Joe Paterno, American Football Coach (1924–)

Due to the devastating impact of recent disasters on so many individuals, perhaps one of the best known voluntary health agencies in the world is the

American Red Cross. Since its founding in 1881 by Clara Barton, the American Red Cross (ARC) has been the nation's premier emergency response organization. As part of a worldwide movement that offers neutral humanitarian care to the victims of war, the American Red Cross distinguished itself by also aiding victims of devastating natural disasters. Over the years, the organization has expanded its services, always with the aim of preventing and relieving suffering. Although not a government agency, in 1905 the Red Cross was chartered by Congress to "carry on a system of national and international relief in time of peace and apply the same in mitigating the sufferings caused by pestilence, famine, fire, floods, and other great national calamities, and to devise and carry on measures for preventing the same." The charter is not only a grant of power, but also an imposition of duties and obligations to the nation, to disaster victims, and to the people who generously support its work with their donations (American Red Cross, 2005).

Today, the American Red Cross is a leader in disaster relief such as the September 11, 2001 terrorist attacks, the 2004 tsunami in Asia, and the 2005 devastating hurricane season in the United States. In addition to domestic disaster relief, the American Red Cross offers compassionate services in five other areas:

1. Community services that help the needy
2. Support and comfort for military members and their families
3. The collection, processing, and distribution of lifesaving blood and blood products
4. Educational programs that promote health and safety (for example, first aid, CPR, water safety)
5. International relief and development programs

The Red Cross is not a government agency; it relies on donations of time, money, and blood to do its work. In all their work, Red Cross volunteers and employees abide by the organization's seven fundamental principles: humanity, impartiality, neutrality, independence, voluntary service, unity, and universality.

Each year, the American Red Cross responds immediately to more than 70,000 disasters, including house or apartment fires (the majority of disaster responses), hurricanes, floods, earthquakes, tornadoes, hazardous materials spills, transportation accidents, explosions, and other natural and man-made disasters. Nearly one million volunteers and 35,000 employees of the Red Cross offer comfort and assistance throughout the world.

Through nearly 900 locally supported chapters, more than 15 million people gain the skills they need to prepare for and respond to emergencies in their homes, communities, and the world. All Red Cross assistance is given free of charge, made possible by the generous contribution of people's time, money, and skills.

As the most visible division of Biomedical Services at the ARC, Blood Services touches more lives than ever before. The use of current medical technologies allows them to provide the nation with a variety of blood products that are as safe as possible.

Today's American Red Cross uses the latest in computer and telecommunications technology to send communications on behalf of family members who are facing emergencies or other important events to members of the US Armed Forces serving all over the world. Both active duty and community-based military can count on the Red Cross to provide emergency communications that link them with their families back home, access to financial assistance, counseling, and assistance to veterans. Red Cross Armed Forces Emergency Services personnel work in nearly 900 chapters in the United States, on 74 military installations around the world, and with our troops in Kuwait, Afghanistan, and Iraq.

For nearly a century, the American Red Cross has prepared people to save lives through health and safety education and training. From first aid, CPR, and blood-borne pathogens training to swimming and life guarding, to HIV/AIDS education and babysitter's training, American Red Cross Preparedness programs help people lead safer and healthier lives. Today's innovative programs also include teaching laypersons and professionals how to use automated external defibrillators (AEDs) to save victims of sudden cardiac arrest.

The American Red Cross also helps vulnerable people around the world to prevent, prepare for, and respond to disasters, complex humanitarian emergencies, and life-threatening health conditions. The American Red Cross accomplishes this goal by working within the International Red Cross and Red Crescent Movement—the world's largest humanitarian network, with 181 national Red Cross and Red Crescent Societies and more than 100 million volunteers.

American Cancer Society – Web site: http://www.cancer.org

*Chandler: Hey, you know, I have had it with you guys and your
"cancer" and your "emphysema" and your "heart disease."
The bottom line is smoking is cool and you know it.*
Episode of *Friends* (American television situation comedy)

Most voluntary organizations would disagree with Chandler from *Friends*. Smoking is the underlying cause of many of our leading health concerns today. The American Cancer Society (ACS) is the nationwide community-based voluntary health organization dedicated to eliminating cancer as a major health problem by preventing cancer, saving the lives of cancer patients, and diminishing suffering from cancer through research, education, advocacy, and service. The American Cancer Society's international mission concentrates on capacity building in developing cancer societies and on collaboration with other cancer-related organizations throughout the world in carrying out shared strategic directions.

Originally founded in 1913 as the American Society for the Control of Cancer (ASCC) by 15 prominent physicians and business leaders in New York City, the American Cancer Society, Inc. today consists of a national Society, with chartered Divisions throughout the country. The national Society is responsible for overall planning and coordination of public and professional education; providing technical help and materials to Divisions and Units; and administering programs of research, medical grants, and clinical fellowships. The National Board of Directors includes representatives from the Divisions and from the general public. More than 3,400 local Units are organized to cover the counties and communities in the United States. More than two million volunteers carry out the ACS mission of eliminating cancer and improving quality of life for those facing the disease.

The aim of the ACS research program is to determine the causes of cancer and to support efforts to prevent and cure the disease. The Society is the largest source of private, nonprofit cancer research funds in the United States, second only to the federal government in total dollars spent. In 2004, the Society spent nearly $131 million in research. Since 1946, the Society has invested more than $2.8 billion in cancer research. The research program consists of three components: extramural grants, intramural epidemiology and surveillance research, and the intramural behavioral research center. The research program focuses primarily on peer-reviewed projects initiated by beginning investigators working in leading medical and scientific institutions across the country. The ACS has funded 38 Nobel Prize winners early in their careers.

Knowing the facts about cancer can save lives and education is one focus of the ACS. With both prevention and early detection information, people can take an active role in how cancer affects them. Primary cancer prevention means taking the necessary precautions to prevent the occurrence of cancer. The ACS develops prevention programs to help adults and children make healthy lifestyle choices that continue throughout life. The Society's programs focus primarily on:

- Tobacco control
- Relationship between diet and physical activity and cancer
- Comprehensive school health education

- Skin cancer reduction
- Regular medical checkups and recommended cancer screenings

The Society publishes a large number of patient education brochures and pamphlets, books, and professional journals to help patients, families, and healthcare professionals. These include books on specific cancer types, coping issues, and prevention; cookbooks; and textbooks and other specialized cancer-related topics for healthcare professionals. Three clinical journals (*Cancer, Cancer Cytopathology,* and *CA-A Cancer Journal for Clinicians*) are also available.

Because cancer takes a toll on the person diagnosed as well as family and friends, the American Cancer Society offers direct support and service programs to try to lessen the impact. These programs cover a wide range of needs from connecting patients with survivors to providing a place to stay when treatment facilities are far from home. Patient services of the American Cancer Society provide a wide range of emotional and practical support for patients, their families, their caregivers, and their communities from the time of diagnosis to the end of the cancer experience.

Cancer is a medical, social, psychological, and economic issue, and it is a political issue as well. Policymakers at all levels of government make decisions every day that impact the lives of nearly nine million cancer survivors, their families, and all potential cancer patients. The Society's advocacy efforts strive to influence public policies at all levels, with special emphasis on laws or regulations relating to

- The use, sale, distribution, marketing, and advertising of tobacco products, particularly to youth.
- Improved access for all Americans, particularly poor and underserved Americans, to a range of healthcare services for the prevention, early detection, diagnosis, and treatment of cancer.
- Increased federal funding and incentives for private sponsorship of cancer research to prevent and cure cancer.
- The rights of cancer survivors.

American Cancer Society advocacy volunteers, as part of a community-based grassroots network, drive these successful initiatives. This network also includes other collaborators who have influenced or supported laws and regulations furthering the fight against cancer. In concert with its cancer research, prevention, and control initiatives, the Society's lobbying and advocacy initiatives strive to influence public policies with special emphasis on laws or regulations to:

- Finance cancer research initiatives.
- Ensure access to quality health care.
- Reform managed care and protect patients.

- Allow scientists to conduct potentially beneficial genetic and biore-search with appropriate review and controls in place.
- Prevent and reduce tobacco use.
- Increase access to and participation in clinical trials.
- Improve the management of cancer pain and symptoms.
- Reduce cancer incidence rates and deaths among the medically underserved.
- Provide early detection and treatment options for site-specific cancers.

American Heart Association – Web site: http://www.americanheart.org/

Except for the occasional heart attack, I never felt better.
Dick Cheney, 42nd Vice President of the United States
under George W. Bush (1941–)

*Coronary heart disease is a silent disease and
the first manifestation frequently is sudden death.*
Unknown author

Heart disease is leading cause of death in the United States. The American Heart Association (AHA) is a national voluntary health agency whose mission is to reduce disability and death from cardiovascular diseases and stroke. In 1924, six cardiologists representing several groups founded the American Heart Association in New York. The American Heart Association made its public debut in late 1948 during a network radio contest, "The Walking Man," on the *Truth or Consequences* program hosted by Ralph Edwards. Millions of Americans sent contributions to the AHA along with guesses on the walking man's identity. The effort netted $1.75 million before Jack Benny was identified as the "Walking Man." (American Heart Association, 2005). Since 1949, the American Heart Association has grown rapidly in size, financial resources, involvement with medical and non-medical volunteers, and influence—both nationally and internationally.

The AHA moved the National Center from New York City to Dallas in 1975 to better serve affiliates and local divisions nationwide. The volunteer-led affiliates and their divisions form a national network of local AHA organizations involved in providing research, education, and community programs and in raising money to support the association's work. The network continues to gain strength as it expands at the grass-roots level.

The AHA focuses its planning in three areas: cardiovascular science, cardiovascular education and community programs, and fund raising efforts. Despite strong opposition from the tobacco industry, the American Heart Association continues to be an advocate for the American public, especially children.

March of Dimes – Web site http://www.marchofdimes.com/

A baby will make love stronger, days shorter, nights longer,
bankroll smaller, home happier, clothes shabbier,
the past forgotten, and the future worth living for.
Anonymous

The mission of the March of Dimes (MOD) is to improve the health of babies by preventing birth defects, prematurity, and infant mortality. It carries out this mission through research, community services, education, and advocacy to save babies' lives. March of Dimes researchers, volunteers, educators, outreach workers, and advocates work together to give all babies a fighting chance against the threats to their health: prematurity, birth defects, and low birth weight.

When I worked on the polio vaccine, I had a theory. I guided
each [experiment] by imagining myself in the phenomenon
in which I was interested. The intuitive realm . . .
the realm of the imagination guides my thinking.
Jonas Salk, American Microbiologist (1914–1995)

The first great polio epidemic in the United States was in 1916. The disease infected mostly children, killing thousands and leaving many more paralyzed. On a summer day in 1921, Franklin D. Roosevelt became one of its victims and 17 years later the March of Dimes was born. The March of Dimes has the unique distinction of being one of a few organizations that achieved its original mission, to conquer polio. The polio vaccine, one of the great health achievements of the last century, may not have happened if not for the funds raised by the MOD to support research and care for polio patients.

Since its inception, the March of Dimes' investment in research has led to the world's highest honor in science, a Nobel Prize, being awarded to 11 scientists whose original work was supported by March of Dimes research grants. Through life-saving research they beat polio, but volunteers continue efforts to help children today by working to save babies from the silent crisis of premature birth.

Nearly half a million babies are born prematurely each year in the United States. Premature babies can suffer lifelong consequences such as mental retardation, blindness, chronic lung disease, and cerebral palsy. The March of Dimes Prematurity Campaign is a multimillion-dollar research, awareness, and education campaign to help families have healthier babies that is expected to continue through 2010. The March of Dimes goal is to reduce the rate of prematurity from 12.1% in 2002 to 7.6% in 2010, in accordance with the US Public Health Service *Healthy People 2010* objective. The campaign includes efforts to advocate, provide education, and research the cause and prevention of prematurity by

- Funding research to find the causes of premature birth.
- Educating women about the risk-reduction strategies, including the signs and symptoms of premature labor.
- Providing support to families affected by prematurity.
- Expanding access to healthcare coverage so that more women can get prenatal care.
- Helping healthcare providers learn ways to help reduce the risk of early delivery.
- Advocating for access to insurance to improve maternity care and infant health outcomes.

Additional Health Agencies

The following additional examples of voluntary health agencies and organizations (with Web addresses for additional information) help illustrate the breadth of health concerns addressed by organizations at the national and international level. This list is by no means exhaustive; there are many more respected organizations dealing with healthcare issues. This list is a sample representation. For more information on organizations that deal with specific health issues or populations, use one of the search engines identified in Chapter 5.

Agency/Organization	Web Address
Alzheimer's Association	http://www.alz.org
American Association of Retired Persons	http://www.aarp.org/
American Diabetes Association	http://diabetes.org
American Disability Association	http://www.adanet.org/
American Foundation for Suicide Prevention	http://www.afsp.org
American Lung Association	http://www.lungusa.org
American Stroke Association	http://www. strokeassociation.org
Arthritis Foundation	http://www.arthritis.org
Epilepsy Foundation of America	http://www.efa.org
Muscular Dystrophy Association	http://www.mdausa.org/
National Kidney Foundation	http://www.kidney.org/
National Osteoporosis Foundation	http://www.nof.org/
National Safe Kids Campaign	http://www.safekids.org
National Women's Health Foundation	http://www. nationalwomenshealth.org/
Oxfam International (International)	http://www.oxfam.org/
Project HOPE (Health Opportunities for People Everywhere)	http://www. projhope.org/(International)

SUMMARY

The government and voluntary health agencies mentioned in this chapter are offered as examples and resources for health education, research, and advocacy on behalf of patients in local, state, regional, or national areas. From helping communities cope with disasters, to providing information to individual patients about specific health conditions, these organizations generally help the public and health professionals improve the quality and quantity of life for all Americans.

REFERENCES

Centers for Disease Control and Prevention (CDC). (2005). CDC's health protection goals. Retrieved September 21, 2005, from http://www.cdc.gov/about/goals/.

American Red Cross. (2005). Federal charter of the American Red Cross. Retrieved September 21, 2005, from http://www.redcross.org/museum/charters.html.

American Heart Association. (2005). History of the American Heart Association. Retrieved September 12, 2005, from http://www.americanheart.org/presenter. jhtml?identifier=10860.

Chapter 7

Physician

Stephanie Chisolm

OBJECTIVES

After studying this chapter, the student should be able to

1. Explain the role of the physician in the healthcare system.
2. Describe the difference between allopathic and osteopathic medicine.
3. Describe the educational preparation and certification required for physicians.
4. Identify resources for additional information on the role of physicians.

INTRODUCTION

*The art of medicine consists in amusing the patient
while nature cures the disease.*
Voltaire (1694–1778)

The term "doctor" refers to a professional skilled or specializing in healing arts, also known as a physician, surgeon, or many other titles based on specialized training. While Voltaire may have been correct considering medical knowledge two hundred years ago, today's medical doctors are highly skilled practitioners, specializing in a wide array of healing arts after an exhaustive amount of academic and clinical training. Physicians serve a fundamental role in our society and have an effect upon all our lives. They diagnose illnesses and prescribe and administer treatment for people suffering from injury or disease. Physicians examine patients, obtain medical histories, and order, perform, and interpret diagnostic tests. They counsel patients on diet, hygiene, and preventive health care. Essentially, physicians function within primary, secondary, and tertiary levels of prevention mentioned at the beginning of this text. Because birth, death, illness, and injury do not subscribe to the time constraints of the typical workday, physicians may perform their duties any hour, day or night, 365 days of the year.

The Role of the Physician

When you first seek medical care, the process most widely used by physicians to tell whether and why you are sick is to ask questions about your health and past medical history. After "taking a history," an appropriate physical examination determines how well the body is functioning and whether there are signs of disease. Doctors also use a variety of tests such as lab tests, x-rays, other imaging techniques, and additional procedures to evaluate your health and identify any diseases or other health problems which may be present. Some of these diagnostic procedures (for example, cardiac catheterization, CT scan, biopsy of internal tissues) are complicated and require many years of training in order to use them safely and accurately.

After the diagnostic process is completed, the doctor recommends treatment if needed. Treatment may involve medication, surgery (there are many types of surgical specialists), or other procedures. A general physician may refer a patient to a specialist to address specific problems. Some specialists are primary care doctors, such as family physicians, general internists, and general pediatricians. Other specialists concentrate on certain body systems, specific age groups, or complex scientific techniques developed to diagnose or treat certain types of disorders. Specialties in medicine developed because of the rapidly expanding body of knowledge about health and illness and the constantly evolving new treatment techniques for disease.

A subspecialist is a physician who has completed training in a general medical specialty and then takes additional training in a more specific area of that specialty called a subspecialty. This training increases the depth of knowledge and expertise of the specialist in that particular field. For example, cardiology is a subspecialty of internal medicine and pediatrics, pediatric surgery is a subspecialty of surgery, and child and adolescent psychiatry is a subspecialty of psychiatry. The training of a subspecialist within a specialty requires an additional one or more years of full-time education (ABMSb, 2005).

Allopathic and Osteopathic Medicine

There are two overall types of physicians: MD—Doctor of Allopathic Medicine—and DO—Doctor of Osteopathic Medicine. MDs also are known as allopathic physicians. While both MDs and DOs may use all accepted methods of treatment, including drugs and surgery, DOs place special emphasis on the body's musculoskeletal system, preventive medicine, and holistic patient care. DOs are more likely than MDs to be primary care specialists although they can be found in all specialties. About half of DOs practice general or family medicine, general internal medicine, or general pediatrics. MDs may be general practitioners or may specialize in a wide variety of health issues after earning their medical degrees.

It takes many years of education and training to become a physician: four years of undergraduate school, four years of medical school, and three to eight years of internship and residency, depending on the specialty selected. A few medical schools offer a combined undergraduate and medical school program that lasts six, rather than the customary eight, years.

Physicians work in one or more of several specialties. These include, but are not limited to, anesthesiology, family and general medicine, general internal medicine, general pediatrics, obstetrics and gynecology, psychiatry, and surgery. Often, due to the volume of information we have about various systems in the human body, those areas have their own specialized physicians, such as endocrinologists, neurologists, cardiologists, or pulmonologists to name just a few. Several of these specialties are described in the following paragraphs.

Anesthesiologists. Anesthesiologists focus on the care of patients in surgery and on pain relief. Like other physicians, they evaluate and treat patients and direct the efforts of those on their staffs. Anesthesiologists confer with other physicians and surgeons about appropriate treatments and procedures before, during, and after operations. These critical specialists are responsible for maintenance of the patient's vital life functions—heart rate, body temperature, blood pressure, breathing—through continual monitoring and assessment during surgery. The American Society of Anesthesiologists, founded in 1905, is an educational, research, and scientific association of physicians, organized to raise and maintain the standards of the medical practice of anesthesiology and improve the care of the patient (for additional information, see http://www.asahq.org/).

Family and general practitioners. Family and general practitioners are often the first point of contact for people seeking health care, acting as the traditional family doctor. They assess and treat a wide range of conditions, ailments, and injuries, from sinus and respiratory infections to broken bones and scrapes. Family and general practitioners typically have a patient base of regular, long-term visitors. Family and general practitioners typically refer patients with more serious conditions to specialists or other health care facilities for more intensive care. The American College of Osteopathic Family Physicians (http://www.acofp.org) and the American Academy of Family

Physicians (http://www.aafp.org/) are resources for additional information about this medical specialty.

General internists. General internists diagnose and provide nonsurgical treatment for diseases and injuries of internal organ systems. They provide care mainly for adults who have a wide range of problems associated with the internal organs, such as the stomach, kidneys, liver, and digestive tract. Internists use a variety of diagnostic techniques to treat patients through medication or hospitalization. Like general practitioners, general internists are primary care specialists. They have patients referred to them by other specialists, in turn referring patients to yet other specialists when more complex care is required. The American Board of Internal Medicine (ABIM) is the US board that sets the standards and certifies the knowledge, skills, and aptitude of physicians who practice in Internal Medicine, its subspecialties and areas of added qualifications (http://www.abim.org/).

General pediatricians. Providing care from birth to early adulthood, pediatricians are concerned with the health of infants, children, and teenagers. They specialize in the diagnosis and treatment of a variety of ailments specific to young people and track their patients' growth to adulthood. Like most physicians, pediatricians work with different healthcare workers, such as nurses and other physicians, to assess and treat children with various ailments, such as asthma, chicken pox, and ear infections. Most of the work of pediatricians, however, involves treating day-to-day illnesses that are common to children—minor injuries, infectious diseases, and immunizations—much as a general practitioner treats adults. Some pediatricians specialize in serious medical conditions and pediatric surgery, and treat autoimmune disorders or serious chronic ailments. The American Academy of Pediatrics (AAP) is an organization of 60,000 pediatricians committed to the attainment of optimal physical, mental, and social health and well-being for all infants, children, adolescents, and young adults (http://www.aap.org).

Obstetricians and gynecologists. Obstetricians and gynecologists (ob/gyns) are specialists whose focus is women's health. They are responsible for care related to pregnancy and the reproductive system and may also provide general medical care for women. Like general practitioners, ob/gyns are concerned with the prevention, diagnosis, and treatment of general health problems, but they focus on ailments specific to the female anatomy, such as breast and cervical cancer, urinary tract and pelvic disorders, and hormonal disorders. Ob/gyns also specialize in childbirth, treating and counseling women throughout their pregnancy, from prenatal diagnosis to delivery and postpartum care. Ob/gyns track the health of, and treat, both mother and fetus as the pregnancy progresses. The American

College of Obstetricians and Gynecologists (ACOG), founded in 1951, is the nation's leading group of professionals providing health care for women (http://www.acog.org).

Psychiatrists. Psychiatrists are the primary physician caregivers in the area of mental health. They assess and treat mental illnesses through a combination of psychotherapy, psychoanalysis, hospitalization, and medication. Psychotherapy involves regular discussions with patients about their problems; the psychiatrist helps them find solutions through changes in their behavioral patterns, the exploration of their experiences, and group and family therapy sessions. Psychoanalysis involves long-term psychotherapy and counseling for patients. In many cases, psychiatrists can administer medications to correct chemical imbalances that may be causing emotional problems. Psychiatrists may also administer electroconvulsive therapy to those of their patients who do not respond to, or who cannot take, medications. The American Psychiatric Association is a medical specialty society where member physicians work together to ensure humane care and effective treatment for all persons with mental disorders, including mental retardation and substance-related disorders (http://www.psych.org).

Surgeons. Surgeons are physicians who specialize in the treatment of injury, disease, and deformity through operations. Using a variety of instruments, and with patients under general or local anesthesia, a surgeon corrects physical deformities, repairs bone and tissue after injuries, or performs preventive surgeries on patients with debilitating diseases or disorders. Although a large number perform general surgery, many surgeons choose to specialize in a specific area. One of the most prevalent specialties is orthopedic surgery: the treatment of the skeletal system and associated organs. Others include neurological surgery (treatment of the brain and nervous system), ophthalmology (treatment of the eye), otolaryngology (treatment of the ear, nose, and throat), and plastic and reconstructive surgery. Like primary care and other specialist physicians, surgeons also examine patients, perform and interpret diagnostic tests, and counsel patients on preventive health care. The American College of Surgeons is a scientific and educational association of surgeons, founded in 1913 to improve the quality of care for the surgical patient by setting high standards for surgical education and practice (http://www.facs.org).

A number of other medical specialists work in clinics, hospitals, and private offices. The following descriptions provide only a glimpse of the diverse specialty areas in the allopathic and osteopathic medical professions. For each, additional training in the form of residency is required before seeking board certification in the specialty area.

Table 7.1 *2006 AMGA Physician Compensation Survey*

Specialty	All Physicians	Starting	Eastern	Western	Southern	Northern
Allergy and Immunology	$227,080	$180,520	$230,500	$236,846	$182,074	$208,000
Anesthesiology	$337,654	$279,922	$297,088	$339,359	$311,600	$342,610
Cardiac & Thoracic Surgery	$470,000	$347,573	$449,800	$478,997	$355,569	$539,999
Cardiology	$363,081	$268,286	$277,503	$368,633	$397,500	$374,494
Colon & Rectal Surgery	$366,687	$288,933	$325,000	$344,940	****	$368,991
Critical Care Medicine	$234,503	$209,850	$271,587	$339,875	****	$243,935
Dermatology	$306,935	$238,103	$253,125	$315,516	$330,727	$280,979
Diagnostic Radiology - Interventional	$424,992	$388,318	$366,400	$419,083	$505,321	$424,992
Diagnostic Radiology - Non-Interventional	$400,000	$340,000	$349,575	$404,877	$384,960	$415,753
Emergency Care	$248,721	$213,326	$205,313	$258,567	$215,066	$248,412
Endocrinology	$194,243	$159,705	$172,748	$207,519	$181,800	$206,253
Family Medicine	$178,366	$143,359	$151,043	$189,204	$180,014	$173,190
Family Medicine - with Obstetrics	$186,451	$149,449	$156,164	$173,950	$159,013	$197,135
Gastroenterology	$344,200	$283,842	$289,414	$356,771	$333,564	$329,495
General Surgery	$310,736	$241,005	$269,635	$308,095	$303,073	$341,400
Geriatrics	$162,541	$135,322	$159,000	$186,759	$150,000	$163,979
Gynecological Oncology	$356,756	$284,540	$337,747	$378,893	****	$365,000
Gynecology	$224,134	$178,391	$227,294	$221,000	$214,323	$224,632
Gynecology & Obstetrics	$271,273	$220,635	$240,968	$274,102	$266,467	$282,679
Hematology & Medical Oncology	$263,284	$215,163	$235,419	$286,699	$256,132	$261,501
Hospitalist	$189,677	$163,917	$166,997	$198,718	$202,355	$180,066
Hypertension & Nephrology	$229,992	$195,640	$187,616	$256,648	$238,923	$219,992
Infectious Disease	$194,750	$160,713	$166,803	$214,665	$171,679	$196,950
Intensivist	$245,293	$224,733	****	$245,254	****	****
Internal Medicine	$183,840	$149,567	$172,070	$193,406	$181,870	$174,572
Neonatology	$246,872	****	****	****	****	****

Table 7.1 *2006 AMGA Physician Compensation Survey (continued)*

Specialty	All Physicians	Starting	Eastern	Western	Southern	Northern
Neurological Surgery	$476,260	$360,110	$423,950	$562,521	$475,274	$476,480
Neurology	$211,995	$172,264	$189,549	$232,782	$195,685	$211,995
Nuclear Medicine (M.D. only)	$300,000	$225,975	****	$304,128	****	$300,000
Obstetrics	$251,787	$196,797	$238,940	$260,615	$269,028	$254,402
Occupational/ Environmental Medicine	$202,063	$173,197	****	$203,495	****	$201,622
Ophthalmology	$281,112	$220,001	$234,500	$279,981	$261,188	$312,741
Oral Surgery	$317,634	$229,370	****	****	$308,300	$343,497
Orthopedic Surgery	$409,518	$331,156	$365,266	$418,641	$364,757	$412,003
Orthopedic -Medical	$262,170	$145,860	****	****	$239,733	$261,085
Orthopedic Surgery - Joint Replacement	$476,446	$407,037	****	$524,306	****	$458,740
Orthopedic Surgery - Hand	$387,626	$316,500	$375,000	$350,002	****	$403,376
Orthopedic Surg.- Pediatrics	$355,758	$302,246	****	****	****	****
Orthopedic Surgery - Spine	$554,054	$395,524	****	$557,630	****	$582,215
Otolaryngology	$315,000	$248,948	$271,699	$318,330	$314,643	$324,835
Pathology (M.D. only	$274,792	$212,351	$236,192	$288,120	$249,634	$284,315
Pediatric Allergy	$163,338	$143,543	****	****	****	****
Pediatric Cardiology	$231,754	$184,941	$194,915	$277,853	$222,132	$238,992
Pediatric Endocrinology	$180,153	$155,341	****	$200,831	****	$170,758
Pediatric Gastroenterology	$216,000	$168,238	$197,341	$236,859	$170,503	$238,992
Pediatric Hematology/ Oncology	$200,260	$165,955	****	$244,909	$192,786	$190,199
Pediatric Intensive Care	$201,901	$158,240	$197,991	****	$168,600	$202,500

continues

Table 7.1 *2006 AMGA Physician Compensation Survey (continued)*

Specialty	All Physicians	Starting	Eastern	Western	Southern	Northern
Pediatric Nephrology	$178,181	$149,706	****	****	****	****
Pediatric Neurology	$197,282	$174,804	****	$211,281	****	$198,782
Pediatric Pulmonary Disease	$175,440	$146,439	****	****	****	****
Pediatric Surgery	$322,969	$249,061	****	****	$248,577	****
Pediatrics & Adolescent	$182,186	$148,529	$174,541	$188,766	$181,612	$170,974
Pediatric Infectious Disease	$179,919	$135,419	****	$228,326	****	$169,227
Perinatology	$341,933	$298,347	****	$348,280	****	$338,995
Physical Medicine & Rehabilitation	$207,004	$167,593	$188,889	$213,624	$200,877	$207,004
Plastic & Reconstruction	$345,000	$274,476	$279,505	$361,982	$344,215	$384,255
Psychiatry	$186,786	$153,415	$161,717	$212,760	$157,873	$181,510
Psychiatry - Child	$214,873	$168,927	****	$237,330	****	$168,927
Pulmonary Disease	$238,450	$194,500	$208,102	$246,650	$282,162	$249,417
Radiation Therapy (M.D. only)	$356,097	$274,706	$285,586	$398,644	$319,289	$377,510
Reproductive Endocrinology	$316,241	$267,210	****	$332,114	****	****
Rheumatologic Disease	$204,166	$159,066	$183,515	$216,975	$181,367	$198,469
Sports Medicine	$245,920	$162,786	****	****	****	$244,161
Surgical Pathology (M.D. only)	****	****	****	****	****	****
Surgical Sports Medicine	$417,106	****	****	****	****	****
Transplant Surgery - Kidney	$351,031	$240,620	****	****	****	$389,496
Transplant Surgery - Liver	$379,409	$321,000	****	****	****	$389,496
Trauma Surgery	$353,706	$268,044	$285,179	****	****	$373,340
Urgent Care	$194,687	$155,438	$192,210	$208,335	$204,172	$177,227
Urology	$349,811	$267,628	$283,880	$343,506	$344,480	$367,008
Vascular Surgery	$354,365	$282,325	$309,872	$385,935	$380,000	$350,000

Source: the American Medical Group Association, 2006, http://www.cejkasearch.com/compensation/amga_physician_compensation_survey.htm, retrieved 11/9/06

Premedical and Medical Education

Premedical students must complete undergraduate work in physics, biology, mathematics, English, and inorganic and organic chemistry. Students also take courses in the humanities and the social sciences. Some students volunteer at local hospitals or clinics to gain practical experience in the health professions. While most medical school applicants are science majors, a particular major is not necessary. Medical schools are less concerned with students' majors than the quality and scope of their work. They must perform well in the required science courses. As long as undergraduates take the *required* perquisite science courses and perform well, students can choose any major in which they are interested.

Thanks to the American Medical College Application Service (AMCAS®) and American Association of Colleges of Osteopathic Medicine Application Service (AACOMAS), applying to medical school is not as complicated as it used to be. Most of the accredited medical schools in the United States participate in these application programs. Students fill out an application and send it with one set of official transcripts to the service of their choice (allopathic or osteopathic). After the service verifies the information provided, it distributes the applications to the school(s) selected. For the few schools not participating in AMCAS or AACOMAS, contact the admissions office directly for application procedures and materials. To start or explore the application process, students can go to http://www.aamc.org/ or https://aacomas.aacom.org/.

The predominant assessment test used to judge qualification for admission to medical school is the Medical College Admission Test (MCAT), a standardized, multiple-choice examination designed to assess problem solving, critical thinking, and writing skills in addition to the examinee's knowledge of science concepts and principles prerequisite to the study of medicine. Scores are reported in each of the following areas: Verbal Reasoning, Physical Sciences, Writing Sample, and Biological Sciences. Medical college admission committees consider MCAT scores as part of their admission decision process.

Almost all US medical schools require applicants to submit MCAT scores during the application process. Many schools may not accept MCAT scores if taken more than three years ago. MCAT registration packets are available online at www.aamc.org.

The minimum educational requirement for entry into a medical school is three years of college; most applicants, however, have at least a bachelor's degree, and many have advanced degrees. There are 146 medical schools in the United States—126 teach allopathic medicine and award a Doctor of

Medicine (MD) degree; 20 teach osteopathic medicine and award the Doctor of Osteopathic Medicine (DO) degree. Acceptance to allopathic and osteopathic medical school is highly competitive. Applicants must submit transcripts, scores from the Medical College Admission Test (MCAT), and letters of recommendation. After submitting an application, many schools ask for additional information such as a secondary application, letters of recommendation, and a statement as to specific interest in their programs. Schools also consider applicants' character, personality, leadership qualities, and participation in extracurricular activities. Most schools require an interview with members of the admissions committee.

Generally, students spend most of the first two years of medical school in laboratories and classrooms, taking courses such as anatomy, biochemistry, physiology, pharmacology, psychology, microbiology, pathology, medical ethics, and laws governing medicine. They also learn to take medical histories, examine patients, and diagnose illnesses. During their last two years, students work with patients under the supervision of experienced physicians in hospitals and clinics, learning acute, chronic, preventive, and rehabilitative care. Through rotations in internal medicine, family practice, obstetrics and gynecology, pediatrics, psychiatry, and surgery, they gain experience in the diagnosis and treatment of illness. Following medical school, almost all MDs and DOs enter a residency—graduate medical education in a specialty that takes the form of paid on-the-job training, usually in a hospital.

A physician's training is costly. More than 80% of medical students borrow money to cover their expenses. People who wish to become physicians must have a desire to serve patients, be self-motivated, and be able to survive the pressures and long hours of medical education and practice. Physicians also must have a good bedside manner, emotional stability, and the ability to make decisions in emergencies. Appreciating concepts of cultural competency and diversity are invaluable to those seeking medical careers today, especially for physicians wishing to practice in states with large minority populations. Due to the ever-expanding medical knowledge base, prospective physicians must be willing to study throughout their career in order to keep up with medical advances.

Medical Residency

A medical residency program, also known as graduate medical education, is usually arranged through a national matching program. It provides newly graduated MDs three to seven years or more of professional training under the supervision of senior physician educators. The National Resident Matching Program (NRMP) is a private, not-for-profit corporation established in 1952 to provide a uniform date of appointment to positions in graduate medical education (GME). The NRMP is not an application-processing service; rather, it provides an impartial venue for matching applicants' and programs' preferences for each other consistently. Each year, approximately 16,000 US medical school students participate in the residency match. In addition, another 17,000 "independent" applicants compete for the approximately 24,000 available residency positions. Independent applicants include former graduates of US medical schools, US osteopathic students, Canadian students, and graduates of foreign medical schools (NRMP, 2005). The length of residency training varies depending on the *specialty* chosen: family practice, internal medicine, and pediatrics, for example, require three years of training; general surgery requires five years. One to three years of additional training in a subspecialty is an option for some doctors who want to become highly specialized in a particular field, such as gastroenterology, a subspecialty of internal medicine and of pediatrics, or child and adolescent psychiatry, a subspecialty of psychiatry ("Your Doctor's Education," 2000).

Licensing and Certification

All states, the District of Columbia, and US territories license physicians. Physicians must graduate from an accredited medical school, pass a three-step licensing examination, and complete one to seven years of graduate medical education. Step 1 of the United States Medical Licensing Examination assesses whether medical school students or graduates understand and can apply important concepts of the sciences basic to the practice of medicine. Step 2 assesses whether medical school students or graduates can apply medical knowledge, skills, and understanding of clinical science essential for provision of patient care under supervision. Step 3 of the medical licensing examination assesses whether medical school graduates can apply medical knowledge and an understanding of biomedical and clinical science essential for the unsupervised practice of medicine. Although physicians licensed in one state usually can get a license to practice in another without further examination, some states limit reciprocity. Graduates of foreign medical schools generally can qualify for licensure after passing an examination and completing a US residency (www.USMLE.org).

MDs and DOs seeking board certification in a specialty may spend up to seven years in residency training, depending on the specialty. A final examination immediately after residency or after one or two years of practice also is necessary for certification by the American Board of Medical Specialists or the American Osteopathic Association. The majority of physicians also choose to become board certified, which is an optional, voluntary process. Certification ensures that the doctor has been tested to assess his or her knowledge, skills, and experience in a specialty and is deemed qualified to provide quality patient care in that specialty. There are two levels of certification through 24 specialty medical boards—doctors can be certified in 36 general medical specialties and in an additional 88 subspecialty fields. Most certifications must be renewed after six to ten years, depending on the specialty ("Your Doctor's Education," 2000).

Where Do Physicians Practice?

Many physicians—primarily general and family practitioners, general internists, pediatricians, ob/gyns, and psychiatrists—work in small private offices or clinics, often assisted by a small staff of nurses and other administrative personnel. Increasingly, physicians are practicing in groups or healthcare organizations that provide backup coverage and allow for more time off. These physicians often work as part of a team coordinating care for a population of patients; they are less independent than solo practitioners. A growing number of physicians are partners or salaried employees of group practices. Organized as clinics or as associations of physicians, medical groups can afford expensive medical equipment and realize other business advantages.

Surgeons and anesthesiologists typically work in well-lighted, sterile environments while performing surgery and often stand for long periods. Most work in hospitals or in surgical outpatient centers. Many physicians and surgeons work long, irregular hours. Almost one third of physicians worked 60 hours or more a week in 2002. Physicians and surgeons must travel frequently between office and hospital to care for their patients. Those who are on call deal with many patients' concerns over the phone and may make emergency visits to hospitals or nursing homes.

Employment Opportunities and Outlook

Few fields offer a wider variety of opportunities. Most doctors spend their professional lives caring for people and continuously learning more about the human body. Every day, in communities around the country, doctors work in neighborhood clinics, hospitals, offices, even homeless shelters and schools, to care for people in need. However, physicians also do many other things.

Physician researchers trained as medical scientists are at work today developing exciting new treatments for cancer, genetic disorders, and infectious diseases like AIDS. Academic physicians share their skills and wisdom by teaching medical students and residents. Others work with health maintenance organizations, pharmaceutical companies, medical device manufacturers, health insurance companies, or in corporations directing health and safety programs.

Physicians and surgeons held about 583,000 jobs in 2002; approximately one out of six was self-employed. About half of salaried physicians and surgeons were in office-based practice, and almost a quarter employed by hospitals. Others practiced in federal, state, and local government; educational services; and outpatient care centers.

The New England and Middle Atlantic States have the highest ratio of physicians to population; the South Central States have the lowest. DOs are more likely than MDs to practice in small cities and towns and in rural areas. MDs tend to locate in urban areas, close to hospitals and education centers.

Employment of physicians and surgeons will grow about as fast as the average for all occupations through the year 2012 due to continued expansion of the health services industries. The growing and aging population will drive overall growth in the demand for physician services, as consumers continue to demand high levels of care using the latest technologies, diagnostic tests, and therapies.

Demand for physicians' services is highly sensitive to changes in consumer preferences, healthcare reimbursement policies, and legislation. For example, if changes to health coverage result in consumers facing higher out-of-pocket costs, they may demand fewer physician services. Demand for physician services may be tempered by patients relying more on other healthcare providers—such as physician assistants, nurse practitioners, optometrists, and nurse anesthetists—for some healthcare services. In addition, new technologies will increase physician productivity. Telemedicine will allow physicians to treat patients or consult with other providers remotely. Increasing use of electronic medical records, test and prescription orders, billing, and scheduling will also improve physician productivity.

Opportunities for individuals interested in becoming physicians and surgeons should remain favorable. Reports of shortages in some specialties or geographic areas may attract new entrants, encouraging schools to expand programs and hospitals to expand available residency slots. However, because physician training is so lengthy, employment change happens gradually. In the short term, to meet increased demand, experienced physicians may work longer hours, delay retirement, or take measures to increase productivity, such as using more support staff to provide services. Opportunities should be particularly good in rural and low-income areas, because some physicians find these areas unattractive due to lower earnings potential, isolation from medical colleagues, or other reasons.

Unlike their predecessors, newly trained physicians face radically different choices of where and how to practice. New physicians are much less likely to enter solo practice and more likely to take salaried jobs in group medical practices, clinics, and health networks.

Physician Earnings

Physicians generally have among the highest earnings of any occupation. According to the Medical Group Management Association's Physician Compensation and Production Survey, median total compensation for physicians in 2006 varies by specialty, as shown in Table 7.1.

Self-employed physicians—those who own or are part owners of their medical practice—generally have higher median incomes than salaried physicians. Earnings vary according to number of years in practice, geographic region, hours worked, skill, personality, and professional reputation. Self-employed physicians and surgeons must provide for their own health insurance and retirement.

Medical Specialty Boards

The American Board of Medical Specialties (ABMS) is the umbrella organization for the 24 approved medical specialty boards in the United States. Established in 1933, the ABMS serves to coordinate the activities of its Member Boards and to provide information to the public, the government, the profession, and its members concerning issues involving specialization and certification in medicine. The mission of the ABMS is to maintain and improve the quality of medical care in the United States by assisting the Member Boards in their efforts to develop and utilize professional and educational standards for the evaluation and certification of physician specialists (ABMSa, 2005).

SUMMARY

Whether pursuing a career in allopathic or osteopathic medicine, it takes many years of education and training to become a physician. Some doctors choose to specialize in one particular organ or disease, such as nephrologists or oncologists. Others, such as pediatricians or gerontologists, focus their learning on caring for particular populations. Regardless of the area of practice, the learning process does not end with graduation from medical school, or even completion of a residency training program. The field of medicine is ever evolving as new research finds cures or easier ways to diagnose and treat the full spectrum of health conditions. MDs and DOs—in fact all healthcare practitioners—must keep up with new knowledge and skills to best help their patients fulfill the *Healthy People 2010* objectives of increased quantity and quality of life.

ADDITIONAL RESOURCES

For a list of medical schools and residency programs, as well as general information on premedical education, financial aid, and medicine as a career, contact

> Association of American Medical Colleges, Section for Student Services, 2450 N St. NW., Washington, DC 20037-1126. Internet: http://www.aamc.org

> American Association of Colleges of Osteopathic Medicine, 5550 Friendship Blvd., Suite 310, Chevy Chase, MD 20815-7231. Internet: http://www.aacom.org

For general information on physicians, contact

> American Medical Association, Department of Communications and Public Relations, 515 N: State St., Chicago, IL 60610. Internet: http://www.ama-assn.org

> American Osteopathic Association, Division of Public Relations, 142 East Ontario St., Chicago, IL 60611. Internet: http://www.aoa-net.org

For information about various medical specialties, contact

> American Society of Anesthesiologists, 520 N. Northwest Hwy., Park Ridge, IL 60068-2573. Internet: http://www.asahq.org

> American Board of Anesthesiology, 4101 Lake Boone Trail, Suite 510, Raleigh, NC 27607-7506. Internet: http://www.abanes.org

> Society of General Internal Medicine, 2501 M St. NW., Suite 575, Washington, DC 20037. Internet: http://www.sgim.org

> American Academy of Pediatrics, 141 Northwest Point Blvd., Elk Grove Village, IL 60007-1098. Internet: http://www.aap.org

> American Board of Obstetrics and Gynecology, 2915 Vine St., Dallas, TX 75204. Internet: http://www.abog.org

American College of Obstetrics and Gynecologists, 409 12th St. SW, P.O. Box 96920, Washington, DC 20090-6920. Internet: http://www.acog.org

American Psychiatric Association, 1000 Wilson Blvd., Suite 1825, Arlington, VA 22209-3901. Internet: http://www.psych.org

American College of Surgeons, 633 North Saint Clair St., Chicago, IL 60611-3211. Internet: http://www.facs.org

American Board of Medical Specialties, 1007 Church Street, Suite 404, Evanston, IL 60201-5913. Internet: http://www.abms.org

REFERENCES

American Board of Medical Specialties (ABMS). (2005a). About ABMS, Retrieved August 10, 2005, from http://www.abms.org/about.asp.

American Board of Medical Specialists (ABMS). (2005b). Which medical specialist for you? Retrieved August 10, 2005, from http://www.abms.org/which.asp.

National Residency Match Program (NRMP). (2005). About the NRMP. Retrieved September 27, 2005, from http://www.nrmp.org/about_nrmp/index.html.

United States Medical Licensing Examination (USMLE). (2005). USMLE home page. Retrieved September 27, 2005, from http://www.usmle.org/.

Your Doctor's Education. (2000). *Journal of the American Medical Association.* JAMA Patient Page, *284*(9).

Chapter 8

Physician Assistant

James B. Hammond

OBJECTIVES

After studying this chapter, the student should be able to

1. Explain the role of the physician assistant in the healthcare system.
2. Explain the historical development process of physician assistants.
3. Describe the educational preparation and certification required for physician assistants.
4. Identify resources for additional information on the role of physician assistants.

INTRODUCTION

If they look like a doctor, act like a doctor, and have a white coat and a stethoscope, they must be a physician, right? Not necessarily. If you were ill or injured and saw a healthcare professional trained to conduct physical exams, diagnose and treat illnesses, counsel on preventive care, assist in surgery, and even write prescriptions in virtually all states, you may well have been seen by a Physician Assistant, or PA as they are commonly called. PAs may be the principal care providers in rural or inner city clinics, where a physician is present for only 1 or 2 days each week. Practicing medicine under the supervision of physicians and surgeons, a PA should not be confused with medical assistants, who perform routine clinical and clerical tasks.

What Is a Physician Assistant?

The PA is a healthcare professional licensed to practice medicine with physician supervision. As part of their comprehensive training, PAs are educated in the medical model designed to complement physician training; in some schools, they attend many of the same classes as medical students. One of the main differences between PA education and physician education is not the core content of the curriculum, but the amount of time spent in formal education. The average medical school education is 155 weeks; the average PA education is 111 weeks. In addition to time in school, physicians are required to do an internship, and the majority complete a residency in a specialty following that. PAs do not have to undertake an internship or residency. A physician has complete responsibility for the care of the patient. PAs share that responsibility with the supervising physicians.

Physician assistants (PAs) are healthcare professionals licensed to practice medicine with physician supervision, in all areas of medicine. According to the American Academy of Physician Assistants, they practice in the areas of primary care medicine—family medicine, internal medicine, pediatrics, and obstetrics and gynecology—as well as in surgery and the surgical subspecialties, and even emergency medicine (AAPA, 2005b). Within the physician-PA relationship, physician assistants exercise autonomy in medical decision-making and provide a broad range of diagnostic and therapeutic services. A PA's practice may also include education, research, and administrative services.

The Development of the Physician Assistant

Multiple social forces contributed to the establishment of the physician assistant profession in the 1960s. Healthcare services expanded rapidly as coverage from Medicare and Medicaid and employer paid health insurance increased access to health care. Advances in medications, as well as new diagnostic and treatment technologies, made it possible to help people with many additional medical problems. Physicians and educators recognized there was a shortage and uneven distribution of primary care physicians. In several areas of the country, physicians looking for a way to extend the services they offered, despite a shortage of physicians, created a new profession to handle many of the common medical conditions they treated. With less training than required for physicians, this new professional would assist physicians in caring for patients within the physician's practice. Dr. Eugene Stead, of the Duke University Medical Center in North Carolina, put together the first class of PAs in 1965. He selected Navy corpsmen who received considerable medical training during their military service and during the war in Vietnam but who had no comparable civilian employment. He based the curriculum of the PA program in part on his knowledge of the fast-track training of doctors during World War II.

The physician assistant is a professional with substantial responsibility who focuses on working with patients to determine what health problems they have and how to treat them. PAs work with closely with physicians, performing the same types of clinical and diagnostic tasks traditionally done only by physicians. They interview patients about their health problems, perform physical examinations, order diagnostic laboratory tests, interpret the test results, decide on appropriate treatments, and prescribe treatments, including medications. They also educate patients about their illnesses, treatments employed, and ways to prevent or reduce illness. This allows the clinical practice to care for a greater number of patients and for the physician to devote more time to more complicated clinical conditions while the PA handles the more common conditions. PA education and training is broad-based, focusing on primary care medicine for all age groups. As they work with physicians throughout their careers, PAs' knowledge and skills grow and their responsibilities expand. Many healthcare analysts believe physician assistants, who typically deliver quality routine health care less expensively than doctors, are an important part of the American health care system, as they are in Canada and some European countries.

While the early mission of PAs focused on primary care medicine, physician specialists also found PAs to be beneficial to their practices, thus their role has expanded. According to the American Academy of Physicians, today 44% work in primary care specialties—family practice (30%), general internal medicine (8%), obstetrics/gynecology (3%), and general pediatrics (3%). The remainder work within the many specialties and subspecialties of medical and surgical care. Initially, as in physician practice, there were more men than women in the PA profession. Over the years, the ratio has changed. Today about 60% of PAs are women.

Since the mid 1990s the profession has been growing rapidly. The number of PA educational programs has grown from 55 to over 130. Currently there are about 60,000 PAs working throughout the United States. PAs are licensed to practice in all 50 states. Forty-eight states allow PAs to prescribe medications (AAPA, 2005c).

The Physician Assistant as a Healthcare Professional

PAs work in virtually all the specialties of medicine. As the following table illustrates, about half of PAs work in primary care (family medicine, general internal medicine, and general pediatrics) and the other half are divided among the other specialties and subspecialties of medicine. Table 8.1 shows the distribution of PAs across medical specialties, with a description of principle duties in each specialty.

PAs work in many settings—private offices, hospitals, clinics, nursing homes, the military, state and federal prisons, public health departments, etc. They also work in all geographic settings—inner city, urban, suburban, small towns, rural, and remote areas. Many work in the same locations as the physician(s) supervisors they work with; others work in locations separate from the

Table 8.1   *Specialties Employing Physician Assistants*

Specialty	Percentage of PAs Working in Specialties*	Common Responsibilities
Family Medicine	39.1	Diagnose and treat common illnesses, educate patients of all ages on health promotion and disease prevention.
Medicine	18.2	Diagnose and treat common illnesses, educate adult patients on health promotion and disease prevention.
Surgery	15.56	Preoperative evaluation, first assist on operations, monitor and treat postoperative problems, educate patients on recovery.
Emergency Medicine	10.4	Diagnose and treat common illnesses in the Emergency Room, assist physicians with more complicated emergency problems.
Medical Subspecialties	4.0	Diagnose and treat common illnesses within the specialty, educate adult patients on health promotion and disease prevention, perform some specialized testing.
Pediatrics	3.8	Diagnose and treat common illnesses, educate patients and parents on health promotion and disease prevention for children.
Obstetrics/Gynecology	3.2	Prenatal and postnatal health care. Diagnose and treat common illnesses afflicting women, provide pregnancy care, educate women on health promotion and disease prevention.
Occupational Medicine	3.0	Work with corporations to provide safe working environments, prevent and treat injuries and illness of the workplace.
Surgical Subspecialties	2.7	Preoperative evaluation, first assist on operations, monitor and treat postoperative problems within the specialty, educate patients on recovery.

*Percentages are from the 2003-2004 NCCPA survey of certified PAs.
Source: NCCPA, 2005

physician(s), communicating with them by phone or electronically by e-mail, fax, or telecommunication (two-way, live video, and audio connections). PAs serve people with physical illnesses, mental illnesses, those who are well-educated and those who are less educated, the well-off and the poor, the strong and the vulnerable, the fortunate and the underserved. Table 8.2 illustrates the variety of settings in which PAs work.

Depending on the specialty and setting in which they work, PAs and the physician(s) they work with determine the PA's specific role and tasks within the practice. PAs who work in primary care outpatient settings typically see patients as much as the physician does. People coming in with common acute, undiagnosed conditions as well as those returning for follow-up of chronic conditions will sometimes see the PA rather than the physician.

In surgical practices, PAs typically assist with preoperative testing or evaluation. They assist the surgeon during the operation and they monitor the patients postoperatively. This allows the physician to care for additional people and to devote more time to more complex or critical patients. PAs working in non-primary care medical specialties often spend a good deal of time conducting diagnostic tests (such as stress tests in cardiology) to gather the data the physician needs to make a diagnosis. They also monitor patients, ordering laboratory tests and adjusting medications to assure that treatments are having the desired result.

Table 8.2   *PA Employment Settings*

Hospitals		**34%**
Emergency rooms	10%	
Inpatient units	9%	
Outpatient units	8%	
Operating rooms	7%	
Physician Group Practices		**29%**
Single-specialty group	20%	
Multi-specialty group	9%	
Solo practice physician offices		**13%**
Federally Qualified Health Centers or Community Health Centers		**8%**

Note: Percentages are from the 2003-2004 NCCPA survey of certified PAs.
Source: NCCPA, 2005

Pre-physician Assistant Preparation

PAs are needed from a wide variety of cultural and ethnic backgrounds to serve a widely diverse population. Nationally, over 130 colleges and universities offer physician assistant educational programs. Because PAs perform the traditional physician tasks of diagnosing and treating patients, physicians are heavily involved in training physician assistants in educational programs patterned after medical school education. The majority of programs are master's level programs. Others are quickly transitioning to the master's level. The focus of PA education is primary care medicine. This broad education provides a base from which graduates practice in primary care and other medical specialties. Candidates applying to PA programs generally come from two groups—those seeking to become a PA as a first career and those seeking to change careers. Those seeking second careers as a PA come from professions including, but not limited to

EMT or Paramedic	Athletic Trainer
Cardiology Technician	Medical Technologist
Registered Nurse	Licensed Practical Nurse
Surgical Technologist / Technician	Exercise Physiologist
Rehabilitation Technician	Mental Health Counselor

Most undergraduate students obtain a Bachelor of Science or Bachelor of Arts degree while completing the prerequisites for admission to PA programs. Programs do not generally require a specific undergraduate major, but they do require specific prerequisite courses. These courses vary from one PA certification program to another. It is important that early in their undergraduate years candidates research the requirements of the PA program/(s) that interest them. Early planning is critical to success and students planning professional health careers should discuss these goals with their academic advisers. It is important to begin this planning process early in an academic program.

Admissions information presented here is only a general guide when planning a pre-physician assistant curriculum. It is important to check with individual PA programs to learn their unique admission requirements, program mission, or policies that might affect a candidate's choice of schools. The course requirements for PA programs typically include study in anatomy, physiology, microbiology, chemistry, and sometimes genetics, statistics, and medical terminology. The Graduate Record Examination (GRE) is the most commonly required standardized test. Schools recognize the desirability of students having a breadth of interests and a diversity of backgrounds. Applicants are urged to obtain a broad cultural background in such fields as literature, social science, psychology, and the fine arts.

Many programs require or prefer healthcare experience prior to entry. Each program defines the type and amount of experience it requires. The average amount is about 1000 hours of direct-contact, patient-care experience. It may take some time to acquire the experience, so advanced planning is important.

PA programs, like many other graduate or certification programs, generally require two to four letters of recommendation as part of the application. Letters from people who can comment on the applicant's academic preparation and healthcare experience are usually preferable to those from personal friends. Students should establish relationships with professionals at the university and in the workplace early on, as they may later serve as references.

In the admissions process, academic performance is a critical criterion for evaluating applicants. Typically, programs review the overall Grade Point Average (GPA) and the GPA for science courses. Some programs require a minimum GPA of applicants. They may also examine the transcript for evidence of academic consistency, course load, and improvement in grade performance. Most programs will interview the leading candidates. Programs look for academic ability particularly in the sciences, comfort working with patients, maturity, judgment, an accurate concept of the types of work PAs perform, and planning for the intensity of PA education. Depending on their mission, some programs prefer candidates seeking to be a PA as a first career; others prefer second-career candidates, while many make no distinction in their selection process. It is wise for candidates to inquire to learn the selection processes of the programs that interest them.

The Central Application Service for Physician Assistants (CASPA)

In 2001, the Association of Physician Assistant Programs (APAP) launched the Central Application Service for Physician Assistants (CASPA). As of April 2005, 93 of the 137 accredited PA programs had elected to participate in this service. Applying to programs through CASPA allows applicants to complete one on-line application and choose which programs to send their completed applications. For more information, or to apply through this Web-based service, please go to the CASPA Web site at www.caspaonline.org.

APAP compiles the *Physician Assistant Programs Directory* for those considering the PA profession. Available only online by subscription at www.apap.org, the directory provides detailed information about each of the programs and answers prospective students' questions. However, as you consult with programs you are interested in attending, you may wish to ask specific questions such as these:

- Will the program accept credits earned at other institutions?
- What kind of healthcare experience is acceptable?
- How recent should course work be?

Application policies, procedures, and deadlines vary considerably from program to program. The application process depends upon whether the program subscribes to the Central Application Service for Physician Assistants (CASPA). Students must apply through CASPA for those programs that subscribe; non-subscribing programs post applications on their own Web sites. In both cases, applicants should be guided by programs' published application deadlines and complete the application process early. Applicants should be prepared to furnish information on their academic backgrounds, employment experience, plans to finance their education, and reasons for choosing the PA profession. In addition, some admissions committees may be interested in knowing why applicants have chosen their particular programs.

PA programs generally admit one group of students per year. Most programs' annual date to begin a new group is in the fall; others start in summer or winter semester. The due date for applications is typically 6 to 12 months prior to the start of classes. Some programs require that all prerequisites be met at time of application; others require prerequisites to be met by time of enrollment.

The Physician Assistant Preparation

Physician assistant educational programs are generally 24 to 30 months in length. They are typically arranged in two approximately even parts—a classroom educational component and a clinical experience component. The classroom courses consist of basic sciences (such as advanced anatomy, pathophysiology, and pharmacology), clinical sciences (such as physical diagnosis, clinical problem solving, pediatric and adult medicine, women's medicine, surgery, emergency medicine, geriatrics, and behavioral medicine), and courses on the healthcare system and health policy. The clinical experiences include rotating through specialties including family medicine, internal medicine, general surgery, emergency medicine, pediatrics, women's medicine, behavioral medicine, and one or more electives. The dominant characteristic of PA education is intensity. It is high-volume, fast-paced learning.

Certification and Licensure Requirements for PAs

All states require graduation from an accredited PA Program and passage of the national certification examination as the basic criteria for granting a license to practice. To maintain national certification through their careers, PAs must acquire 100 hours of continuing medical education every two years and pass a re-certification examination every six years as required by the National Commission on Certification of Physician Assistants. Some states require PAs to maintain national certification in order to renew state licensure (NCCPA, 2005).

Postgraduate PA Education

PAs working in specialty areas must acquire additional knowledge and skill after graduation from an entry level, primary care program. They do so in one of two ways. Most PAs working in a specialty go to work for a physician(s) in that specialty. They learn the elements of the specialty that they need for their role in the practice from the physician(s) with whom they work. The alternate route to postgraduate specialty knowledge is through attending a formal postgraduate educational residency in a particular specialty. There are 29 such residencies across the United States. They are in the following specialties (APPAP, 2005):

Emergency Medicine	Urology
Rural Medicine	General Surgery
Neurology	Obstetrics/Gynecology
Orthopedics	Cardiothoracic Surgery
Family Medicine	Psychiatry
Dermatology	Pediatrics
Oncology	

Generally each residency accepts only a small number of students (1 to 10). The residencies are typically 12 months in length. Most provide stipends or salaries to the participating students while they are enrolled.

National Professional Organizations for Physician Assistants

There are four major national organizations associated with the profession. Two are organizations of the profession.

The *American Academy of Physician Assistants* (AAPA) is the national organization of physician assistants. Its mission is to "promote quality, cost-effective, accessible health care, and to promote the professional and personal development of physician assistants" (AAPAb, 2005). It has constituent organizations in all states and student organizations in most PA educational programs.

The *Association of Physician Assistant Programs* (APAP) is the national organization of PA education. All PA programs belong to this organization. Its primary mission is to "to pursue excellence, foster faculty development, advance the body of knowledge that defines quality education and patient-centered care, and promote diversity in all aspects of physician assistant education" (APAP, 2005). It offers a Program Directory that is helpful to prospective students as they seek to determine which program/s are best suited to them.

The remaining two national organizations associated with the profession are not organizations of the profession. Rather, they were established to serve the public by assuring high-quality PAs and PA programs.

The *Accreditation Review Commission on Education for the Physician Assistant* (ARC-PA) is "the accrediting agency that protects the interests of the public and PA profession by defining the standards for PA education and evaluating PA educational programs within the territorial United States to ensure their compliance with those standards" (ARC-PA, 2005). All entry-level PA Programs, regardless of the degree they offer, must meet these standards.

The *National Commission on Certification of PAs* (NCCPA) assures "the public that certified physician assistants meet established standards of knowledge and clinical skills upon entry into practice and throughout their careers" (NCCPA, 2005). Graduation from an ARC-PA accredited program and NCCPA certification are the two common credentials required by states for licensure to practice. The letters that commonly follow the name of a PA are "PA-C." The "C" shows that the PA has passed the national certification examination and completed other requirements set forth by NCCPA to maintain certification.

Estimated Salary and Work Environment of the Physician Assistant

The job market for PAs has been strong for many years and is predicted to remain so. PA salaries vary by the specialty and geographic location in which they work. According to the 2004 AAPA Physician Assistant Census Report, the mean annual income from the primary employer for PAs working at least

32 hours per week was $78,257. The comparable figure for PAs who graduated in 2003 was $65,641 (AAPA, 2004). Income varies by specialty, practice setting, geographical location, and years of experience.

Future Trends for Physician Assistants

The future of the PA profession appears to be one of continued strong growth with employment opportunities in primary care and specialties, in inner city, urban, suburban, and rural settings. The Bureau of Labor Statistics of the US Department of Labor rates the career of physician assistant in its highest category of projected growth. Employment of PAs is expected to grow much faster than the average for all occupations through the year 2012, due to anticipated expansion of the health services industry and an emphasis on cost containment, resulting in increasing utilization of PAs by physicians and healthcare institutions. The Bureau defines "grow much faster than average" when growth is projected to "increase 36 percent or more" by 2012. As seen in Figure 8.1, the Bureau projections put PAs near the top of the list of fastest-growing occupations through 2012 (Bureau, 2005).

PA education is moving toward standardization of educational degrees at the masters level. As health care in the United States continues to develop, new fields for employment of PAs arise. Most recently these include geriatric care and hospital-based care. The profession is challenged to attract an adequate number of qualified students and faculty members to meet the continuing need for more PAs.

Internationally, the PA profession is beginning discovered by a growing number of nations faced with challenges to provide access to high-quality, cost-effective medical care. They too are finding that a physician-PA team is a cost-effective and efficient way to expand care while appropriately utilizing the knowledge and skills of all team members.

The PA as Part of the Healthcare Team

Teamwork is at the heart of the PA profession. The physician-PA team is an essential concept of the profession. Because diseases and disorders affect virtually all areas of life, comprehensive health care requires a broader team of medical, nursing, allied health, and social work professionals to provide comprehensive care. PAs work with professionals from all these areas to improve the health of the people they serve. The following case study illustrates this team work.

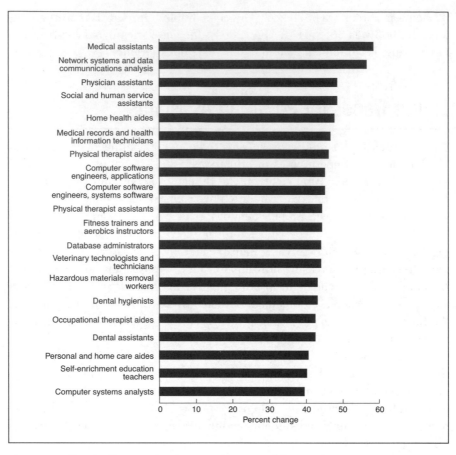

Figure 8.1 *Percent Change in Employment in Occupations Projected to Grow Fastest, 2002–2012*
Source: US BLM (2005)

Case Study: *A day in a life of a primary care PA*

Ms. Shirley Briggs is a PA working with Dr. Sam Helms in the Midwest Family Practice in Smalltown, U.S.A. Midwest Family Practice is a full-serve Family Medicine practice providing obstetrical, pediatric, adult, and geriatric service. It also provides occupational medical support for the local paper mill, care for patients in the local nursing home, and admits patients to the small local hospital. Ms. Briggs' day begins at the hospital.

7:00 AM. Ms. Briggs goes to the newborn nursery to check up on an infant who was born last evening. Dr. Helms had come in for the delivery. She examines the infant and speaks with the nurse about the infant's activity level and the status of some routine tests done on all newborns. She then speaks with the mother about the amount of help available at home when the infant and mother go home later today. Before leaving the nursery, Ms. Briggs makes sure the social worker will speak with the mother about the availability of services through the Women Infant and Children program offered by the public health department.

7:30 AM. Ms. Briggs joins Dr. Helms on the adult medical floor of the hospital. They make rounds on the five patients they have in the hospital. One of the patients, Mr. Waters, was admitted through the emergency room during the night with a flare-up of his chronic lung disease. After rounds, Dr. Helms heads for the office where he will begin seeing patients at 9:00 AM. Ms. Briggs remains in the hospital to conduct a more extensive interview and examination of Mr. Waters to be sure they have current information on all of his health problems, not just his current respiratory situation. She adjusts the medical orders for medications he takes for his hypertension and diabetes and dictates the complete medical history and physical examination of Mr. Waters for the hospital record.

9:30 AM–12 Noon. Ms. Briggs sees outpatients in the office. Ms. Dolan, a worker from the local paper mill, has sustained a small cut on her arm while at work. Ms. Briggs cleans and sutures the laceration. Later, Johnny Evans, a 35-year-old with adult hypertension, is seen. Dr. Helms had been seeing him for his hypertension that had been under good control, but now seems to be out of control. Ms. Briggs examines Mr. Evans and concludes that a significant change in medications is needed. Before prescribing the new medication, she consults with Dr. Helms to be sure the new treatment regimen will not conflict with Dr. Helms' long-term plan for managing the hypertension.

The last patient of the morning is Sally Falls, a fairly new diabetic. After checking her blood tests and speaking with Ms. Falls, it is apparent to Ms. Briggs that Sally is ready for additional information to help her and her family understand this life-long disease. Ms. Briggs arranges for Ms. Falls to meet with a Diabetic Educator.

1:00–5:00 PM. This is the day for Ms. Briggs' twice-a-month visit to the nursing home in which Midwest Family Practice has patients. She sees about 15 residents this afternoon. Several of them receive physical and occupational therapy to help them cope with and recover from various ailments. Ms. Briggs reads the notes the therapists have left in the chart. She stops by the physical therapist's office in the nursing home to discuss the progress of a couple of the residents. After seeing each of the nursing home residents, Ms. Briggs writes orders to adjust medications and initiate or change other therapies depending on what she has learned during her examinations. She discusses the situation of each resident with the nurse. She learns that two of the residents are complaining about the meals and not eating well. She asks that the dietician see these patients and alter their diets to accommodate their preferences where possible while maintaining a diet consistent with alleviating their healthcare problems.

Though the job description of PAs varies widely, Ms. Briggs' role in the Midwest Family Practice illustrates that PAs interact with professionals from many other healthcare disciplines as they go about their daily duties.

SUMMARY

Today, the Physician Assistant plays a valuable role in the healthcare system. Able to counsel patients regarding primary prevention of diseases and injuries, diagnose, and treat those same health conditions, the PA plays a direct role in all levels of prevention. In the United States, PAs are mid-level practitioners licensed to practice medicine with physician supervision. They can treat patients and, in most states, prescribe medicine. PAs in surgical practices also serve as first assists in surgery. PAs provide medical services that are reimbursed under Medicare and third-party insurances. Working in a variety of healthcare settings, the PA maintains expertise through professional certification, in a broad array of medical areas and can change his or her area of practice as their needs or desires arise. This allows for more flexibility in the career of the physician assistant. The projected growth of the profession to help augment the services of physicians and the diverse areas of practice make being a physician assistant an appealing career option for many individuals who want to make a difference in health care.

ADDITIONAL RESOURCES

www.aapa.org – This is the site of the American Academy of Physician Assistants—the national organization of PAs. It is a large, well-mapped site that includes a great deal of information on the PA profession, issues challenging the profession, laws governing PAs, and more. It also has links to PA organizations in all states, interest groups of PAs working in most specialties, international PAs, and the other PA organizations.

www.apap.org – The Association of Physician Assistant Programs is the national organization of PA educational programs. The site contains links to PA programs and to the Centralized Application Service for PAs (CASPA). It is an excellent source of information about PA Education.

www.appap.org – The Association of Postgraduate PA Programs' site provides information about further education for PAs after they complete an entry-level PA program. It has links to the programs that offer specialty education.

www.nccpa.net – The National Commission for Certification of Physician Assistants is the national organization that administers the national board examination for PA graduates. The site explains the certification process and provides general information on the practice of PAs.

www.arc-pa.org – The Accreditation Review Commission on Education for the Physician Assistant is the national organization that sets and enforces the standards for PA educational programs. It provides quality assurance for PA educational programs. The site provides information about accreditation standards and accreditation status of PA Programs.

STUDY QUESTIONS

1. What types of medical tasks do PAs perform?
2. What medical specialties employ PAs?
3. With what other medical profession is PA most closely linked?
4. Approximately what percentage of PAs work in primary care medicine? In other medical specialties?
5. Why is it important for candidates to research and select the PA program(s) they are most interested in applying to *before* they plan their pre-PA studies?
6. What are the typical characteristics programs are looking for when they interview candidates?
7. What types of courses are generally included in the education of PAs?
8. What two credentials are required of all PAs seeking a state license to practice?
9. What national organizations can provide additional information about PAs and PA education through their Web sites?
10. What are the prospects for PA jobs in the coming years?

REFERENCES

Accreditation Review Commission on Education for the Physician Assistant, Inc. (ARC-PA). (2005). Home page. Retrieved June 28, 2005, from http://www.arc-pa.org.

American Academy of Physician Assistants (AAPA). (2005a). 2004 AAPA Physician Assistant Census Report: Annual Income. Data retrieved June 9, 2005, from www.aapa.org/research/04census-intro.html.

American Academy of Physician Assistants (AAPA). (2005b). Mission statement. Retrieved June 28, 2005, from www.aapa.org/mission.html.

American Academy of Physician Assistants (AAPA). (2005c). Where physician assistants are authorized to prescribe. Retrieved June 27, 2005, from www.aapa.org/gandp/rxchart.html.

Association of Physician Assistant Programs (APAP). (2005). Mission. Retrieved June 28, 2005, from www.apap.org/aboutapap.htm.

Association of Postgraduate Physician Assistant Programs (APPAP). (2005). APPAP programs by specialty. Retrieved June 28, 2005, from http://www.appap.org/prog_specialty.html.

National Commission on Certification of Physician Assistants (NCCPA). (2005). About us: Purpose and mission. Retrieved June 28, 2005, from http://www.nccpa.net/AboutUs.aspx.

Chapter 9

Nursing

Vicki C. Martin

OBJECTIVES

After studying this chapter, the student should be able to

1. Explain the role of the nurse in the healthcare system.
2. Describe the difference between a registered nurse and licensed practical nurse.
3. Describe the educational preparation and certification required for nurses.
4. List various healthcare settings where nurses are employed.
5. Identify resources for additional information on the role of nurses.

INTRODUCTION

*Constant attention by a good nurse may be just
as important as a major operation by a surgeon.*
Dag Hammarskjold, Swedish Statesman
and United Nations official (1905–1961)

N ursing is a discipline focused on assisting individuals, families, and communities in attaining, re-attaining, and maintaining optimal health and functioning. Nursing is considered a science and an art. It focuses on promoting quality of life as defined by persons and families from womb to tomb, in every aspect of the lifespan. In pre-modern times, nuns and the military often provided nursing services. The religious and military roots of modern nursing remain in evidence today. For example, in Britain, nurses are known as "sisters." Traditional nursing caps (now rarely seen in the healthcare community) were worn in recognition of these early beginnings.

However, the attire worn by nurses is not the only thing that has changed in recent years. It is an exciting time to be a nurse! Each new day brings with it challenges, opportunities, and experiences often unmatched by any other profession. It is through these challenges, opportunities, and experiences that nurses make a difference every day in the lives of clients.

There is no one career path in nursing and there is virtually no limit to the number of avenues you can pursue in the field of nursing. At a glance, nursing can be described as a dynamic profession built upon foundational characteristics of human caring, intellectual competency, integrity, autonomy, collaboration, and ethical principles. These characteristics, as well as many others not mentioned, shape who nurses are as individuals and as a profession, dictating how nurses provide for those in their care. Nurses aim to provide holistic, competent care that impacts all aspects of life for individuals, families, and communities. Nurses are at hand to usher in life, to celebrate accomplishments and set-backs throughout life, and to lend comfort at the end of life.

Description of the Profession

Entry into the profession of nursing exists at two levels: Registered Nurse (RN) and Licensed Practical Nurse (LPN). Each level has prescribed educational and licensing requirements as well as career advancement capabilities. Let's look at the uniqueness of both levels and how each is instrumental within the healthcare system.

Registered Nurses

Regardless of the practice setting, RNs are critical liaisons between the healthcare team (physicians, physical therapists, nutritionists, etc.) and the client. The RN is aware of and involved in all aspects of care for clients and their family, advocating and providing for healthcare needs, providing education while coordinating care and services. Higher educational training yields greater opportunities and responsibilities in each of these areas. When positioned to give direct care, RNs assess clients for signs and symptoms related to illness or disease; collaborate with physicians and ancillary healthcare team members to plan care that will assist with the management of the illness or disease; evaluate the effectiveness of the treatment plan and suggest revisions as needed; educate clients and their families about health promotion and disease prevention; and administer medications and treatments as ordered by the physician. The focus of care is on the client, while paying particular attention to the emotional, psychological, and social implications of the healthcare need. Registered Nurses also provide important input into policy development and implementation within hospital or outpatient settings that promote positive healthcare outcomes for clients and families.

Registered nurses are able to practice nursing in a wide variety of settings. Cross-training allows for nurses to change settings as frequently as they wish. Over the course of their careers, nurses may change settings several times. This enables nurses to enjoy a number of benefits: increased job satisfaction and career advancement, changes in physical demands when needed, flexibility in scheduling, and increased challenge and opportunity to learn different jobs within the field of nursing. The job possibilities in nursing are endless. Let's explore a few of the practice settings that are common to nursing.

Hospital

The hospital setting is the most well-known setting for nursing practice. Many nurses are staff nurses who provide care to clients on medical-surgical, pediatric, maternity, psychiatric, and cancer floors, for example. They may also work in specialty areas such as intensive care units, operating rooms, emergency rooms, cardiac cath labs, special x-ray procedure labs, and transplant clinics. Duties within these settings vary as does rank. Registered nurses who are educated at the baccalaureate level (BSN) will often advance more readily that will an RN educated at the associate degree or diploma level. For example, baccalaureate nurses will be able to hold management positions as a head nurse of a unit within a hospital setting. Most hospitals incorporate a career ladder into their hiring and advancement policies. Educational training is but one requirement for advancement within the clinical ladder format. Other requirements may include such things as a willingness to serve on hospital committees, willingness to mentor new nurses, involvement in continuing education, and active involvement in professional organizations.

Community Health

Nurses may work in a variety of community agencies, providing both direct care or managing services rendered in clinics or with home-bound clients. Examples of this type of nursing would include conducting clinics for a particular population of interest, such as the diabetic client, women and children, or the HIV client. The focus of care is not only to meet clients' immediate health needs, but also to educate clients on how to improve their health and prevent complications of illness or disease. Nurses within these community settings are highly engaged with other community leaders such as physicians, teachers, and parents to ensure that health needs of the community are addressed through education. Community nurses may also be involved in giving direct care to clients who are home-bound and in need of follow-up nursing care. Many of these clients may have recently been discharged from a hospital but still may need to have medications administered, wounds managed, or be in need of follow-up with nutritional needs, new baby care, or pain management. Home health nurses must be able to assess the client's progress and provide care independently.

School Nurses

School nursing is a more recent addition to the opportunities afforded registered nurses. This role has traditionally been fulfilled by licensed practical nurses (LPNs). Nationwide, children with low-risk disabilities and health disorders are attending public schools in greater numbers. More and more, the qualifications for school nurse positions include being a registered nurse with educational preparation at the baccalaureate level. School nurses are involved with administering medications and providing emergency care to all school-age children. They also are heavily involved in health education and maintaining the health-related policies within the school setting. Federal grant money through the US Department of Education has been allocated and distributed to baccalaureate nursing programs to promote school nursing as a practice option upon graduation.

Occupational Health

Nurses within the industrial sector provide invaluable care to individuals at the worksite. These nurses provide health screening, emergency care for work site injuries, health promotion and disease prevention education, and assess work environments for potential hazards to the health of employees and customers. Occupational health nurses are also involved in formulating work-related policies to help prevent site injuries as well as monitor federal OSHA regulations for the work place.

Offices

Nurses provide outpatient care for clients within physician offices, ambulatory surgical centers, and walk-in healthcare centers. They perform routine assessments of the client's chief healthcare concern, assist with treatments and minor surgery, administer medications, perform routine laboratory tests, prepare for and assist with examinations, and provide for client education. Nurses within various office settings may manage client services and referrals as well as provide healthcare counseling.

Nursing Homes and Rehabilitative Care Facilities

Within each of these settings, registered nurses provide limited direct client care. Responsibilities of the registered nurse encompass management of client services, planning care, supervising care, and performing administrative duties such as ensuring that federal regulations are enforced within the facility regarding health care. Direct client care is performed primarily by licensed practical nurses and nursing assistants.

Other registered nurses, with educational preparation beyond the baccalaureate level, may practice as *nurse practitioners, clinical nurse specialists, certified nurse midwives,* and *certified nurse anesthetists.* With each specialty, additional licensing or certification requirements exist which are often state specific.

Licensed Practical Nurses

Licensed Practical Nurses (LPNs) often receive their educational preparation within vocational or technical schools. The basic training program generally lasts 12 to 18 months. While practice policy varies with different states and institutions, LPNs generally perform basic care duties under the supervision of registered nurses and physicians.

Job responsibilities include delivering basic hygiene care, assessing the health status of the client, administering basic treatments and procedures, administering most medications, providing basic wound care, performing routine laboratory tests, and collecting samples for laboratory testing. LPNs also engage in client and family teaching with basic illnesses and care. LPNs supervise the care given to clients by nursing assistants. Practice settings include hospitals, nursing homes, offices, and schools. LPNs are not generally able to practice within community health settings as they are not able to work independently and must be supervised by a registered nurse. State law dictates the overall responsibilities and practice policies that govern the licensed practical nurse.

History and Background of the Nursing Profession

Nursing as we know it today has evolved out of necessity during periods of global and national stress. War has played a significant role throughout nursing history by creating the need for care that could be provided by nurses. While references to informal nursing can be found throughout history, Florence Nightingale has been honored as the founder of professional nursing.

Nightingale began her nursing training at the Institution of Deaconesses in Germany in 1851 prior to the Crimean War and began training other nurses herself in 1854 in London (Small, 1998). In October 1854, Nightingale was asked by the British Secretary of War to lead a group of nurses to care for wounded soldiers during the Crimean War. Over the course of the next year, Nightingale worked to provide sanitary conditions for the treatment of the soldiers, which resulted in a decrease in the mortality rate from 42% to 2%. She established special diets for the soldiers to aid in their healing, as well as statistical record keeping to monitor health improvement and death rates. Nightingale provided spiritual care, music, and recreation to encourage and comfort the soldiers (Small, 1998). By the end of the Crimean War, Nightingale had trained over 125 nurses to care for the wounded and ill soldiers (Small, 1998). After the war, Nightingale established the first nursing school in England. By 1873, graduates of this program migrated to the United States to become supervisors in the first hospital-based (diploma) nursing schools: Massachusetts General Hospital in Boston, Bellevue Hospital in New York, and the New Haven Hospital in Connecticut (Small, 1998).

By this time, nursing in the United States was also being shaped by war. Conditions of the Civil War were similar to those experienced by Florence Nightingale—primitive working conditions, poor sanitation, lack of food and water, and lack of record keeping mechanisms to track illness progression and death. Unfortunately, there were fewer than 2000 nurses to care for more than six million soldiers, with half a million surgical cases (Fitzpatrick, 1997). Two well-known nurses, Harriet Tubman, known as the "Conductor of the Underground Railroad" and Clara Barton, who eventually founded the Red Cross in 1882, cared for the sick and injured during the Civil War (Carnegie, 1995). When the war ended, numerous nurse training schools opened their doors, emphasizing on-the-job training rather than formal education. The first nursing textbook was published in 1876 and titled *A Manual of Nursing* (Cherry & Jacob, 2005). Because of lingering segregation and discrimination, African-American men and women were not allowed to attend established nurse training schools. Consequently, in 1886 John D. Rockefeller funded the first school of nursing for African-American women at the Atlanta Baptist Seminary (Jones, 2004).

Again, between 1900 and 1945, the United States was at war—this time abroad. Women were given the right to vote, were moving into the workforce rapidly, and were once again called to care for soldiers wounded in battle. Medications such as insulin and penicillin were improving health and preventing premature death due to infection (Stanhope & Lancaster, 2004). Community health nursing also rose in prominence during this era, with nurses caring mostly for disadvantaged women and children. Given the demand for nurses in all sectors of life, admission into nurse training schools increased, as did the resultant number of graduate nurses available as a healthcare resource. However, there was no way to determine the minimal standards of competency of the graduates from nurse training programs across the nation. In 1901, permissive licenses were available but were not mandated for all nurses. By 1923, all states had instituted examinations for permissive licensure (Kalisch & Kalisch, 1995).

During the Great Depression of the 1930s many nursing jobs were lost. Nursing, however, did not remain stagnant during that time. The licensure issue remained a national concern and in the mid 1930s standardized nursing examinations, developed by each state, led to mandatory licensing of all nurses in 1947 (Kalisch & Kalisch, 1995). The passage of the Social Security Act in 1935 provided avenues for payment for nursing care and new nursing jobs were once again created (Connelly, 2004). Similarly, WWII caused the military to recognize that nurses were scarce and that federal funds were needed to expand nursing education (Stanhope & Lancaster, 2004). It was during WWII that nurses were finally recognized as an integral part of military service and were enabled to attain officer ranks within the army and navy. Colonel Julie O. Flikke was the first army nurse to be promoted to colonel in the US Army and served as superintendent of the Army Nurse Corps from 1937 to 1942 (Robinson & Perry, 2001).

Three decades after WWII saw the emergence of nursing as a true profession. Minimal national standards for nursing education were established and by 1950 all state boards of nursing were utilizing a single standardized examination for licensure of nurses. Nursing education continued to improve in quality and quantity with increased numbers of baccalaureate programs and associate degree programs (Kalisch & Kalisch, 1995). The educational focus was less directed toward on-the-job training and reflected an emphasis on research and theory development to guide nursing practice. In 1943, the Nurse Training Act was enacted to provide federal funding for nursing education. Shortly thereafter, the passage of the Hill-Burton Act in 1946 provided the largest commitment of federal money to the construction of hospitals and healthcare facilities nationwide. Together, these two federal acts created increased demand for nurses, pulling them from traditional community settings into hospital practice (Connelly, 2004).

Federal legislation, once again, had a profound impact on nursing during the 1960s. The Community Mental Health Centers Acts of 1963 and the passage of the Medicare and Medicaid Acts of 1965 increased federal funding to outpatient mental health facilities and extended insurance coverage to all individuals covered by Social Security and those whose incomes were at or below poverty levels (Baer et al., 2001). As a result, increased numbers of nurses were needed to further staff hospitals, as hospital insurance coverage was now possible for many and to staff home health agencies as Medicare now provided for essential skilled home nursing care (Stanhope & Lancaster, 2004). The home healthcare movement was one of the first practice settings that provided nurses with the option to work only weekday shifts.

The 1970s heralded the women's rights movement and it was this movement that caused nurses to focus not only upon providing quality patient care but to also demand salaries and benefits that reflected that excellence. Nursing was instrumental in establishing hospice programs, birthing centers, and elder daycare facilities. At the same time, nurse practitioner programs expanded, requiring a master's degree in nursing as well as certification to practice (Buhler-Wilkerson, 2001). Professionally, nursing was focused on scholarly pursuits of education, research, and practice.

Dramatic changes in health care and economic growth within the United States resulted in increasing demands for nurses and a drastic decrease in nursing enrollments. Healthcare costs soared but nursing salaries did not. Medical and technological advances flourished, leading to new specialties, outpatient services, and increased opportunities for nurse practitioners. In 1983, DRGs (diagnostic related groups) were developed to curtail the soaring costs of healthcare. DRGs standardized care and reimbursed hospitals only what was considered to be a standard cost for the diagnosis of the patient. As a result, nurse practitioners increased in popularity as a means to provide cost-effective care that focused on the prevention, rather than just merely the treatment, of illness (Stanhope & Lancaster, 2004). There were dramatic decreases in nursing school enrollments nationwide as students pursued careers with higher potential earnings. The lack of salary equity, complexities in the healthcare system, and lack of overall professional recognition yielded a serious national nursing shortage in all areas of healthcare delivery (Ellis & Hartley, 2004).

Sluggish economic growth plagued the 1990s, sending more women with families back into the workforce. Nurse employers were faced with the need to be creative and flexible with scheduling that enabled more nurses to be attracted into the workforce and still be able to meet demanding family obligations. Creative shifts such as 10-hour/4 day-per-week or 12-hour/3 day-per-week schedules became commonplace in hospitals and other healthcare facilities. Higher shift differential pay was added as well and the ability to forfeit benefits for higher salaries became standard (Cherry & Jacob, 2005). Nursing priorities shifted to include increased emphasis upon preventive health care, health promotion education to individuals and families, case management of complex healthcare services, and increased use of community healthcare services to limit expensive hospital care. Nursing research continued to be paramount to ensure that nursing care was sound, efficient, and outcomes based—known as evidence-based practice. While licensing continued to be mandated for all nurses entering nursing practice as well as for nurse practitioners, growing concern mounted over improved methods of ensuring continued competence in a field that was ever changing. National certifying agencies were established to provide criterion-based certification of all nurse practitioners and clinical nurse specialists with periodic re-certifications required (Cherry & Jacob, 2005).

Today, the nursing profession continues to struggle with many of the same issues of the past. The need to advocate for higher wages, increased autonomy, sufficient staffing, and appropriate participation in healthcare decision-making are among the battles that continue to ravage the nursing profession. Similarly, nurses must continue to advocate for patients' rights to access affordable, cost-effective, quality health care and for healthcare providers to be accountable in their delivery of care. These challenges, along with the challenges of changing medical technology and an aging society, will require the commitment and proactive approach that are demonstrated strengths of the nursing profession. Just as in the past, nurses will continue to be at the forefront of medicine, patient care, healthcare advocacy, and excellence in service.

Educational Requirements for Nursing

Registered Nurses

The baccalaureate degree in nursing, the associates degree in nursing, or the diploma in nursing are all basic educational avenues that will prepare students for licensure as an RN but are very different in their educational approach.

Baccalaureate or Bachelors of Science Degree in Nursing (BSN): Case Western Reserve established the first true four-year nursing program in 1924. Today, there are more than 569 basic BSN programs and 620 that offer accelerated BSN tracks for RNs from associates degree or diploma programs in nursing (Berlin, Stennett, & Bednash, 2003). Students desiring a baccalaureate degree must enroll in a four-year college or university and complete two years of general education courses as well as two years of nursing-specific courses. The general education courses are concentrated in the liberal arts and sciences, giving students a strong critical-thinking foundation prior to specialization in the nursing curriculum. Nursing courses reflect the fundamentals of nursing, which include care of the patient with medical, surgical, psychiatric, pediatric, and maternity conditions. Unlike other types of programs, baccalaureate education also includes emphasis upon community health, beginning management and leadership skills, research, healthcare policy, and professional involvement in nursing organizations. Students also will learn to manage care of individuals, families, and communities through experiences with case management. BSN graduates are prepared to not only pass the NCLEX (licensure examination) but are equipped to enter graduate programs in their chosen specialty area. The baccalaureate degree in nursing is required in many areas across the nation for entry into various specialty areas of practice and for certification in those specialties.

Associates Degree in Nursing (ADN): In the late 1950s, with a growing nursing shortage after WWII, associate degree programs in nursing quickly developed at the community college level. RNs prepared at the associate degree level continue to be the largest group of practicing nurses today. Today, there are over 885 ADN programs nationwide (Cherry & Jacob, 2005). The original concept behind the creation of the associate degree in nursing was that technical nurses (ADNs) would work with professional nurses (BSNs) as a team. In reality, associate degree nurses have forged a new career path in nursing. This fast track to nursing allows for quicker, more affordable entry into the practice setting and also enables nurses to work as RNs while returning to obtain their baccalaureate degrees on a full-time or part-time basis if they so choose. Students are required to complete two full years with fewer courses in the liberal arts and sciences and condensed nursing content. The nursing content contains the foundational courses in medical, surgical, pediatric, maternity, and psychiatric conditions. Practice essentials are emphasized without being able to explore more advanced concepts of community health nursing, healthcare policy, or management and leadership. Career advancement within the practice arena is generally dependent upon further educational preparation at the baccalaureate level. Associate degree nurses sit for the NCLEX licensure examination as well as various certification exams with specialty areas of nursing such as pediatrics, gerontologic, medical-surgical, cardiovascular, and psychiatric nursing.

Diploma in Nursing: Diploma programs are the oldest and most traditional of the nursing education programs that prepare students for RN licensures. These programs were initially developed in the late 1800s and were hospital-based training facilities. At their peak in the 1950s and 1960s, there were more than 1300 diploma programs in nursing. As society and health care have changed, fewer than 86 diploma programs exist today (Cherry & Jacob, 2005). Diploma nursing programs continue to have strong ties to hospitals and adhere more to a hands-on approach to nursing education. Many programs have linked with community colleges to require some arts and science courses. Diploma programs today generally require two full academic years of study and do not award any college degree. Nursing content focuses on the foundations of medical, surgical, pediatric, maternity, and psychiatric conditions without additional content in broader areas of nursing responsibility. Diploma nurses are equipped to sit for the NCLEX licensure examination and to be licensed as an RN, however, additional educational preparation is required for job opportunities outside of the traditional staff nurse role. Certifications also exist for diploma nurses desiring to work in a specialty area of nursing such as cardio-vascular, gerontologic, medical-surgical, pediatrics, and psychiatry.

Licensed Practical Nurses (LPN's)

Practical nurse programs are the shortest and most restricted options for individuals who wish to practice as a licensed nurse (Cherry & Jacob, 2005). Most programs range in length from 9–12 months and are housed in vocational or technical schools. No college credit is given for completion of the program but the individual may sit for the LPN licensure. More than 1100 LPN programs exist nationwide, although their numbers are decreasing (NLN, 1997).

Advanced Nursing Education

Beyond the baccalaureate level, a nurse may pursue higher education at the masters and doctoral levels.

Masters in Nursing: Masters programs in nursing increased in the 1960s and 1970s as the need for highly trained, competent educators, administrators, and clinicians emerged due to increasing complexities in the healthcare arena (Cherry & Jacob, 2005). Today, there are more than 398 Masters in Nursing programs nationwide (Berlin, Stennett, & Bednash, 2003). Generally, programs require an additional one to two years of advanced preparation beyond the baccalaureate degree to fulfill requirements at the masters level. Students may study in a variety of specialties which may include advance practice as a clinical nurse specialist or nurse practitioner, or education. Clinical nurse specialists prepare in selected areas such as pediatrics, cardiology, anesthesia, midwifery, and oncology and are generally required to pass a certification examination prior to practicing. Nurse practitioners also select the area of specialty practice that they desire, which may include family, adult, pediatric, and gerontology. Nurse practitioners are required to sit for an additional licensure examination that enables them to practice with physicians and manage their own clients' needs, including prescribing appropriate medications, laboratory tests, etc. Specialty certification may also be obtained by sitting for an examination in areas such as diabetes management and advanced end of life care. Most nurse educators, managers, and administrators are also required to complete a master's or doctoral degree.

MSN programs offer different options for study. Most programs are specifically designed for the BSN prepared nurse but several offer master's degree programs for non-nursing, second degree seeking individuals. Programs range from on campus curriculums, to Web-enhanced or completely online curriculums designed to suit the needs of working individuals.

Doctoral Programs: In 1934, Columbia University developed the first Doctor of Education degree (EdD) in nursing education and New York University offered the first PhD program for nurses (Cherry & Jacob, 2005). Today approximately 83 nursing doctoral programs exist (Berlin, Stennett, & Bednash, 2003). There are four basic types of doctoral degrees available in nursing. The doctoral of philosophy (PhD) prepares nurses for research; the doctor of nursing science (DNS) prepares nurses for advanced clinical nursing practice; the doctor of nursing (ND) prepares non-nurses for careers in leadership; and the doctorate in clinical nursing practice (DNP) is designed primarily for advanced practice nurses, such as nurse practitioners. Most university nursing programs require a terminal degree, the doctoral degree, for all nurse educators.

Role of Professional Nursing Organizations

Active participation in a professional organization is critical to the role development of a nurse. Nurses rely on the strength of their supporting organizations to inform, educate, and empower them to collectively make positive changes in the nursing profession and the healthcare arena. The American Nurses Association, founded in 1911, is the foundation for all professional aspects of nursing. Since its inception, the ANA has been an active voice for nurses in healthcare policy, the standardization of nursing practice and education, and assuring the welfare of all nurses nationwide. Since 1994, the ANA has maintained position statements on a wide variety of key national issues such as assisted suicide, active euthanasia, childhood immunizations, long-term care, cessation of tobacco, work redesign, and informal care giving (Schwirian, 1998). These position statements contribute to the national debate on the future of health care and contribute to the professional stature of nursing.

Student nurses also have a voice in nursing education, practice, and healthcare reform through the National Student Nurses Association. Since its inception in 1953, student nurses from across the nation, at all levels of nursing education, have actively worked toward a unified position on healthcare issues and have aligned themselves with the American Nurses Association to give strength to the voice of future nurses.

Specialty organizations such as the American Association of Medical-Surgical Nurses or the American Association of Critical-Care Nurses have gained prominence within nursing as they were a better fit for nurses involved in full-time nursing practice. While these specialty organizations are involved in healthcare policy debate, their primary emphasis is to provide an increased avenue for networking and continuing education common to each specialty area of nursing practice. Similar to the ANA, specialty organizations engage in professional development at the local chapter level as well as nationally.

Sigma Theta Tau International is the honor society for nursing scholars in all venues of the nursing profession. STTI's mission is to create a global community of nurses who lead in using scholarship, knowledge, and technology to improve the health of the world's people. Membership into STTI requires a baccalaureate degree in nursing or higher as well as demonstrated scholarly ability as a student or as a community leader. Nursing scholarship, often in the form of research, is disseminated throughout the nursing community via conferences, workshops, and sponsored publications available to all members.

Nurses in the Workforce

Work Environment

In general, most nurses work in comfortable healthcare settings. A considerable amount of walking and standing is required for most nursing positions, especially within the hospital setting. While nursing care is generally needed 24 hours a day in an institutional setting, community health, office, and occupational health nurses are able to work regular daylight hours. Because of the high demand for nurses, they are often on call or asked to work extra shifts and holidays to ensure coverage for patient care. More than one in five RNs worked part-time in 2002 (Bureau of Labor Statistics, 2005).

Nurses may also find themselves at risk for back injuries, needle sticks, and exposure to radiation and hazardous materials. Just as with any high-risk occupation, healthcare agencies maintain standardized guidelines and annual training sessions which help to minimize environmental, job-related harm to nurses. Similarly, exposure to infectious diseases is a risk that nurses must protect against. Nurses are educated within their initial nursing programs and through annual continuing education to guard against potential exposure to diseases and other dangers within their practice settings.

Earnings

According to the Bureau of Labor Statistics (2005), the median annual income of registered nurses was $48,090 with the highest 10% of nurses earning more than $69,670. Higher earnings were reported by nurses with advanced degrees. In 2000, the earnings of a master's prepared nurse averaged $61,262 while a doctorally prepared nurse averaged $63, 522 (Spratley, Johnson, Sochalski, Fritz, & Spencer, 2000). Recent trends have demonstrated steady increases in salary capabilities for nurses at all levels of preparation and practice setting, largely due to the national nursing shortage. Attractive benefits of many employers may include on-site child care, flexible work schedules, educational benefits for the attainment of higher education, and lucrative bonuses. Many hospitals offer higher hourly wages in lieu of benefits for nurses who are covered under spousal healthcare insurance plans. Nurses may also elect to be cross-trained in several practice areas within a hospital and work only when needed to earn significantly higher hourly wages without benefits.

Future Professional Trends for Nursing

The Nursing Shortage

As the largest occupation, job opportunities for RNs are expected to continue to be very good, especially during the current nursing shortage. Future employment is expected to grow faster than any other occupation through at least 2012, which will allow for the creation of many new jobs. Currently, professional nurses over the age of 40 represent nearly 60% of the workforce (Buerhaus, Staiger, & Auerbach, 2000). Similarly, RNs under 30 years of age represent only 10% of the total nurse population (Buerhaus, Staiger, & Auerbach, 2000). Because of the aging nursing population, it is projected that by 2010 one million more registered nurses will be needed than are available in the United States. By 2020, the demand will exceed 40%, with only a 6% increase in the supply of available nurses (Spratley et al., 2000). Imbalances between the supply and demand for qualified nurses should cause employers to creatively address workload, compensation, continuing education, and working conditions in order to attract and retain nurses (Bureau of Labor Statistics, 2005).

The Nursing Faculty Shortage

Likewise, an aging faculty pool, with an average age of 48.8 for masters-prepared and 53.3 for doctoral-prepared faculty, is adding to the nursing shortage crisis. Forty-one percent of schools cited that faculty shortage was the number one reason for the declining numbers of students gaining admission to nursing schools. In fact, in 2002, an AACN survey determined that 5283 students were not admitted to nursing programs due to inadequate numbers of qualified faculty to teach (Berlin, Stennett, & Bednash, 2003). Lack of appropriate federal and state funding for nursing education makes it difficult to attract potential faculty members by luring them away from higher salaries within clinical sites (AACN, 2003).

Areas of job growth include hospital outpatient facilities as well as community health agencies and nursing care facilities. Because of limits placed upon hospital stays by insurance providers, fewer patients will receive in-hospital care for longer than 24 to 48 hours at a time. Therefore, the need for in-home care will increase as will the need for additional nursing staff required to provide care. Similarly, patients who do find themselves with lengthy hospital stays will generally be sicker and require a greater intensity of specialty nursing care. The result will likely be that there will be an increased need for nurses to care for fewer, but sicker patients.

Educational Changes

The changing healthcare system will require an educational and skill mix to handle increasingly complex demands. Therefore, the projected demand will be for more baccalaureate-prepared nurses with critical thinking, leadership, case management, and health promotion skills who are capable of delivering care across a variety of structured and unstructured healthcare settings (Cherry & Jacob, 2005). Research has demonstrated that nurses prepared at the baccalaureate level provide care that has been associated with lower patient mortality rates (Aiken, 2002). This trend will require, as never before, that healthcare organizations consider quality of patient care and patient outcomes, as well as the financial implications of using nurses with varying degrees of educational preparations. Individuals considering nursing should carefully weigh the advantages and disadvantages of enrolling in a baccalaureate program as career advancement opportunities are generally more available to those with a BSN.

A New Role: The Clinical Nurse Leader

The American Association of Colleges of Nursing (AACN) in collaboration with a variety of nurse leaders in practice settings are being tasked with creating a new role for nursing. The new role is designed to better address the complexities of current healthcare delivery by providing practitioners who are equipped to ensure excellence of care across all practice settings. The new role, known as the *Clinical Nurse Leader*, will assume accountability for patient outcomes through the use of research-based practice which will help to design, implement, and evaluate patient care. The call for the new nursing role will force nursing to address all of the current educational levels of nursing by revisiting the way the field educates, licenses, and defines the scope of practice for each level (AACN, 2003). As nurses examine new ways to define the education and practice of nursing, we must continue to strive to enhance the quality of healthcare provision and to ensure patient safety.

SUMMARY

The historical nature of nursing provides encouragement for the healthcare system in that nursing thrives during times of challenge. The very nature of patient care has evolved during times of war, with its despicable sanitation and tremendous shortages of adequate personnel to care for those in need. The future forecasts of severe shortages of adequately prepared nurses to care for a graying society has already served to ignite new ways of thinking about, educating, and advocating for nursing. The nurse of today, portrayed as a highly intelligent, technologically savvy, astute practitioner, will continue to attract young individuals into nursing. Additional funding of nursing programs in higher educational settings by federal and state officials will multiply the applicant pools of colleges and universities nationwide, allowing for an increased supply of new nurses to combat the increased demand. Nurses are advocating for themselves in greater numbers than ever before through their professional organizations and elected governmental officials. No longer the silent majority, nurses are becoming active in designing and implementing new models for healthcare delivery and shared governance of their own practice environments. Through active participation in the shaping of nursing's future, nurses will realize an increased sense of autonomy, job satisfaction, career mobility, and financial compensation. Ultimately, the patient will benefit the most through improvement in care received, more seamless transitions through the complexities of the healthcare system, and greater understanding of their own health and wellness potential. Are there challenging roads ahead for nursing? Certainly! Are nurse up to the challenge? Absolutely!

ADDITIONAL RESOURCES

American Nurses Association — www.nursingworld.org
American Association of Colleges of Nursing — www.aacn.nche.edu
National Council of State Boards of Nursing — www.ncsbn.org
National League for Nursing — www.nln.org
National Student Nurses Association — www.nsna.org
Sigma Theta Tau International Honor Society — www.nursingsociety.org

REFERENCES

Aiken, L. (2002). Hospital nurse staffing and patient mortality, nurse burnout, and job dissatisfaction. *Journal of the American Medical Association, 288*(16), 1987–1993.

American Association of Colleges of Nursing (AACN). (2003). *Increase in nursing school enrollments for the third consecutive year: Increase falls below projected need to reverse the nursing shortage.* Unpublished manuscript from www.aacn.nche.edu/Media/NewsRelease/2003Dec10.htm.

Baer, E. D., D'Antoini, P., Rinker, S., & Lynaugh, J. E. (2001). *Enduring issues in American nursing.* New York: Springer Publishing.

Berlin, L. E., Stennett, J., & Bednash, G. (2003). *2002–2003 enrollment and graduations in baccalaureate and graduate programs in nursing.* Washington, DC: American Colleges of Nursing.

Buerhaus, P., Staiger, D., & Auerbach, D. (2000). Implications of an aging registered nurse workforce. *Journal of the American Medical Association, 283*(22), 2948–2954.

Buhler-Wilkerson, K. (2001). *No place like home: A history of nursing and home care in the United States.* Baltimore: Johns Hopkins.

Bureau of Labor Statistics, US Department of Labor. (2005). *Occupational outlook handbook: Registered nurses* (2004–2005 ed.). Washington, DC: US Department of Labor. Retrieved September 27, 2005, from http://www.bls.gov/oco/ocos083.htm.

Carnegie, M. E. (1995). *The path we tread: Blacks in nursing worldwide: 1854–1994* (3rd ed.). New York: National League for Nursing.

Cherry, B. & Jacob, S. R. (2005). *Contemporary nursing: Issues, trends, & management* (3rd ed.). St. Louis, MO: Elsevier Mosby.

Connolly, C. (2004). Beyond social history: New approaches to understanding the state of and the state in nursing history. *Nursing History Review, 12,* 5–24.

Ellis, J. R. & Hartley, C. L. (2004). *Nursing in today's world: Challenges, issues, and trends.* (8th ed.). Philadelphia: J. B. Lippincott.

Fitzpatrick, M. F. (1997). The mercy brigade. *Civil War Times, 36*(3), 34–40.

Jones, Z. (2004). Knowledge systems in conflict: The regulation of African-American midwifery. *Nursing History Review, 12,* 167–184.

Kalisch, P. & Kalisch, B. (1995). *The advance of American nursing* (3rd ed.). Philadelphia: J. B. Lippincott.

National League for Nursing (NLN). (1997). *Trends in contemporary nursing education* (1st ed.). New York: National League for Nursing.

Robinson, T. M. & Perry, P. M. (2001). *Cadet nurse stories: The call for and response of women during World War II.* Indianapolis, IN: Center Nursing Press.

Schwirian, P. M. (1998). *Professionalization of Nursing: Current issues and trends.* Philadelphia: J. B. Lippincott.

Small, H. (1998). In Small H. (Ed.), *Florence Nightingale: Avenging Angel* (1st ed.). London, England: Constable.

Spratley, E., Johnson, A., Sochaliski, F. M., & Spencer, W. (2000). *The registered nurse population: Findings from the national sample survey of registered nurses.* Washington, DC: US Department of Health and Human Services.

Stanhope, M. & Lancaster, J. (2004). *Community and public health nursing.* St Louis, MO: Mosby.

Chapter 10

Dentistry

Stephanie Chisolm

OBJECTIVES

After studying this chapter, the student should be able to

1. Explain the role and function of dental professionals, including dentists, dental hygienists, and dental technicians.
2. Explain the difference between the various areas of specialization for dentists.
3. Describe the educational preparation and certification required for dental professionals.
4. Summarize the estimated earning and career potential of various dental professionals.
5. Identify resources for additional information on dentistry as a profession.

INTRODUCTION

> *Trips to the dentist—I like to postpone that kind of thing.*
> Johnny Depp

When not flashing a gold tooth as Captain Jack Sparrow in the *Pirates of the Caribbean*, actor Johnny Depp, like many people, prefers to postpone visits to the dentist. However, most of us understand the importance and value of a healthy mouth and teeth. Our teeth not only add flash to our smile, but aid in eating and speaking.

Oral Health As a Global Concern

In September 2005, the first-ever global child dental health taskforce was established. The taskforce will initiate pan-European and wider global action between now and 2025 to make tangible improvements in child oral health. The World Health Organization (WHO), the World Dental Federation, and over 40 chief dental officers and leading dental figures from across the world, back the initiative. Although oral health has steadily improved over the last 30 years, dental disease is still the number one disease affecting children, occurring five to eight times more frequently than asthma, the second most common chronic disease. In industrialized countries, the majority of schoolchildren are affected by dental decay, disease levels being highest in the underprivileged groups. Dental disease levels are also increasing rapidly in the developing countries (WHO, 2005).

Millions of elderly people across the globe are not getting the oral health care they need because governments are not aware enough of the problem. By 2025, there will about 1200 million people aged 65 years according to UN estimates. Failure to address oral health needs today could develop into a costly problem tomorrow. Although the poor are more vulnerable to this and other problems, the oral health problems of the elderly cross class lines. Low awareness, lack of access to oral health services, and the misconception that older people will not benefit from health education and preventive measures such as fluoridation, conspire to deprive the elderly of crucial care.

Oral disease is the fourth most expensive ailment to treat in most industrialized countries, according to WHO's World Oral Health Report 2003. The burden of oral disease is likely to grow in many developing countries because of unhealthy diets rich in sugars and high consumption of tobacco according to WHO experts. Industrialized countries spend 5 to 10% of their national public health resources on dental care a year, but most developing countries allocate no budget at all for the control of oral disease (WHO Oral Health, 2005).

Healthy People and Oral Health

One of the *Healthy People 2010* objectives is to reduce the proportion of young children, adolescents and adults with untreated dental decay in permanent teeth. The goals of objective 21-2 are to reduce this proportion to no more than 21% of children and 15% of adolescents and adults. Cavities are holes in our teeth created by the wear, tear, and decay of tooth enamel. Dental cavities have been repaired or filled with a variety of materials throughout history, including stone chips, turpentine resin, gum, and metals. In the practice of dentistry, the dentist, along with the dental hygienist and dental technologists, work within primary, secondary, and tertiary prevention areas to reduce the proportion of people with untreated dental decay. As oral health becomes an essential, recognized factor in America's public health agenda, the importance of dental healthcare team members grows.

Diversity in Dentistry

Dentistry is the practical application of the knowledge of dental science (the science of placement, arrangement, and function of teeth and their supporting bones and soft tissues) to human beings. A dentist is a professional practitioner of dentistry. Dentists maintain the health of teeth, gums, and other tissues of the oral cavity through prevention, diagnosis, and treatment of oral diseases and disorders. They remove decay, fill cavities, examine x-rays, place protective plastic sealants on children's teeth, straighten teeth, and repair fractured teeth. They also perform corrective surgery on gums and supporting bones to treat gum diseases. Dentists extract teeth and make models and measurements for dentures to replace missing teeth. A dentist may administer anesthetics and write prescriptions for antibiotics and other medications. Dentistry requires diagnostic ability and manual skills. Dentists provide instruction on diet, brushing, flossing, the use of fluorides, and other aspects of oral hygiene. Dental care will continue to focus more on prevention in the future, including teaching people how to take better care of their teeth. Dentists will increasingly provide care aimed at preventing the loss of teeth—rather than simply providing treatments, such as fillings. Improvements in dental technology also allow dentists to offer more effective and less painful treatment to their patients.

Dentists should have good visual memory, excellent judgment regarding space and shape, a high degree of manual dexterity, and scientific ability. In addition to the actual skills required to practice dentistry, many dentists working in private practice also oversee a variety of administrative tasks, including bookkeeping and buying equipment and supplies. They may employ and supervise dental hygienists, dental assistants, dental laboratory technicians, and receptionists. Good business sense, self-discipline, and good communication skills are helpful for success in private dental practice.

The majority of dentists are general practitioners, handling a variety of dental needs. Others practice in any of nine specialty areas recognized by the American Dental Association.

Orthodontists, the largest group of specialists, straighten teeth by applying pressure to the teeth with braces or retainers. Orthodontic treatment can be carried out for purely aesthetic reasons—improving the general appearance of patients' teeth for cosmetic reasons—but treatment is often prescribed for practical reasons, providing the patient with a functionally improved bite (bringing the opposing surfaces of the teeth of the two jaws into contact or occlusion) and/or muscle comfort.

The next largest group, *oral and maxillofacial surgeons*, operate on the mouth and jaws, typically performing dental extractions and facial surgery. Historically, dental extractions have been used to treat a variety of illnesses. Before the discovery of antibiotics, chronic tooth infections created a variety of health problems, and therefore removal of a diseased tooth was a common treatment for various medical conditions. Instruments used for dental extractions date back several centuries. Today, maxillofacial surgery is done as a treatment, but also for improving function and appearance. The remainder of dentists may specialize in a variety of areas. Specialists in all of these fields must satisfy certain local and national (US "Board Certified") registry requirements.

Pediatric dentists are the pediatricians of dentistry. A pediatric dentist has two to three years specialty training following dental school and limits his/her practice to treating children. Pediatric dentists are primary and specialty oral care providers for infants and children through adolescence, including those with special health needs. According to the American Academy of Pediatric Dentistry, the pediatric dental community is continually doing research to develop new techniques for preventing dental decay and other forms of oral disease. Studies show that children with poor oral health have decreased school performance, poor social relationships, and less success later in life. Children experiencing pain from decayed teeth are distracted and unable to concentrate on schoolwork.

Periodontists treat the gums and bone supporting the teeth. Periodontics is the study of clinical aspects of the supporting structures of the teeth, including the gingiva, alveolar (jaw) bone, root cementum, and the periodontal ligament, in health and disease. Periodontal disease takes on many different forms, but is usually considered to be a chronic, bacterial infection of the gums. Untreated, it often leads to tooth loss and alveolar bone loss.

Prosthodontists specialize in the diagnosis and treatment of complex oral-related disease and conditions. Prosthodontics requires three to four years of additional formal training in an American Dental Association (ADA) approved program. Specialty programs consist of extensive training in head and neck anatomy, preservation and restoration of oral health, materials science, esthetic tooth replacement, TMD-related disorders, traumatic injury to facial structures, sleep disorders, and the restoration of the jaws and teeth after treatment for head and neck cancer. Maxillofacial prosthodontics is a subspecialty in which additional training has been pursued for treatment and restoration of missing head and neck structures such as ears, eyes, and nose by prosthetic means.

Endodontics is a subspecialty of dentistry, that deals with the tooth pulp or dentine complex. The most common procedure done in endodontics is root-canal therapy. The root canal is the hollow area at the center of a tooth. In dentistry, a pulpectomy is an endodontic treatment to cure an infection of the root canal; informally, a *root canal*. For patients, root canal therapy is one of the most feared procedures in all of dentistry; contrary to popular belief, however, root canal treatment is usually painless due to effective pain control techniques used by the dentist while the treatment is being performed and the (optional) use of pain control medication after treatment.

Public health dentists work to promote good dental health and prevent dental diseases within the community. Public health dentists study dental epidemiology and social health policies. They may treat patients within the public healthcare system such as prisons or Indian Health Services (see Chapter 18 on Public Health for more information).

Oral pathologists study oral diseases. Oral pathology, also known in the United States as *oral and maxillofacial pathology,* is the specialty of dentistry and pathology which deals with the nature, identification, and management of diseases affecting the oral and maxillofacial regions. It is a science that investigates the causes, processes, and effects of these diseases. The practice of oral and maxillofacial pathology includes research and diagnosis of diseases using clinical, radiographic, microscopic, biochemical, or other examinations, and in many instances involves the management of patients. *Oral and maxillofacial radiologists* diagnose diseases in the head and neck using imaging technologies.

Other dental education exists where no post-graduate formal university training is required: cosmetic dentistry, dental implant therapy, and temporal-mandibular joint therapy. These usually require attendance at additional training courses. There are restrictions on allowing these dentists to call themselves specialists in these fields. The specialist titles are registrable titles and controlled by the local dental-licensing bodies. While not a recognized specialty, some dentists spend additional time learning the science of forensic odontology, consisting of the gathering and use of dental evidence in law. Any dentist with experience or training in this field may perform this function. The role of the forensic dentist is primarily documentation and verification of identity, often of victims of a crime.

Employment of Dentists

Most dentists work four or five days a week. Some work evenings and weekends to meet their patients' needs. Most full-time dentists work between 35 and 40 hours a week, but others work more. Initially, dentists may work more hours as they establish their practice. Experienced dentists often work fewer hours. A considerable number continue in part-time practice well beyond the usual retirement age. Most dentists are solo practitioners, meaning that they own their own businesses and work alone or with a small staff. Some dentists have partners, and a few work for other dentists as associate dentists.

According to the Bureau of Labor Statistics, dentists held about 153,000 jobs in 2002. About two in five dentists were self-employed. A major portion of dentists work in private practice. Approximately 80% of dentists in private practice are sole proprietors, and 13% belong to a partnership. A small number of salaried dentists work in hospitals and offices of physicians (BLS, Dentist).

All 50 states and the District of Columbia require licensure for dentists. To qualify for a license in most states, a candidate must graduate from one of the 55 dental schools accredited by the ADA's Commission on Dental Accreditation in 2002 and they must pass written and practical examinations involving treatment on actual patients. Candidates may fulfill the written part of the state licensing requirements by passing the National Board Dental Examinations. Individual states or regional testing agencies administer the written or practical examinations. Many states require varying amounts of continuing education to keep dental certifications current.

Job prospects should be good as new dentists take over established practices or start their own. Demand for dental care overall should grow substantially through 2012. As members of the baby-boom generation advance into middle age, a large number will need maintenance on complicated dental work, such as bridges. In addition, elderly people are more likely to retain their teeth than were their predecessors, so they will require much more care than in the past. The younger generation will continue to need preventive checkups despite treatments such as fluoridation of the water supply and sealants, which decrease the incidence of tooth decay. However, employment of dentists is not expected to grow as rapidly as the demand for dental services, because, as their practices expand, dentists are likely to hire more dental hygienists and dental assistants to handle routine services.

The median annual earnings of salaried dentists were $123,210 in 2002. Earnings vary according to number of years in practice, location, hours worked, and specialty. Self-employed dentists in private practice tend to earn more than salaried dentists. A relatively large proportion of dentists are self-employed. Like other business owners, these dentists must provide their own health insurance, life insurance, liability insurance, and retirement benefits.

Becoming a Dentist

Dental schools require a minimum of two years of college-level pre-dental education, regardless of the major chosen. Only a small number of applicants enter dental school after two or three years of college and complete their bachelor's degree while attending dental school. However, most dental students have at least a bachelor's degree. Pre-dental education emphasizes course work in science, and many applicants to dental school major in a science such as biology or chemistry, while other applicants major in another subject and take many science courses as well. All dental schools require applicants to take the Dental Admissions Test (DAT). The Dental Admissions Test is a standardized, multiple-choice exam required by all dental schools. It covers the following areas:

- Knowledge of natural sciences (biology, general chemistry, organic chemistry)
- Perceptual ability (two- and three-dimensional problem-solving: angle discrimination, form development, cubes, orthographic projections, apertures, and paper folding)
- Reading comprehension (basic sciences and dental)
- Quantitative reasoning (algebraic equations, fractions, conversions, percentages, exponential notation, probability and statistics, geometry, trigonometry, and applied mathematics problems)

When selecting students, schools consider scores earned on the DAT, applicants' grade point averages, and information gathered through recommendations and interviews. Competition for admission to dental school is keen. According to the ADA, which administers the DAT, applicants can take the test after completing at least one year of college and the aforementioned science courses. Many students take the test their junior year. The computer-administered test scores are valid for 12 months.

Like other health professional graduate education programs, the ADA sponsors the American Association of Dental Schools Application Service (AADSAS). The AADSAS is a centralized application service that allows applicants to submit one application form (including a personal essay and transcripts) to the AADSAS, which forwards the information in a standardized format to the dental schools indicated on the application. Fifty of fifty-five US dental schools participate in AADSAS. Students wishing to apply to one of the five non-AADSAS schools, requesting advanced standing, transferring from another school, applying for a combined degree program, or enrolling as a foreign student need to contact their chosen school directly for application details.

Dental school usually lasts four academic years. Studies begin with classroom instruction and laboratory work in basic sciences, including anatomy, microbiology, biochemistry, and physiology. Beginning courses in clinical sciences, including laboratory techniques, also are provided at this time. During the last two years, students treat patients, usually in dental clinics, under the supervision of licensed dentists. Most dental schools award the degree of Doc-tor of Dental Surgery (DDS). The rest award an equivalent degree, Doctor of Dental Medicine (DMD). Either the DDS or DMD degree is required to become a dentist. Despite the difference in name, they are equivalent degrees. Both use the same curriculum requirements set by the American Dental Asso-ciation's Commission on Dental Accreditation. Most dentists go through eight years of schooling—four years of undergraduate education and four years of dental school—to become a general practitioner. Some dental school gradu-ates continue their clinical training for an additional one to two years through a General Practice Residency (GPR) or an Advanced Education in General Dentistry (AEGD). Those pursuing one of the specialties in dentistry will have an additional one to four years of schooling.

What Is a General Practice Residency (GPR)?

A GPR offers post-doctoral students more advanced instruction and clinical training in general dentistry—particularly with intensive hospital experi-ence. GPR residents provide care for a wide range of ambulatory and hospi-talized patients. General practice residents also rotate through different areas of service, including general medicine, general surgery, and anesthesiology. The training and experience offered through a GPR enables dentists to obtain privileges at local hospitals once they are in private practice. Like AEGD programs, GPR programs also involve advanced training in preventive den-tistry, periodontics, restorative dentistry, endodontics, and oral surgery. Although training in orthodontics and pediatric dentistry is desirable, it is not mandatory for GPR programs. The GPR program is usually one or two years in length. A GPR leads to a post-graduate certificate.

What Is an Advanced Education in General Dentistry (AEGD)?

An AEGD is designed for graduates who are interested in becoming general practitioners and improving their scientific knowledge and clinical skills in diagnosis, treatment planning, and decision-making during treatment. The AEGD program involves advanced training in preventive dentistry as well as specialty areas such as periodontics, restorative dentistry, endodontics, oral surgery, orthodontics, and pediatric dentistry. This experience prepares grad-uates to provide a full range of general dental care and refer patients to the appropriate specialists when necessary. The AEGD program also offers more hands-on experience in managing a practice. It is usually one year, with an optional second year, and leads to a post-graduate certificate.

What Is the Difference Between the AEGD and the GPR Programs?

The major difference between the AEGD and GPR programs is the emphasis that the AEGD program places on clinical dentistry compared to the emphasis on medical management in the GPR program. Also, AEGD programs generally do not have affiliations with hospitals, whereas all GPR programs are sponsored by a hospital or a hospital-affiliated institution such as a dental school or Veterans Administration facility.

Currently, about 17 states license or certify dentists who intend to practice in a specialty area. Requirements include two to four years of post-graduate education and, in some cases, the completion of a special state examination. Most state licenses permit dentists to engage in both general and specialized practice. Dentists who want to teach or conduct research usually spend an additional two to five years in advanced dental training, in programs operated by dental schools or hospitals. According to the American Dental Association (ADA), each year about 12% of new graduates enroll in postgraduate training programs to prepare for a dental specialty.

Additional Resources for Dentistry

Persons interested in practicing dentistry should obtain the requirements for licensure from the board of dental examiners of the state in which they plan to work. For information on dentistry as a career and a list of accredited dental schools, as well as a list of state boards of dental examiners, contact

> American Dental Association, Commission on Dental Accreditation
> 211 E. Chicago Ave.
> Chicago, IL 60611
> Phone: 312-440-2500
> Internet: http://www.ada.org

> Academy of General Dentistry
> 211 East Chicago Ave., Suite 900
> Chicago, IL 60611-1999
> Phone: 888.AGD.DENT (888.243.3368)
> Internet: http://www.agd.org/

American Academy of Pediatric Dentistry
211 East Chicago Avenue, Suite 700
Chicago, IL 60611-2663
Phone: (312) 337-2169
Internet: http://www.aapd.org/

American Dental Association
211 East Chicago Ave.
Chicago, IL 60611-2678
Phone: 312-440-2500
Internet: http://www.ada.org/

American Student Dental Association
211 E. Chicago Ave., Suite 1160
Chicago, IL 60611-2687
Phone: (800) 621-8099, ext. 2795 or 312-440-2795 (direct)
Internet: http://www.asdanet.org/

For information on admission to dental schools, contact:

American Dental Education Association
1400 K Street, NW, Suite 1100
Washington, DC 20005
Phone: 202-289-7201
Internet: www.adea.org

Dental Hygienists

A *dental hygienist* is a licensed dental professional who specializes in preventive care. Some hygienists are licensed to administer local anesthesia, depending on the applicable regulations in their area. Dental hygienists remove soft and hard deposits from teeth, instruct patients how to practice good oral hygiene, and provide other preventive dental care. Hygienists examine patients' teeth and gums, recording the presence of diseases or abnormalities. They remove calculus, stains, and plaque from teeth; perform root planing as a periodontal therapy; take and develop dental x-rays; and apply cavity-preventive agents such as fluorides and pit and fissure sealants. In some states, hygienists administer anesthetics; place and carve filling materials, temporary fillings, and periodontal dressings; remove sutures; and smooth and polish metal restorations. Although hygienists may not diagnose diseases, they can prepare clinical and laboratory diagnostic tests for the dentist to interpret. Hygienists sometimes work chair-side with the dentist during treatment. Dental hygienists also help patients develop and maintain good oral health. For example, they may explain the relationship between diet and oral health or inform patients how to select toothbrushes and show them how to brush and floss their teeth. Dental hygienists use hand and rotary instruments and ultrasonics to clean and polish teeth, x-ray machines to take dental radiographs, syringes with needles to administer local anesthetics, and models of teeth to explain oral hygiene. Dental hygienists should work well with others and must have good manual dexterity, because they use dental instruments within a patient's mouth, with little room for error.

Flexible scheduling is a distinctive feature of this job. Full-time, part-time, evening, and weekend schedules are widely available. Important health safeguards include strict adherence to proper radiological procedures, and the proper use of appropriate protective devices such as safety glasses, surgical masks, and gloves to protect themselves and patients from infectious diseases.

Dental hygienists must be licensed by the state in which they practice. To qualify for licensure, a candidate must graduate from an accredited dental hygiene school and pass both a written and clinical examination. The American Dental Association Joint Commission on National Dental Examinations administers the written examination, which is accepted by all states and the District of Columbia. State or regional testing agencies administer the clinical examination. In addition, most states require an examination on the legal aspects of dental hygiene practice.

In 2002, the Commission on Dental Accreditation accredited about 265 programs in dental hygiene. Most dental hygiene programs grant an associate degree, although some also offer a certificate, a bachelor's degree, or a master's degree. A minimum of an associate degree or certificate in dental hygiene is required for practice in a private dental office. A bachelor's or master's degree usually is required for research, teaching, or clinical practice in public or school health programs. About half of the dental hygiene programs prefer applicants who have completed at least one year of college. However, requirements vary from one school to another. Schools offer laboratory, clinical, and classroom instruction in subjects such as anatomy, physiology, chemistry, microbiology, pharmacology, nutrition, radiography, histology (the study of tissue structure), periodontology (the study of gum diseases), pathology, dental materials, clinical dental hygiene, and social and behavioral sciences.

Dental hygienists held about 148,000 jobs in 2002 (BLS, Dental Hygienists). Because multiple jobholding is common in this field, the number of jobs exceeds the number of hygienists. More than half of all dental hygienists worked part-time—fewer than 35 hours a week. Almost all jobs for dental hygienists were in dentists' offices. A very small number worked for employment services or in the offices of physicians.

Employment of dental hygienists is growing much faster than the average for all occupations through 2012, in response to increasing demand for dental care and the greater utilization of hygienists to perform services previously performed by dentists. While many states have restrictions as to how many hygienists each dentist can employ, job prospects are expected to remain excellent. In fact, the Bureau of Labor Statistics expects dental hygienists to be one of the fastest growing occupations through the year 2012.

Population growth and greater retention of natural teeth will continue to stimulate demand for dental hygienists. Older dentists, who have been less likely to employ dental hygienists, are leaving the occupation and the recent graduates taking over their practices are more likely to employ one or even two hygienists. In addition, as dentists' workloads increase, they are likely to hire more hygienists to perform preventive dental care, such as cleaning, so that they may devote their own time to more profitable procedures.

Earnings vary by geographic location, employment setting, and years of experience. Dental hygienists may be paid on an hourly, daily, salary, or commission basis. Median hourly earnings of dental hygienists were $26.59 in 2002. The middle 50% earned between $21.96 and $32.48 an hour. The lowest 10% earned less than $17.34, and the highest 10% earned more than $39.24 an hour. Benefits vary substantially by practice setting and may be contingent upon full-time employment. According to the American Dental Association, almost all full-time dental hygienists employed by private practitioners received paid vacation. The ADA also found that 9 out of 10 full-time and part-time dental hygienists received dental coverage. Dental hygienists who work for school systems, public health agencies, the federal government, or state agencies usually have substantial benefits.

Additional Resources for Dental Hygienists

For information on a career in dental hygiene, including educational requirements, contact

> Division of Education, American Dental Hygienists' Association
> 444 N. Michigan Ave., Suite 3400
> Chicago, IL 60611
> Internet: http://www.adha.org

For information about accredited programs and educational requirements, contact:

Commission on Dental Accreditation, American Dental Association
211 E. Chicago Ave., Suite 1814
Chicago, IL 60611
Internet: http://www.ada.org

American Dental Hygienists' Association
444 North Michigan Avenue, Suite 3400
Chicago, IL 60611
Phone: (312) 440-8900
Internet: http://www.adha.org/

Dental Technicians

A *dental technician* is part of the dental team who fabricates dental appliances, dentures, crown and bridgework, and other prosthetic devices such as mouth guards and splints. The technician will be skilled in working with gold, precious metals, dental porcelain, acrylics, and, recently CAD/CAM (the combination of computer-aided design and computer-aided manufacturing) software, in order to custom manufacture devices that will exactly fit a patient. The profession attracts artistic, detail-oriented individuals who have a flare for this unique combination of science, art, and digital dexterity.

Dentists send a specification of the item to be manufactured, along with an impression (mold) of the patient's mouth or teeth. The dental technician creates a model of the patient's mouth by pouring plaster into the impression and allowing it to set. The model serves as the basis of the prosthetic device. Technicians examine the model, noting the size and shape of the adjacent teeth, as well as gaps within the gum line. Based upon these observations and the dentist's specifications, technicians build and shape a nearly exact replica of the lost tooth or teeth. Dental laboratory technicians can specialize in five areas: orthodontic appliances, crowns and bridges, complete dentures, partial dentures, or ceramics. The work is extremely delicate and time consuming. Salaried technicians usually work 40 hours a week, but self-employed technicians frequently work longer hours.

Dental laboratory technicians held about 47,000 jobs in 2002 (BLS, Dental Technician). Around 7 out of 10 technician positions were in medical equipment and supply manufacturing laboratories, which usually are small, privately owned businesses with fewer than five employees. However, some laboratories are large; a few employ more than 50 technicians. Some dental laboratory technicians work in offices of dentists. Others work for hospitals providing dental services, including US Department of Veterans Affairs hospitals. Some technicians work in dental laboratories in their homes, in addition to their regular job.

Most dental laboratory technicians learn their craft on the job. Becoming a fully trained technician requires an average of three to four years, depending upon the individual's aptitude and ambition, but it may take a few years more to become an accomplished technician. Training in dental laboratory technology also is available through community and junior colleges, vocational-technical institutes, and the US Armed Forces. Formal training programs vary greatly both in length and in the level of skill they impart.

In 2002, the Commission on Dental Accreditation in conjunction with the American Dental Association (ADA) approved 25 programs in dental laboratory technology. These programs provide classroom instruction in dental materials science, oral anatomy, fabrication procedures, ethics, and related subjects. In addition, each student receives supervised practical experience in a school or an associated dental laboratory. Accredited programs normally take two years to complete and lead to an associate degree. A few programs take about four years to complete and offer a bachelor's degree in dental technology. Graduates of two-year training programs need additional hands-on experience to become fully qualified. Each dental laboratory owner operates in a different way, and classroom instruction does not necessarily expose students to techniques and procedures favored by individual laboratory owners. The National Board for Certification, an independent board established by the National Association of Dental Laboratories, offers certification in dental laboratory technology.

A high degree of manual dexterity, good vision, and the ability to recognize very fine color shadings and variations in shape are necessary. An artistic aptitude for detailed and precise work also is important. High school students interested in becoming dental laboratory technicians should take courses in art, metal and wood shop, drafting, and sciences. Courses in management and business may help those wishing to operate their own laboratories.

In large dental laboratories, technicians may become supervisors or managers. Experienced technicians may teach or may take jobs with dental suppliers in such areas as product development, marketing, and sales. Still, for most technicians, opening one's own laboratory is the way toward advancement and higher earnings.

Median hourly earnings of dental laboratory technicians were $13.70 in 2002. The middle 50% earned between $10.51 and $18.40 an hour. The lowest 10% earned less than $8.16, and the highest 10% earned more than $23.65 an hour. Median hourly earnings of dental laboratory technicians in 2002 were $13.78 in medical equipment and supplies manufacturing firms and $12.98 in the offices of dentists. Technicians in large laboratories tend to specialize in a few procedures, and, therefore, tend to be paid a lower wage than those employed in small laboratories who perform a variety of tasks.

For a list of accredited programs in dental laboratory technology, contact

Commission on Dental Accreditation
American Dental Association
211 E. Chicago Ave., Chicago, IL 60611
Internet: http://www.ada.org

For information on requirements for certification, contact

National Board for Certification in Dental Technology
325 John Knox Rd. #L103
Tallahassee, FL 32303
Internet: http://www.nbccert.org

For information on career opportunities in commercial laboratories, contact

National Association of Dental Laboratories
1530 Metropolitan Blvd.
Tallahassee, FL 32308
Internet: http://www.nadl.org

General information on grants and scholarships is available from dental technology schools.

Dental Assistants

Dental assistants perform a variety of patient care, office, and laboratory duties. They work chair-side as dentists examine and treat patients in situations sometimes referred to as "Four-Handed Dentistry." They make patients as comfortable as possible in the dental chair, prepare them for treatment, and obtain their dental records. Assistants hand instruments and materials to dentists and keep patients' mouths dry and clear by using suction or other devices. Assistants also sterilize and disinfect instruments and equipment, prepare trays of instruments for dental procedures, and instruct patients on postoperative and general oral health care. Some dental assistants prepare materials for impressions and restorations, take dental x-rays, and process x-ray film as directed by a dentist. They also may remove sutures, apply topical anesthetics to gums or cavity-preventive agents to teeth, remove excess cement used in the filling process, and place rubber dams on the teeth to isolate them for individual treatment.

Those dental assistants with laboratory duties make casts of the teeth and mouth from impressions, clean and polish removable appliances, and make temporary crowns. Dental assistants with office duties schedule and confirm appointments, receive patients, keep treatment records, send bills, receive payments, and order dental supplies and materials. About half of dental assistants have a 35- to 40-hour workweek, which may include work on Saturdays or evenings.

Dental assistants held about 266,000 jobs in 2002. Almost all jobs for dental assistants were in offices of dentists. A small number of jobs were in offices of physicians, educational services, and hospitals. About a third of dental assistants worked part-time, sometimes in more than one dental office.

Most assistants learn their skills on the job, although an increasing number are trained in dental-assisting programs offered by community and junior colleges, trade schools, technical institutes, or the Armed Forces. Assistants must be a second pair of hands for a dentist; therefore, dentists look for people who are reliable, can work well with others, and have good manual dexterity. High school students interested in a career as a dental assistant should take courses in biology, chemistry, health, and office practices.

The American Dental Association's Commission on Dental Accreditation approved 259 dental-assisting training programs in 2002. Programs include classroom, laboratory, and preclinical instruction in dental-assisting skills and related theory. In addition, students gain practical experience in dental schools, clinics, or dental offices. Most programs take one year or less to complete and lead to a certificate or diploma. Two-year programs offered in community and junior colleges lead to an associate degree. All programs require a high school diploma or its equivalent, and some require science or computer-related courses for admission. A number of private vocational schools offer four to six month courses in dental assisting, but the Commission on Dental Accreditation does not accredit these programs.

Most states regulate the duties that dental assistants perform through licensure or registration. Licensure or registration may require passing a written or practical examination. States offering licensure or registration have a variety of schools offering courses—approximately 10 to 12 months in length—that meet their state's requirements. Many states require continuing education to maintain licensure or registration. A few states allow dental assistants to perform any function delegated to them by the dentist. Individual states have adopted different standards for dental assistants who perform certain advanced duties, such as radiological procedures. The completion of the Radiation Health and Safety examination offered by the Dental Assisting National Board (DANB) meets those standards in more than 30 states. Some states require the completion of a state-approved course in radiology as well.

Certification is available through DANB and is recognized or required in more than 30 states. Other organizations offer registration, most often at the state level. Certification is an acknowledgment of an assistant's qualifications and professional competence and may be an asset when one is seeking employment. Candidates may qualify to take the DANB certification examination by graduating from an accredited training program or by having two years of full-time, or four years of part-time, experience as a dental assistant. In addition, applicants must have current certification in cardiopulmonary resuscitation. For annual recertification, individuals must earn continuing education credits.

Without further education, advancement opportunities are limited. Some dental assistants become office managers, dental-assisting instructors, or dental product sales representatives. Others go back to school to become dental hygienists. For many, this entry-level occupation provides basic training and experience and serves as a stepping-stone to more highly skilled and higher paying jobs.

Job prospects for dental assistants should be excellent. Employment is expected to grow much faster than the average for all occupations through the year 2012. In fact, dental assistants are expected to be one of the fastest growing occupations through the year 2012. In addition to job openings due to employment growth, numerous job openings will arise out of the need to replace assistants who transfer to other occupations, retire, or leave the labor force for other reasons. Many opportunities are for entry-level positions offering on-the-job training.

Median hourly earnings of dental assistants were $13.10 in 2002. The middle 50% earned between $10.35 and $16.20 an hour. The lowest 10% earned less than $8.45, and the highest 10% earned more than $19.41 an hour. Benefits vary substantially by practice setting and may be contingent upon full-time employment. According to the American Dental Association, almost all full-time dental assistants employed by private practitioners received paid vacation time. The ADA also found that 9 out of 10 full-time and part-time dental assistants received dental coverage.

Additional Resources for Dental Assistants

Information about career opportunities and accredited dental assistant programs is available from

> Commission on Dental Accreditation
> American Dental Association
> 211 E. Chicago Ave., Suite 1814
> Chicago, IL 60611
> Internet: http://www.ada.org

For information on becoming a Certified Dental Assistant and a list of State boards of dentistry, contact:

> Dental Assisting National Board, Inc.
> 676 North Saint Clair, Suite 1880
> Chicago, IL 60611
> Internet: http://www.danb.org

For more information on a career as a dental assistant and general information about continuing education, contact:

> American Dental Assistants Association
> 35 East Wacker Drive, Suite 1730
> Chicago, IL 60601
> Internet: http://www.dentalassistant.org

For more information about continuing education courses, contact:

> National Association of Dental Assistants
> 900 S. Washington Street, Suite G-13
> Falls Church, VA 22046

SUMMARY

Dental professions are as wide as the smiles the professionals treat. Applying the knowledge of dental science, dentists may specialize in a variety of areas: oral and maxillofacial surgery, pediatric dentistry, periodontics, endodontics, public health dentistry, oral pathology, and radiology. Teeth are essential components to overall health, as they impact nutrition as well as speech. Maintaining good oral health is an important part of improving quality of life for individuals throughout their lifespan, the overarching goal of *Healthy People 2010* objectives.

ACKNOWLEDGEMENTS

Special thanks to Douglas Wright, DDS and staff, Harrisonburg, VA.

REFERENCES

Bureau of Labor Statistics, US Department of Labor, *Occupational Outlook Handbook, 2004–05 Edition*, Dentists, on the Internet at http://www.bls.gov/oco/ocos072.htm (visited September 07, 2005).

Bureau of Labor Statistics, US Department of Labor, *Occupational Outlook Handbook, 2004–05 Edition*, Dental Hygienists, on the Internet at http://www.bls.gov/oco/ocos097.htm (visited September 07, 2005).

Bureau of Labor Statistics, US Department of Labor, *Occupational Outlook Handbook, 2004–05 Edition*, Dental Laboratory Technicians, on the Internet at http://www.bls.gov/oco/ocos238.htm (visited September 07, 2005).

Bureau of Labor Statistics, US Department of Labor, *Occupational Outlook Handbook, 2004–05 Edition*, Dental Assistants, on the Internet at http://www.bls.gov/oco/ocos163.htm (visited September 07, 2005).

World Health Organization (WHO). (2005, September). Special theme: Oral health *Bulletin of the World Health Organization, 83*(9).

Chapter 11

Pharmacy

Stephanie Chisolm

OBJECTIVES

After studying this chapter, the student should be able to

1. Explain the role of the pharmacist in the healthcare system.
2. Describe the difference between a pharmacist and the pharmacy technician and aides.
3. Describe the educational preparation and certification required to become a pharmacist.
4. Identify the various healthcare environments where pharmacists may be employed.
5. Identify resources for additional information on the role of pharmacists.

INTRODUCTION

> *The desire to take medicine is perhaps the greatest*
> *feature which distinguishes man from animals.*
> Sir William Osler (1849–1919),
> In H. Cushing, *Life of Sir William Osler* (1925)

Pharmacy is the art, practice, or profession of preparing, preserving, compounding, and dispensing drugs. A *pharmacist* is a person licensed to engage in pharmacy. Pharmacists dispense drugs prescribed by physicians and other health practitioners and provide information to patients about medications and their use. They advise healthcare providers on the selection, dosages, interactions, and side effects of medications. Pharmacists also monitor the health and progress of patients in response to drug therapy to ensure safe and effective use of medication. Pharmacists must understand the use, clinical effects, and composition of drugs, including their chemical, biological, and physical properties.

American Pharmacists

In early colonial days, the community apothecary would use a variety of herbs and substances to compound medications for individuals. Compounding—the actual mixing of ingredients to form powders, tablets, capsules, ointments, and solutions—is a small part of the pharmacist's practice today, because most medicines are produced by pharmaceutical companies in a standard dosage and drug delivery form.

Like the apothecary of colonial America, most pharmacists work in a community setting. Today, this includes the retail drugstore, a healthcare facility, such as a hospital, nursing home, mental health institution, or a neighborhood health clinic. Pharmacists counsel patients and answer questions about prescription and over-the-counter drugs, including questions regarding possible side effects or interactions among various drugs. They also may give advice about diet, exercise, or stress management, or about durable medical equipment and home healthcare supplies. A recent study of patient counseling provided in community pharmacies found that the amount and quality of counseling varied significantly according to the state regulations requiring patient counseling, the business of the pharmacy, and even the age of the pharmacist, with younger pharmacists offering more counseling (Svarstad, Bultman, & Mount, 2004). In a consumer survey, providing printed materials, explanations of how medications work, and possible side effects, were viewed as important services provided by pharmacists (LoBuono, 2002).

The Role of the Pharmacist

Pharmacists also may complete third-party insurance forms and other paperwork. Those who own or manage community pharmacies may sell non-health-related merchandise, hire and supervise personnel, and oversee the general operation of the pharmacy. Some community pharmacists provide specialized services to help patients manage conditions such as diabetes, asthma, smoking cessation, or high blood pressure. A growing number of community pharmacists have certification to administer vaccinations in their businesses.

Pharmacists in healthcare facilities dispense medications, may make sterile solutions and purchase medical supplies, and also assess, plan, and monitor drug programs or regimens. Pharmacists counsel patients on the use of drugs while in the hospital and on their use at home after discharge. Pharmacists may also evaluate the patterns and outcomes of drug/medication use for patients within hospitals or managed care organizations.

Clinical pharmacists are usually more directly involved in patient care than retail pharmacists. The average hospital-based clinical pharmacist makes rounds with doctors, suggests drug therapies, and monitors patient responses. If the patient has an adverse reaction to a drug, then it is the clinical pharmacist's responsibility to notify the doctor and suggest a better treatment. Clinical pharmacists also monitor dosages to make sure patients are getting enough—but not too much—of the drug therapy.

Pharmacists who work in home health care monitor drug therapy and prepare infusions—solutions injected into patients—and other medications for use in the home. Some pharmacists specialize in specific drug therapy areas, such as intravenous nutrition support, oncology (cancer), nuclear pharmacy (used for chemotherapy), geriatric pharmacy, and psychopharmacotherapy (the treatment of mental disorders with drugs).

Whatever the venue, more doors are opening for clinical pharmacists as healthcare providers increasingly rely on pharmacists to help manage growing patient loads, and insurance companies look to them to scrutinize drug expenses. The hours vary more than in the retail environment, but the pay is comparable and the satisfaction levels are higher for pharmacists who enjoy the challenge of the healthcare environment.

Most pharmacists keep confidential computerized records of patients' drug therapies to ensure that harmful drug interactions do not occur. Pharmacists are responsible for the accuracy of every prescription they fill, but they often rely upon *pharmacy technicians* and *pharmacy aides* to assist them in the dispensing process. Thus, the pharmacist may delegate prescription-filling and administrative tasks while supervising their completion. They also frequently oversee pharmacy students serving as interns in preparation for graduation and licensure.

Pharmacy Beyond the Corner Drug Store

Nontraditional pharmacy work includes research for pharmaceutical manufacturers, developing new drugs and therapies, and testing their effects on people. Other pharmacists work in marketing or sales, providing expertise to clients (healthcare practitioners) on a drug's use, effectiveness, and possible side effects. Some pharmacists also work for health insurance companies, developing pharmacy benefit packages and carrying out cost-benefit analyses on certain drugs. Other pharmacists work for the government and pharmacy associations.

Finally, some pharmacists are employed full-time or part-time as college faculty, teaching classes and performing research in a wide range of areas.

Pharmacogenomics is having an ever-increasing impact on drug discovery and development. Pharmacogenomics refers to the use of techniques to describe the inherited factors influencing drug concentrations and/or effects among individuals or populations. Absorption, distribution, metabolism, elimination, and efficacy are subject to genetic variability. Defining which genetic determinants influence a given drug's effects, particularly those in clinical development, remains a challenge for the pharmaceutical industry. Pharmacogenomics is the field exploring these differences, providing new knowledge and tools to treat people on an individual basis known as "personalized" or "targeted medicine."

Current clinical trials do not commonly address inherent genetic variability, or statistically assess drug response as a function of genetic traits (Weinstein, 2005). However, recognizing the goal of "personalized medicine," the Food and Drug Administration has also launched a new Web site dedicated to this topic (www.fda.gov/cder/genomics). From a therapeutic perspective, this evolving knowledge of pharmacogenomics affords clinicians novel insight into a patient's unique biochemical makeup. Diagnostic genetic information will help predict not only a patient's drug response, but also the likelihood of interactions and adverse effects—enabling true individualization of drug and dose selection.

Herceptin for the treatment of breast cancer is an example of targeted therapy. The drug is effective only in situations where the cancerous tissue carries a specific genetic marker. If that marker is not present, the patient receives no benefit from treatment and is exposed to unnecessary potential risk associated with drug treatment (FDA, 2005). Pharmacogenomics allows us to identify sources of an individual's profile of drug response and predict the best possible treatment option for this individual. The use of genomic information, accelerated by the sequencing of the human genome and the advent of new tools and technologies, has opened new possibilities in drug discovery and development. With the implementation of the Health Insurance Portability and Accountability Act (HIPAA) of 1996 (see Chapter 4), one aspect of this genetic awareness often overlooked in our quest for knowledge is the ethical consequence of this patient-sensitive information (FDA, 2005).

New opportunities are emerging for pharmacists in managed-care organizations, where they may analyze trends and patterns in medication use for their populations of patients, and for pharmacists trained in research, disease management, and pharmacoeconomics—determining the costs and benefits of different drug therapies. Pharmacists also will have opportunities to work in research and development, as well as sales and marketing for pharmaceutical manufacturing firms. New breakthroughs in biotechnology will increase the potential for drugs to treat diseases and expand the opportunities for pharmacists to conduct research and sell medications.

Job opportunities for pharmacists in patient care will rise as cost-conscious insurers and health systems continue to emphasize the role of pharmacists in primary and preventive health services. Health insurance companies realize that the expense of using medication to treat diseases and various health conditions often is considerably less than the potential costs for patients whose conditions go untreated. Pharmacists also can reduce the expenses resulting from unexpected complications due to allergic reactions or medication interactions.

Education and Training to Become a Pharmacist:

Pharmacy programs grant the degree of Doctor of Pharmacy (Pharm.D.), which requires postsecondary study and the passing of the licensure examination of a state board of pharmacy. Pharmacy curricula begin with at least a year of concentrated study in the basic sciences (chemistry, anatomy, physiology, microbiology, etc.) followed by two years of pharmacology (the study of drug mechanisms of action), therapeutics (rational use of drugs) and pharmacokinetics (drug absorption, distribution, metabolism, excretion). Scattered across curricula are courses to teach students how to dispense prescriptions, communicate effectively with patients and other healthcare providers, and use medical literature to improve patient care. Students also learn professional ethics. In addition to classroom study, students receive in-depth exposure to and actively participate in a variety of pharmacy practice settings under the supervision of licensed pharmacists. The Pharm.D. degree has replaced the Bachelor of Pharmacy (B.Pharm.) degree, as of 2005.

The Pharm.D. is a four-year program that requires at least two years of college study prior to admittance, although most applicants have three years prior to entering the program. Entry requirements usually include courses in mathematics and natural sciences, such as chemistry, biology, and physics, as well as courses in the humanities and social sciences. Approximately half of all colleges require the applicant to take the Pharmacy College Admissions Test (PCAT).

In 2003, the American Association of Colleges of Pharmacy (AACP) launched the Pharmacy College Application Service, known as PharmCAS, for students interested in applying to schools and colleges of pharmacy. This centralized service allows applicants to use a single Web-based application and one set of transcripts to apply to multiple Pharm.D. degree programs (http://www.pharmcas.org).

According to the American Association of Colleges of Pharmacy's 2004 profile of pharmacy students, there were seven applications for every student slot in Fall 2004 in the nation's 89 pharmacy schools, with females submitting nearly two thirds of the applications (AACP, 2004). High interest in pharmacy is something of a double-edged sword. Up to 10 new schools of pharmacy will be open by 2010, and existing schools are expanding their own enrollments to meet the demand. More students means more pressure on schools to find qualified faculty and preceptor sites where students gain practical hands-on experience under the guidance of a licensed pharmacist.

Preparing for Pharmacy School

Prior to pharmacy school, undergraduate study should consist of mathematics and sciences such as biology, chemistry, and physics, as well as humanities and social sciences. Students need to pay close attention to the curriculum recommended by the college of pharmacy to which they intend to apply, in order to fulfill admissions requirements. In addition to being knowledgeable, a pharmacist will need to have good people skills. Prospective pharmacists should have scientific aptitude, good communication skills, and a desire to help others. They also must be conscientious and pay close attention to detail, because the decisions they make affect human lives.

Interest in pharmacy as a career remains high. In 2004, the nation's pharmacy schools reported a 54% jump in admission applications and awarded a record number of Pharm.D. degrees, according to an annual survey of the profession's educational landscape (Ukens, 2005). Other options for pharmacy graduates who are interested in further training include one- or two-year residency programs or fellowships. Pharmacy residencies are postgraduate training programs in pharmacy practice, and usually require the completion of a research study. Pharmacy fellowships are highly individualized programs designed to prepare participants to work in research careers. Some pharmacists who run their own pharmacies obtain a master's degree in business administration (MBA). Areas of graduate study include pharmaceutics (the study of the relationships between drug delivery, drug disposition and clinical response), and pharmaceutical chemistry (physical and chemical properties of drugs and dosage forms), pharmacology (effects of drugs on the body), and pharmacy administration.

After passing the licensure exam, pharmacists are ready to join the healthcare team in a variety of work settings. In community pharmacies, pharmacists usually begin at the staff level. In independent pharmacies, after they gain experience and secure the necessary capital, some become owners or part owners of pharmacies. Pharmacists in chain drugstores may be promoted to pharmacy supervisor or manager at the store level, then to manager at the district or regional level, and later to an executive position within the chain's headquarters. Hospital pharmacists may advance to supervisory or administrative positions. Pharmacists in the pharmaceutical industry may advance in marketing, sales, research, quality control, production, packaging, or other areas.

Career Opportunities in Pharmacy

Very good employment opportunities are expected for pharmacists over the 2002–2012 period because the number of degrees granted in pharmacy is expected to be less than the number of job openings created by employment growth and the need to replace pharmacists who retire or otherwise leave the occupation. Recently, enrollments in pharmacy programs are rising as high salaries and good job prospects attract more students. Despite this increase in enrollments, pharmacist jobs should still be more numerous than those seeking employment.

Pharmacy professions will grow faster than the average for all occupations through the year 2012, due to the increased pharmaceutical needs of a growing elderly population and increased use of medications. The growing numbers of middle-aged and elderly people, who typically use more prescription drugs, will continue to spur demand for pharmacists in all employment settings. Other factors likely to increase the demand for pharmacists include scientific advances that will make more drug products available, new developments in genome research and medication distribution systems, increasingly sophisticated consumers seeking more information about drugs, and coverage of prescription drugs by a greater number of health insurance plans and by Medicare.

The Work Environment

Pharmacists work in clean, well-lighted, and well-ventilated areas. Many pharmacists spend most of their workday on their feet. When working with sterile or potentially dangerous pharmaceutical products, pharmacists wear gloves and masks and work with other special protective equipment. While salaries for pharmacists are generally high, many community and hospital pharmacies are open for extended hours or around the clock, so pharmacists may work evenings, nights, weekends, and holidays. Consultant pharmacists may travel to nursing homes or other facilities to monitor patients' drug therapy.

According to the Bureau of Labor Statistics, pharmacists held about 230,000 jobs in 2002. About 62% work in community pharmacies that are either independently owned or part of a drugstore chain, grocery store, department store, or mass merchandiser. Most community pharmacists are salaried employees, but some are self-employed owners. About 22% of salaried pharmacists work in hospitals, and others work in clinics, mail-order or on-line pharmacies, pharmaceutical wholesalers, home healthcare agencies, or the federal government.

While their career options have broadened over the years, most pharmacists still work in either retail establishments or hospitals. *Retail pharmacists* prepare and dispense medications, advise customers about how to use medications and warn them about possible drug interactions. Retail pharmacists also consult with customers about over-the-counter medicines, conduct health screenings, administer immunizations, and address general healthcare issues.

Similarly, *hospital pharmacists* provide, prepare, and dispense medicines, special feeding solutions, and diagnostic agents. They may also consult with doctors about the correct dosage and appropriate form and time of administration and make physicians aware of any possible adverse reactions. Some hospital pharmacists now make patient rounds. Pharmacists who are employed by hospitals (25% of the profession), in clinics, and in HMOs dispense prescriptions and work as consultants to the medical team. They also make sterile solutions for use in the ER and in surgical procedures, purchase medical supplies, instruct interns, and perform administrative duties. Some in the hospital and medical field continue their education and conduct research into new medicines and areas of drug therapy, or specialize in certain drug therapies, for example, those used to treat psychiatric disorders.

Hospital pharmacists work with more types of medications than retail pharmacists. They use IV drugs that need a lot of preparation, with a fair amount of calculation, mixing, and checking that does not occur in the community setting. While most hospital pharmacists do not have as much patient contact as their retail counterparts, these pharmacists have significant contact with other healthcare providers, such as nurses, doctors, and dietitians. They may also be involved in deciding which drugs will be used in the pharmacy.

Employment of pharmacists will not grow as fast in hospitals as in other industries, as hospitals reduce inpatient stays, downsize, and consolidate departments. The increase in outpatient surgeries means more patients purchase medications through retail, supermarket, or mail-order pharmacies, rather than through the hospital. An aging population means more pharmacy services are required in nursing homes, assisted living facilities, and home care settings, where the most rapid job growth among pharmacists is expected.

Community pharmacies are taking steps to manage increasing prescription volume. Automation of drug dispensing and greater employment of pharmacy technicians and pharmacy aides will help these establishments to dispense more prescriptions. With its emphasis on cost control, managed care encourages the use of lower cost prescription distributors, such as mail-order firms and online pharmacies, for purchases of certain medications. Prescriptions ordered through the mail or via the Internet, filled in a central location, are shipped to the patient at a lower cost. Mail-order and online pharmacies typically use automated technology to dispense medication and employ fewer pharmacists. If the utilization of mail-order pharmacies increases rapidly, job growth among pharmacists could be limited.

Median annual wage and salary earnings of pharmacists in 2002 were $77,050. The middle 50% earned between $66,210 and $87,250 a year. Median annual earnings in the industries employing the largest numbers of pharmacists in 2002 were as follows:

Grocery stores	$78,270
Health and personal care stores	$76,800
General medical and surgical hospitals	$76,620

Pharmacy Licensure

State licensure requirements are available from each state's Board of Pharmacy. To become a licensed pharmacist, you must meet the requirements of the state or jurisdiction in which you are seeking licensure. The following examinations and other qualifications are prerequisites for licensure in most US jurisdictions. You are encouraged to contact the board of pharmacy of the state in which you wish to practice for their specific licensure requirements (Pharmacist.com, 2005).

The North American Pharmacist Licensure Examination™ (NAPLEX®) is required in all US jurisdictions except California, which administers its own examination. NAPLEX, developed by the National Association of Boards of Pharmacy® (NABP®), is a computer-based test that assesses the candidate's ability to apply knowledge gained in pharmacy school to practice situations. The NAPLEX is a 4 hour and 15 minute examination that consists of 185, 5-option multiple-choice test questions. A majority of the questions are in a scenario-based format (that is, patient profiles with accompanying test questions). To properly analyze and answer the questions presented, individuals must refer to the information provided in the patient profile. Interspersed among these profile-based questions are "stand-alone questions" whose answers are drawn solely from the information provided in the question.

Most states require a drug law examination as a condition of licensure. The Multistate Pharmacy Jurisprudence Examination™ (MPJE®) is currently administered in 45 US jurisdictions that are tailored to assess the pharmacy jurisprudence requirements of individual states. All candidates are tested on their mastery of pharmacy law as outlined in the MPJE Competency Statements. Each participating state board of pharmacy approves those questions that are specific to the federal and state laws of the jurisdictions in which candidates are seeking licensure. Candidates must take a separate exam for each state or jurisdiction in which they are seeking licensure. Some states require candidates for licensure to pass a laboratory or practice examination to ensure that candidates can accurately and safely prepare and dispense medications.

All state boards of pharmacy require candidates to complete an internship or externship before licensure. Such practice experience usually consists of 1,500 hours of experience, gained during pharmacy school (beginning after the first year of training). Some states require that internship hours be completed solely after graduation from pharmacy school and before licensure. The internship process is subject to state board of pharmacy regulations. Each intern, internship site, and preceptor must register with the state board of pharmacy to have the hours counted toward licensure.

Pharmacy Technicians and Aides

Pharmacy technicians help licensed pharmacists provide medication and other healthcare products to patients. Technicians usually perform routine tasks to help prepare prescribed medication for patients, such as counting tablets and labeling bottles. Technicians refer any questions regarding prescriptions, drug information, or health matters to a pharmacist.

Pharmacy aides work closely with pharmacy technicians. They are often clerks or cashiers who primarily answer telephones, handle money, stock shelves, and perform other clerical duties. Pharmacy technicians usually perform more complex tasks than do pharmacy aides, although, in some states, their duties and job titles overlap.

Pharmacy technicians who work in retail or mail-order pharmacies have varying responsibilities, depending on state rules and regulations. Technicians receive written prescriptions or requests for prescription refills from patients. They also may receive prescriptions sent electronically from the doctor's office. They must verify that the information on the prescription is complete and accurate. To prepare the prescription, technicians must retrieve, count, pour, weigh, measure, and sometimes mix the medication. Then, they prepare the prescription labels, select the type of prescription container, and affix the prescription and auxiliary labels to the container. Once the prescription is filled, technicians price and file the prescription, which must be checked by a pharmacist before it is given to a patient. Technicians may establish and maintain patient profiles, prepare insurance claim forms, and stock and take inventory of prescription and over-the-counter medications.

In hospitals, nursing homes, and assisted-living facilities, technicians have added responsibilities. They read patient charts and prepare and deliver the medicine to patients. The pharmacist must check the order before it is delivered to the patient. The technician then copies the information about the prescribed medication onto the patient's profile. Technicians also may assemble a 24-hour supply of medicine for every patient. They package and label each dose separately. The package is stored in the medicine cabinet of each patient until the supervising pharmacist checks it for accuracy before the patient receives it.

Pharmacy technicians held about 211,000 jobs in 2002. Two thirds of all jobs were in retail pharmacies, either independently owned or part of a drugstore chain, grocery store, department store, or mass retailer. About 22% of jobs were in hospitals and a small number were in mail-order and Internet pharmacies, clinics, pharmaceutical wholesalers, and the federal government.

Although most pharmacy technicians receive informal on-the-job training, employers favor those who have completed formal training and certification. However, according to the Bureau of Labor Statistics, there are currently few state and no federal requirements for formal training or certification of pharmacy technicians. Employers who have neither the time nor money to give on-the-job training often seek formally educated pharmacy technicians. Formal education programs and certification emphasize the technician's interest in and dedication to the work. In addition to the military, some hospitals, proprietary schools, vocational or technical colleges, and community colleges offer formal education programs for pharmacy technicians.

Formal education programs for pharmacy technicians require classroom and laboratory work in a variety of areas, including medical and pharmaceutical terminology, pharmaceutical calculations, pharmacy recordkeeping, pharmaceutical techniques, and pharmacy law and ethics. Technicians also are required to learn medication names, actions, uses, and doses. Many training programs include internships, in which students gain hands-on experience in actual pharmacies. Students receive a diploma, a certificate, or an associate degree, depending on the program.

Prospective pharmacy technicians with experience, working as aides in a community pharmacy or volunteering in a hospital, may have an advantage. Employers also prefer applicants with strong customer service and communication skills and with experience managing inventories, counting, measuring, and using computers. Technicians entering the field need strong mathematics, spelling, and reading skills. A background in chemistry, English, and health education also may be beneficial. Some technicians are hired without formal training, but under the condition that they obtain certification within a specified period to retain employment.

The Pharmacy Technician Certification Board administers the National Pharmacy Technician Certification Examination. This exam is voluntary in most states and displays the competency of the individual to act as a pharmacy technician. However, more states and employers are requiring certification as reliance on pharmacy technicians grows. Eligible candidates must have a high school diploma or GED and no felony convictions; those who pass the exam earn the title of Certified Pharmacy Technician (CPhT). Employers, often pharmacists, know that individuals who pass the exam have a standardized body of knowledge and skills. Many employers will also reimburse the costs of the exam as an incentive for certification. Certified technicians must be recertified every two years.

Successful pharmacy technicians are alert, observant, organized, dedicated, and responsible. They should be willing and able to take directions. They must enjoy precise work—details are sometimes a matter of life and death. Although a pharmacist must check and approve all their work, they should be able to work on their own without constant instruction from the pharmacist. Candidates interested in becoming pharmacy technicians cannot have prior records of drug or substance abuse. Strong interpersonal and communication skills are needed because there is a lot of interaction with patients, coworkers, and healthcare professionals. Teamwork is very important because technicians are often required to work with pharmacists, aides, and other technicians.

Good job opportunities are expected for full-time and part-time work, especially for technicians with formal training or previous experience. Job openings for pharmacy technicians will result from the expansion of retail pharmacies and other employment settings, and from the need to replace workers who transfer to other occupations or leave the labor force.

Employment of pharmacy technicians is expected to grow faster than the average for all occupations through 2012 due to the increased pharmaceutical needs of a larger and older population, and to the greater use of medication. Cost-conscious insurers, pharmacies, and health systems will continue to emphasize the role of technicians. As a result, pharmacy technicians will assume responsibility for more routine tasks previously performed by pharmacists. Pharmacy technicians also will need to learn and master new pharmacy technology as it surfaces. For example, technicians must oversee the machines, stock the bins, and label the containers of robotic machines to dispense medicine into containers.

Almost all states legislate the maximum number of technicians who can safely work under a pharmacist at one time. In some states, technicians have assumed more medication-dispensing duties as pharmacists have become more involved in patient care, resulting in more technicians per pharmacist. Changes in these laws could directly affect employment.

According to the Bureau of Labor Statistics, median hourly earnings of wage and salary pharmacy technicians in 2002 were $10.70. The middle 50% earned between $8.74 and $13.19; the lowest 10% earned less than $7.44, and the highest 10% earned more than $15.82. Median hourly earnings in the industries employing the largest numbers of pharmacy technicians in 2002 were as follows:

General medical and surgical hospitals	$12.32
Grocery stores	$11.34
Drugs' and druggists' sundries merchant wholesalers	$10.60
Health and personal care stores	$9.70
Department stores	$9.69

Certified technicians may earn more. Shift differentials for working evenings or weekends also can increase earnings. Some technicians belong to unions representing hospital or grocery store workers.

Pharmacy aides help licensed pharmacists with administrative duties in running a pharmacy. Aides often are clerks or cashiers who primarily answer telephones, handle money, stock shelves, and perform other clerical duties. They work closely with pharmacy technicians. Pharmacy technicians usually perform more complex tasks than do aides, although, in some states, the duties and titles of the jobs overlap. Aides refer any questions regarding prescriptions, drug information, or health matters to a pharmacist.

Aides have several important duties that help the pharmacy to function smoothly. They may establish and maintain patient profiles, prepare insurance claim forms, and stock and take inventory of prescription and over-the-counter medications. Accurate recordkeeping is necessary to help avert a potentially dangerous drug interaction. Because many people have medical insurance to help pay for the prescription, it is essential that pharmacy aides efficiently and correctly correspond with third-party insurance providers to obtain payment. Pharmacy aides also maintain the inventory and inform the supervisor of stock needs so that the pharmacy has the vital medications for those who need them. Some also clean pharmacy equipment, help with the maintenance of equipment and supplies, and manage the cash register.

Pharmacy aides held about 60,000 jobs in 2002. About 80% work in retail pharmacies either independently owned or part of a drug store chain, grocery store, department store, or mass retailer; the vast majority of these are in drug stores. About 1 in 10 work in hospitals and the rest work in mail-order pharmacies, clinics, and pharmaceutical wholesalers.

Most pharmacy aides receive informal on-the-job training, but employers favor those with at least a high school diploma. Prospective pharmacy aides with experience working as a cashier may have an advantage when applying for jobs. Employers also prefer applicants with strong customer service and communication skills and experience managing inventories and using a computer. Aides entering the field need strong spelling, reading, and mathematics skills.

Successful pharmacy aides are organized, dedicated, friendly, and responsible. They should be willing and able to take directions. Candidates interested in becoming pharmacy aides cannot have prior records of drug or substance abuse. Strong interpersonal and communication skills are necessary because there is a lot of interaction with patients, coworkers, and healthcare professionals. Teamwork is very important because aides are often required to work with technicians and pharmacists.

Pharmacy aides usually receive training on the job. They may begin by observing a more experienced worker. After they become familiar with the store's equipment, policies, and procedures, they begin to work on their own. Once they become experienced workers, they are not likely to receive additional training, except when new equipment is introduced or when policies or procedures change.

To become a pharmacy aide, one should be able to perform repetitious work accurately. Aides need good basic mathematics skills and good manual dexterity. Because they deal constantly with the public, pharmacy aides should be neat in appearance and able to deal pleasantly and tactfully with customers. Some employers may prefer people with experience typing, handling money, or operating specialized equipment, including computers.

Advancement usually is limited, although some aides may decide to become pharmacy technicians or to enroll in pharmacy school to become pharmacists. Cost-conscious insurers, pharmacies, and health systems will continue to employ aides. As a result, pharmacy aides will assume some responsibility for routine tasks previously performed by pharmacists and pharmacy technicians, thereby giving pharmacists more time to interact with patients and affording technicians more time to prepare medications. The number of pharmacy aides will not grow as fast as pharmacists and pharmacy technicians, however, because of legal limitations regarding their duties. Many smaller pharmacies that can afford only a small staff will favor pharmacy technicians because of their more extensive training and job skills.

According to the Bureau of Labor Statistics, median hourly wage and salary earnings of pharmacy aides were $8.86 in 2002. The middle 50% earned between $7.41 and $11.00; the lowest 10% earned less than $6.36, and the highest 10% earned more than $13.71. Median hourly earnings of pharmacy aides were $8.33 in health and personal care stores, $11.77 in general medical and surgical hospitals, and $9.08 in grocery stores in 2002.

Many pharmacy aides work evenings, weekends, and holidays. Eighty percent of jobs are in retail pharmacies. Job opportunities are expected to be good, especially for those with related work experience.

Other Career Options

Education and training in the pharmaceutical sciences opens up more career choices than just the practice of pharmacy. Drug manufacturers and wholesalers hire pharmacists as sales and medical service representatives. Drug companies see the advantages of having informed salespeople pitching their products to retail pharmacies and hospitals, and pharmacists provide credible information on new drug products to prospective buyers. A qualified pharmacist can also teach in colleges of pharmacy, supervise the manufacture of pharmaceuticals, or get involved with the research and development of new medicines. With additional academic work, pharmacists can move into pharmacology or become pharmaceutical chemists. The academically minded combine pharmaceutical and legal education to pursue jobs as patent lawyers or consultants on pharmaceutical and drug laws.

SUMMARY

The term "Better Living through Chemistry" has been applied to a wide variety of concepts over the years. However, within the field of pharmacy, individuals truly can live better, healthier lives even with illness and disability. From the big pharmacy chain stores to local supermarkets and from hospitals to research labs, today's pharmacists need scientific, business, and people skills to help provide many of the medicinal treatments that enhance quality and length of life.

ADDITIONAL RESOURCES

American Association of Colleges of Pharmacy
1426 Prince St.
Alexandria, VA 22314
Phone: (703) 739-2330
Web site: http://www.aacp.org/

American Pharmacists Association
2215 Constitution Avenue, NW
Washington, DC 20037-2985
1-800-237-APhA (2742)
Web site: http://www.aphanet.org

Pharmacy Technician Certification Board
2215 Constitution Ave., NW.
Washington, DC 20037
Web site: http://www.ptcb.org

American Society of Health-System Pharmacists
7272 Wisconsin Ave.
Bethesda, MD 20814
Web site: http://www.ashp.org

National Association of Chain Drug Stores
413 N. Lee St.
P.O. Box 1417-D49
Alexandria, VA 22313-1480
Web site: http://www.nacds.org

Information on the North American Pharmacist Licensure Exam (NAPLEX) and the Multistate Pharmacy Jurisprudence Exam (MPJE) is available from

National Association of Boards of Pharmacy
700 Busse Hwy.
Park Ridge, IL 60068
Web site: http://www.nabp.net

REFERENCES

American Association of Colleges of Pharmacy (AACP). (2004). Academic pharmacy's vital statistics. Alexandria, VA: American Association of Colleges of Pharmacy.

Food and Drug Administration (FDA). (2005). Genomics at FDA, Background information on genomics. Retrieved August 6, 2005, from http://www.fda.gov/cder/genomics/background.htm.

Pharmacist.com. (2005). Licensure—licensing info. Retrieved August 7, 2005, from http://www.pharmacist.com/articles/l_t_0001.cfm.

LoBuono, C. (2002). Consumers rate pharmacists. *Drug Topics, 10,* 53.

Svarstad, B. L., Bultman, D. C., & Mount, J. K. (2004, Jan–Feb). Patient counseling provided in community pharmacies: Effects of state regulation, pharmacist age, and business. *Journal of the American Pharmaceutical Association, 44*(1), 22–29.

Ukens, C. (2005, April 4). Pharmacy school enrollment still growing. *Drug Topics.* Retrieved August 6, 2005, from http://www.drugtopics.com/drugtopics/article/articleDetail.jsp?id=153755.

Weinstein, D. (2005, April 18). Pharmacogenomics and you. *Drug Topics.* Retrieved August 7, 2005, from http://www.drugtopics.com/drugtopics/article/articleDetail.jsp?id=156487.

Acknowledgement

Special thanks to
Mary Ann F. Kirkpatrick, RPh, PhD
Associate Professor of Pharmacy Practice
Associate Dean for Student Affairs
Bernard J. Dunn School of Pharmacy
Shenandoah University
1460 University Drive
Winchester, VA 22601

Chapter 12

Nutrition and Dietetics

Tammy Wagner and
Stephanie Chisolm

OBJECTIVES

After studying this chapter, the student should be able to

1. Explain the role of the dietitian in the healthcare system.
2. Describe the difference between a dietitian and nutritionist.
3. Describe the educational preparation and certification required for a registered dietitian.
4. Identify the various healthcare environments where registered dietitians may be employed.
5. Identify resources for additional information on the role of registered dietitians, such as the American Dietetics Association.

INTRODUCTION

> *There is no sincerer love than the love of food.*
> George Bernard Shaw (1856–1950)

Most of us have favorite foods we love. Food has many social and cultural meanings, as well as providing essential nutrients for survival. Dietetics is the science or art of applying the principles of nutrition to the diet. While most people apply the term "diet" to efforts for weight loss, it actually means the kind and amount of food prescribed for a person or animal for a special reason. Nutrition is defined as the sum of the processes by which an animal or plant takes in and utilizes food substances. All of this is a convoluted way to say simply, "you are what you eat," an expression that has never been more applicable than it is today, as we expand our knowledge of health and nutrition. Humans require food substances to supply the components necessary to build tissues, to repair tissues as they wear out and die, to keep the body in good working condition, and to supply fuel for energy. The Morgan Spurlock-directed film, *Super Size Me*, billed as a documentary film of "epic proportions," helped focus attention on the problem of obesity in this country.

According to the American Obesity Association, obesity is a disease that affects nearly one third of the adult American population (approximately 60 million). The number of overweight and obese Americans has continued to increase since 1960, a trend that is not slowing down. The Centers for Disease Control and Prevention report data from the Behavioral Risk Factor Surveillance System that demonstrate a significant increase in the obesity epidemic within the US population over the past decade. In 1991, only 4 of 45 participating states had obesity prevalence rates of 15 to 19% and none had prevalence greater than 20%. By the year 2000, all of the 50 states except Colorado had a prevalence of 15% or greater, with 22 of the 50 states having obesity prevalence as high as 20% or more. In 2001, 20 states had an obesity prevalence of 15–19%; 29 states had a prevalence of 20–24%; and one state reported a prevalence of more than 25%. The prevalence of obesity among US adults increased to 20.9% in 2001, a 74% increase since 1991. Check Figure 12.1 to see where your state weighs in on the obesity scale!

Today, 64.5% of adult Americans (about 127 million) are overweight or obese. Each year, obesity causes at least 300,000 excess deaths in the United States. Healthcare costs of American adults with obesity amount to approximately $100 billion. Obesity is one of the 10 leading health indicators used in monitoring the Healthy People 2010 objectives. The Surgeon General's Call to Action to Prevent and Decrease Overweight and Obesity in 2001 listed the following factors which contribute to the rise in obesity in the United States.

- Overweight and obesity result from an energy imbalance. This involves eating too many calories and not getting enough physical activity.
- Body weight is the result of genes, metabolism, behavior, environment, culture, and socioeconomic status.
- Behavior and environment play a large role in causing people to be overweight and obese. These are the greatest areas for prevention and treatment actions.

For good nutrition, a person should eat a well-balanced diet, one that provides an adequate amount of each of the classes of nutrients each day, furnishing at the same time an adequate but not excessive number of calories for the body's energy needs. The foods required for proper nutrition fall roughly into three major groups: proteins, carbohydrates, and fats; vitamins, minerals, and water are also important. Children require relatively larger amounts of nutrients and calories because of their rapid growth.

State Obesity	1991	1995	1998	1999	2000	2001
Alabama	13.2	18.3	20.7	21.8	23.5	23.4
Alaska	13.1	19.2	20.7	19.2	20.5	21.0
Arizona	11.0	12.8	12.7	11.6	18.8	17.9
Arkansas	12.7	17.3	19.2	21.9	22.6	21.7
California	10.0	14.4	16.8	19.6	19.2	20.9
Colorado	8.4	10.00	14.0	14.3	13.8	14.4
Connecticut	10.9	11.9	14.7	14.5	16.9	17.3
Delaware	14.9	16.2	16.6	17.1	16.2	20.0
District of Columbia	15.2	n/a	19.9	17.9	21.2	19.9
Florida	10.1	16.5	17.4	17.9	18.1	18.4
Georgia	9.2	12.6	18.7	20.7	20.9	22.1
Hawaii	10.4	10.4	15.3	15.3	15.1	17.6
Idaho	11.7	13.8	16.0	19.5	18.4	20.0
Illinois	12.7	16.4	17.9	20.2	20.9	20.5
Indiana	14.8	19.6	19.5	19.4	21.3	24.0
Iowa	14.4	17.2	19.3	20.9	20.8	21.8
Kansas	n/a	15.8	17.3	18.5	20.1	21.0
Kentucky	12.7	16.6	19.9	21.1	22.3	24.2
Louisiana	15.7	17.4	21.3	21.5	22.8	23.3
Maine	12.1	13.7	17.0	18.9	19.7	19.0
Maryland	11.2	15.8	19.8	17.6	19.5	19.8
Massachusetts	8.8	11.1	13.8	14.3	16.4	16.1
Michigan	15.2	17.7	20.7	22.1	21.8	24.4
Minnesota	10.6	15.0	15.7	15.0	16.8	19.2
Mississippi	15.7	18.6	22.0	22.8	24.3	25.9
Missouri	12.0	18.0	19.8	20.8	21.6	22.5

Figure 12.1 *Obesity Prevalence Among US Adults by State. BRFSS Data by Year*

State Obesity	1991	1995	1998	1999	2000	2001
Montana	9.5	12.6	1.7	14.7	15.2	18.2
Nebraska	12.5	15.7	17.5	20.2	20.6	20.1
Nevada	n/a	13.3	13.4	15.3	17.2	19.1
New Hampshire	10.4	14.7	14.7	13.8	17.1	19.0
New Jersey	9.7	14.2	15.2	16.8	17.6	19.0
New Mexico	7.8	12.7	14.7	17.3	17.8	18.8
New York	12.8	13.3	15.9	16.9	17.2	19.7
North Carolina	13.0	16.5	19.0	21.0	21.3	22.4
North Dakota	12.9	15.6	18.7	21.2	19.8	19.9
Ohio	14.9	17.2	19.5	19.8	21.0	21.8
Oklahoma	11.9	13.0	18.7	20.2	19.0	22.1
Oregon	11.2	14.7	17.8	19.6	21.0	20.7
Pennsylvania	14.4	16.1	19.0	19.0	20.7	21.4
Rhode Island	9.1	12.9	16.2	16.01	16.8	17.3
South Carolina	13.8	16.1	20.2	20.2	21.5	21.7
South Dakota	12.8	13.6	15.4	19.0	19.2	20.6
Tennessee	12.1	18.0	18.5	20.1	22.7	22.6
Texas	12.7	15.0	19.9	21.1	22.7	23.8
Utah	9.7	12.6	15.3	16.3	18.5	18.4
Vermont	10.0	14.2	14.4	17.2	17.7	17.1
Virginia	10.1	15.2	18.2	18.6	17.5	20.0
Washington	9.9	13.5	17.6	17.7	18.5	18.9
West Virginia	15.2	17.8	22.9	23.9	22.8	24.6
Wisconsin	12.7	15.3	17.9	19.3	19.4	21.9
Wyoming	n/a	13.9	14.5	16.4	17.6	19.2

Figure 12.1 *Obesity Prevalence Among US Adults by State. BRFSS Data by Year (continued)*
Source: CDC, 2006.

Description of the Profession

The only way to keep your health is to eat what you don't want, drink what you don't like, and do what you'd rather not.
Mark Twain, American Humorist, Writer and Lecturer (1835–1910)

Dietitians are the professionals who plan food and nutrition programs and supervise the preparation and serving of meals. They help to prevent and treat illnesses by promoting healthy eating habits and recommending dietary modifications, such as using less salt for those with high blood pressure or the reduction of fat and sugar intake for those who are overweight. The dietitian is a food and nutrition expert. The professional credential is "RD" for registered dietitian. The term dietitian itself derives from *dieto*, meaning diet or food; diet comes from the Greek *diaita*, meaning "manner of living." Dietitians possess both the scientific knowledge base of nutrition as a science and as an art. They promote nutritional health for the public. Dietitians have the background to blend scientific knowledge with social and cultural factors that influence what people eat, why they eat, and how it affects the body. Dietitians have skills to help individuals in illness and disease prevention; as well as prescribe intakes for performance, fitness, and general health. Dietitians are an integral part of the health team and interact with many other professionals and disciplines.

Dietitian versus Nutritionist: What Is the Difference?

The term "dietitian" and "registered dietitian" are often used interchangeably and are professionally regulated terms. A dietitian has at least a four-year undergraduate degree plus a dietetic internship and/or master's degree in nutrition or a closely related field. A dietitian must pass a national exam and continue to update his/her knowledge of nutrition through ongoing education. By meeting these strict standards, a dietitian is awarded a license to work using the title registered dietitian or RD.

Anyone can use the term *nutritionist*, even without any formal education or training. It's not a professionally regulated term—which means that there are no minimum qualifications for a person to call himself or herself a nutritionist. There are programs that sell certificates in nutrition, but they are not sanctioned by the American Dietetics Association and do not meet the standards for specialized training of a dietitian. A dietitian can work as a "nutritionist," but a "nutritionist" cannot work as a dietitian. State or federal health departments may give their registered dietitians the job title "Public Health Nutritionist" to reflect the focus on a prevention-based approach to health. Companies and health food stores who sell nutritional and diet supplements, and other self-proclaimed "nutritionists" cannot legally call themselves dietitians, because they do not meet the strict criteria for this professional title.

History of the Profession

Awareness of food and its impact on health is even found in ancient history. The first known written dietary recommendation, carved on Babylonian stone around 2500 B.C. stated, "If a man has pain inside, food and drink coming back to his mouth...let him refrain from eating onions for three days." The Book of Judges in the Old Testament prescribes a prenatal diet saying, "Therefore beware, and drink no wine or strong drink, and eat nothing unclean, for lo, you shall conceive and bear a son." The oldest known cookbook, *Apicius*, dates to approximately 100 B.C. Chinese observations about diabetes date all the way to the 3rd century.

In 1896, the US Department of Agriculture published Bulletin 28, the first food composition tables. They defined *dietitian* as a "person who specializes in the knowledge of food and can meet the demands of medical profession for diet therapy." At the turn of the 20th Century, Florence Corbett established the first internship for dietitians in 1903 at the New York Department of Charities. Casimir Funk discovered a chemical substance named *amine* that was essential to life, so he added the prefix *vita*. In 1910, fighting faddism and quackery was an issue.

With the outbreak of World War I, the examination of 2.5 million draftees in Great Britain found 41% to be in poor health, mainly due to malnutrition. The United States enrolled dietitians in the American Red Cross for army duty. Their nutritional expertise provided leadership for the soldiers and the general public at home. In 1917, two dietitians, Lenna Cooper and Lulu Graves, organized a special meeting of hospital dietitians to discuss emergency war needs. Out of this meeting, The American Dietetic Association, discussed later in this chapter, was formed.

In 1946, the National School Lunch Act was passed, which expanded dietetics to school lunch programs, training of personnel in food services and nutrition education. The civil rights movement of the late 1960s highlighted issues of poverty and hunger. The Cooperative Extension Service of the USDA began in 1968 and provided nutrition and food education for low-income families. The USDA food assistance programs to low-income families were established in the 1970s. These programs included food stamps for impoverished families, school lunch and breakfast programs, child care and summer food service for children, supplemental feeding programs for women, infants, and children (WIC), and lastly nutrition for the elderly. In 1977, nutrition education was added to the food stamp program. The Nutrition Education and Training Program was the first federal nutrition program for children.

The 21st century dietetics professional is on the forefront of healthcare reform. There is increased emphasis on nutrition and women's health. Inadequate nutrition education in medical schools is another matter of high priority. Currently 8 out of 10 leading diseases in the United States are linked to nutrition. Another opportunity for dietetic practitioners is the gap between consumer nutrition knowledge and behavior. In 1997, the ADA published the Nutrition Trends Survey that showed the public's exhaustion of conflicting nutrition information, frustration of perceived time to eat healthfully, and lack of faith in the importance of diet and nutrition. Current survey trends include

- Obesity and overweight, with a focus on children
- A focus on special population groups
  - Adolescent Nutrition
  - Child Nutrition
  - Elderly Health and Nutrition
  - Women's Health
  - Men's Health
- Safe, sustainable, and nutritious food supply
- Nutrigenetics and nutrigenomics
- Integrative medicine, including supplements and alternative medicine
- Medical nutrition therapy and nutrition diagnoses

Where Do Dietitians Work?

The majority of registered dietitians work in the treatment and prevention of disease, administering medical nutrition therapy, often part of medical teams. They work in hospitals, HMOs, private practice, or other healthcare facilities. In addition, a large number of dietitians work in food service settings, community and public health settings, academia, and research. A growing number of registered dietitians work in the food and nutrition industry, in business, journalism, sports nutrition, corporate wellness programs, and private practice. Major areas of practice include clinical, community, management, and consultant dietetics.

Clinical dietitians provide nutritional services for patients in institutions such as hospitals and nursing care facilities. They assess patients' nutritional needs, develop and implement nutrition programs, and evaluate and report the results. They also confer with doctors and other healthcare professionals in order to coordinate medical and nutritional needs. Some clinical dietitians specialize in the management of overweight patients or the care of critically ill or renal (kidney) and diabetic patients. In addition, clinical dietitians in nursing care facilities, small hospitals, or correctional facilities may manage the food service department.

Community dietitians counsel individuals and groups on nutritional practices designed to prevent disease and promote health. Working in places such as public health clinics, home health agencies, and health maintenance organizations, community dietitians evaluate individual needs, develop nutritional care plans, and instruct individuals and their families. Dietitians working in home health agencies provide instruction on grocery shopping and food preparation to the elderly, individuals with special needs, and children.

Increased public interest in nutrition has led to job opportunities in food manufacturing, advertising, and marketing. In these areas, dietitians analyze foods, prepare literature for distribution, or report on issues such as the nutritional content of recipes, dietary fiber, or vitamin supplements.

Management dietitians oversee large-scale meal planning and preparation in healthcare facilities, company cafeterias, prisons, and schools. They hire, train, and direct other dietitians and food service workers; budget for and purchase food, equipment, and supplies; enforce sanitary and safety regulations; and prepare records and reports.

Consultant dietitians work under contract with healthcare facilities or in their own private practice. They perform nutrition screenings for their clients and offer advice on diet-related concerns such as weight loss or cholesterol reduction. Some work for wellness programs, sports teams, supermarkets, and other nutrition-related businesses. They may consult with food service managers, providing expertise in sanitation, safety procedures, menu development, budgeting, and planning.

Minimum Education/Certification Requirements

Students interested in becoming a dietitian or nutritionist should take courses in biology, chemistry, mathematics, health, and communications. Dietitians and nutritionists need at least a bachelor's degree in dietetics, foods and nutrition, food service systems management, or a related area. College students in these majors take courses in foods, nutrition, institution management, chemistry, biochemistry, biology, microbiology, and physiology. Other suggested courses include business, mathematics, statistics, computer science, psychology, sociology, and economics.

Of the 46 States and jurisdictions with laws governing dietetics, 30 require licensure, 15 require certification, and 1 requires registration. The Commission on Dietetic Registration of the American Dietetic Association (ADA) awards the Registered Dietitian credential to those who pass a certification exam after completing their academic coursework and supervised experience. Because practice requirements vary by state, interested candidates should determine the requirements of the state in which they want to work before sitting for any exam.

As of 2003, there were about 230 bachelor's and master's degree programs approved by the ADA's Commission on Accreditation for Dietetics Education (CADE). Supervised practice experience can be acquired in two ways. The first requires the completion of a CADE-accredited coordinated program. As of 2003, there were more than 50 accredited programs, which combined academic and supervised practice experience and generally lasted four to five years. The second option requires the completion of 900 hours of supervised practice experience in any of the 264 CADE-accredited/approved internships. These internships may be full-time programs lasting 6 to 12 months or part-time programs lasting two years. Students interested in research, advanced clinical positions, or public health may need an advanced degree.

Experienced dietitians may advance to assistant director, associate director, or director of a dietetic department or may become self-employed. Some dietitians specialize in areas such as renal or pediatric dietetics. Others may leave the occupation to become sales representatives for equipment, pharmaceutical, or food manufacturers.

Entry-level dietitians are knowledgeable in eight areas: communications, physical and biological sciences, social sciences, research, food, nutrition, and management. Registered dietitians must meet the following criteria to earn the RD credential:

- Receive a bachelor's degree from a US regionally accredited university or college and course work approved by the Commission on Accreditation for Dietetics Education (credentialing agency of ADA). Students will study subjects in food and nutrition sciences, food service systems management, business, economics, computer science, culinary arts, sociology, communications, biochemistry, physiology, microbiology, anatomy, and chemistry.

- Complete a CADE-accredited supervised practice program at a health care facility, community agency, or a food service corporation combined with undergraduate or graduate studies. Typically, a practice program will run 6 to 12 months.

- Pass a national examination administered by the Commission on Dietetic Registration.
- Complete continuing professional educational requirements to maintain registration.

The Role of the American Dietetics Association

The American Dietetics Association (ADA, www.eatright.org) is the nation's largest organization of food and nutrition professionals. The ADA was founded in 1917 in Cleveland, Ohio by a group of visionary women, led by Lenna F. Cooper and ADA's first president, Lulu C. Graves. These women were dedicated to food conservation and helping the government improve the public's health and nutrition during World War I. Its role is to serve the public by promoting optimal nutrition, health, and well-being. Currently there are nearly 65,000 members. Today, ADA is led by a Board of Directors consisting of national leaders in nutrition and health. The dietetics profession is governed by a 130-member elected House of Delegates. Its mission is to lead the future of dietetics with the vision to be the most valued source of food and nutrition services. ADA is committed to helping people enjoy healthy lives. ADA serves the public by promoting optimal nutrition, health, and well-being.

Fifty state dietetic associations, plus the District of Columbia, Puerto Rico, and the American Overseas Dietetic Association, are affiliated with ADA, as well as approximately 230 district associations. The Commission on Accreditation for Dietetics Education (CADE) is the credentialing agency of ADA and has sole authority in all matters pertaining to certification.

The Commission on Accreditation for Dietetics Education (CADE) is ADA's accrediting agency for education programs preparing students for careers as registered dietitians or dietetics technicians. CADE exists to serve the public by establishing and enforcing eligibility requirements and accreditation standards that ensure the quality and continued improvement of nutrition and dietetics education programs. Programs meeting those standards are accredited by CADE. It is recognized by the US Department of Education and the Council for Higher Education Accreditation. This affirms that CADE meets national standards and is a reliable authority on the quality of nutrition and dietetic education programs. CADE's vision is that the accredited programs will be valued and respected for preparing competent professionals for entry-level employment and will continue to be updated due to a continually evolving practice. CADE's mission is to serve the public by ensuring quality education in dietetics that reflects the continual evolvement of the dietetics practice. CADE's goals include the following:

- Demonstrate accountability to the public through the establishment and application of market responsive, rigorous standards which require programs to document academic quality and student achievement.
- Provide and communicate clear CADE expectations to assist programs in meeting quality accreditation standards.
- Enhance preparation for entry-level practice by requiring program self-examination to ensure quality improvement and planning for purposeful change.
- Encourage educational innovation and diversity in order to address evolving dietetic practice.
- Continually evaluate accreditation practices and develop and maintain appropriate policies and procedures which ensure fair and consistent decision-making of accreditation decisions.
- Provide opportunities for professional development and educational leadership.

The Commission on Dietetic Registration has the sole and independent authority in all matters pertaining to certification, including, but not limited to, standard setting, establishment of fees, finances, and administration. The CDR protects the public through credentialing processes of dietetics practitioners by identifying knowledgeable and skilled dietitians. There are more than 76,000 dietitians and dietetic technicians. CDR currently awards four separate and distinct credentials: *Registered Dietitian* (RD); *Dietetic Technician, Registered* (DTR); *Board Certified Specialist in Renal Nutrition* (CSR); and *Board Certified Specialist in Pediatric Nutrition* (CSP). The Commission's certification programs are fully accredited by the *National Commission for Certifying Agencies* (NCCA), the accrediting arm of the *National Organization for Competency Assurance* (NOCA) based in Washington, DC. This accreditation reflects achievement of the highest standards of professional credentialing. The Commission consists of 10 members who serve a three-year term. Nine members are elected by credentialed practitioners, RDs, and DTRs. These elected members include seven RDs, one RD Specialist, and one DTR. In addition, a public representative is appointed to the Commission and has full rights and privileges.

Employment and Work Environment

Dietitians and nutritionists held about 49,000 jobs in 2002. More than half of all jobs were in hospitals, nursing care facilities, outpatient care centers, or offices of physicians and other health practitioners. State and local government agencies provided about one job in five—mostly in correctional facilities, health departments, and other public health-related areas. Some dietitians and nutritionists work in special food services, an industry which includes firms that provide food services on contract to facilities such as colleges and universities, airlines, correctional facilities, and company cafeterias. Other jobs were in public and private educational services, community care facilities for the elderly (which includes assisted-living facilities), individual and family services, home health care services, and the Federal Government—mostly in the US Department of Veterans Affairs. Some dietitians were self-employed, working as consultants to facilities such as hospitals and nursing care facilities, or providing dietary counseling to individual clients.

The US Bureau of Labor Statistics (BLS, 2006) expects employment of registered dietitians to grow about as fast as the average for all occupations through the year 2010 because of the increased emphasis on disease prevention, a growing and aging population, and public interest in nutrition. Employment in hospitals is expected to show little change because of anticipated slow growth and patients' reduced lengths of hospital stay. Faster growth is anticipated in nursing homes, residential care facilities, and physicians' clinics. ADA's most recent survey of members shows RDs work in these settings:

Hospitals (inpatient and acute care)	34.0%
Clinics and ambulatory care centers	11.6%
Community and public health programs	11.3%
Extended care facilities	10.9%
Consultation (primarily to health care facilities)	6.3%
College and university faculty	5.5%
Other for-profit organizations and industries	4.7%
Other nonprofit organizations	4.5%
Private practice (primarily to individual clients)	3.5%
School food service (K-12 and college)	3.0%
Consultation, primarily to other organizations	2.0%
HMOs, physician, and other care providers	1.7%
Home care	1.1%

Salary Range and Job Outlook for Registered Dietitians

According to the American Dietetic Association, median annualized wages for registered dietitians in 2005 varied by practice area as follows: $53,800 in consultation and business; $60,000 in food and nutrition management; $60,200 in education and research; $48,800 in clinical nutrition/ambulatory care;

$50,000 in clinical nutrition/long-term care; $44,800 in community nutrition; and $45,000 in clinical nutrition/acute care. Salaries also vary by years in practice, education level, geographic region, and size of the community.

Challenges Faced by the Dietetics Profession

There is very little diversity in the field. A large majority are Caucasian (>85%) women (>95%) between the ages of 26-50 (> 75%) (Bryk and Soto, 2001). ADA has identified some priority public health issues. There is an increasing epidemic of obesity and overweight in adults, adolescents, and children; nutritional concerns of an ever-growing aging population; and lastly treatment of individuals with multiple disease and conditions. There is a more focused concern on mental health and depression issues in a society continually pushed to do more in less time. Stress and its impact on nutritional health is an area that continues to grow.

SUMMARY

With many of today's Leading Health Indicators tied in some way to food and nutrition, the profession of dietetics is an important component of the healthcare system. A comprehensive goal of dietitians is represented in the words on the ADA seal, *Quam Plurimus Prodesse* (to benefit as many as possible). Today there are more than 70,000 dietetic professionals with nearly 65,000 as members of ADA. The future of dietetics encompasses many areas of food service, food science, clinical nutrition, and wellness. One of the Healthy People 2010 objectives is to increase the percentage of adults who are at a healthy weight (defined as a body mass index [BMI] equal to or greater than 18.5 and less than 25). These objectives also aim to increase the proportion of individuals who are counseled about healthy behaviors, such as diet and nutrition. The Registered Dietitian plays a critical role in educating individuals and the general public about the role of food in their life and health.

ADDITIONAL RESOURCES

American Dietetic Association
Headquarters of the American Dietetic Association
120 South Riverside Plaza, Suite 2000
Chicago, Illinois 60606-6995
Phone: (800)/877-1600

American Dietetic Association
1120 Connecticut Avenue NW, Suite 480
Washington, DC 20036
Phone: (800)/877-0877
Internet: www.eatright.org

United States Department of Agriculture Center for Nutrition Policy and Promotion
3101 Park Center Drive
Room 1034
Alexandria, VA 22302-1594

Dietary Guidelines
Phone: 1-888-7PYRAMID (1-888-779-7264)
Internet: http://www.mypyramid.gov/

REFERENCES

Bryk, J.A. & Soto, T.K. (2001). Report on the 1999 Membership Database of the American Dietetics Association, Vol. 101, Issue 8, August 2001 pp. 947–953.

Bureau of Labor Statistics, US Department of Labor, *Occupational Outlook Handbook, 2006–07 Edition*, Dietitians and Nutritionists, on the Internet at http://www.bls.gov/oco/ocos077.htm (visited November 24, 2006).

Centers for Disease Control and Prevention (CDC). (2006). Overweight and obesity: Obesity Trends 1991–2001. Prevalence of obesity among US adults by state. Retrieved April 29, 2006, from http://www.cdc.gov/nccdphp/dnpa/obesity/trend/prev_reg.htm.

Chapter 13

Physical Therapy

Jeff G. Konin

OBJECTIVES

After studying this chapter, the student should be able to

1. Explain the role and function of the physical therapist in the health-care system.
2. Explain the difference between the various areas of specialization for physical therapists.
3. Describe the educational preparation and certification required for physical therapists.
4. Summarize the estimated earning and career potential of physical therapists in various roles and organizations.
5. Identify resources for additional information on physical therapy as a profession.

INTRODUCTION

I am convinced that life in a physical body
is meant to be an ecstatic experience.
Shakti Gawain

Advances in medical technology have enabled people to live longer, and hopefully better, lives over the last few decades. When injury or illness does strike, physical therapists provide services that help restore function, improve mobility, relieve pain, and prevent or limit permanent physical disabilities of patients suffering from injuries or disease. They restore, maintain, and promote overall fitness and health. Their patients include accident victims and individuals with disabling conditions such as low back pain, arthritis, heart disease, fractures, head injuries, and cerebral palsy.

What Is Physical Therapy?

Physical therapy, or physiotherapy, is the treatment of disorders of the muscles, bones, or joints by means of physical agents—heat, light, water, manual and electronic massage, and exercise. Physical therapy is a dynamic and ever-changing field. Physical therapists (PTs) are health professionals who evaluate and treat people with a variety of dysfunctions. They assess joint motion, muscle strength and endurance, cardiac and pulmonary function, development, functional ability, sensation and perception, integrity of the skin, muscle tone and reflexes, and performance of functional activities. They evaluate patients' needs, diagnose physical therapy problems, establish plans of care, and evaluate their effectiveness.

Therapists examine patients' medical histories and then test and measure the patients' strength, range of motion, balance and coordination, posture, muscle performance, respiration, and motor function. They also determine patients' ability to be independent and reintegrate into the community or workplace after injury or illness. Next, physical therapists develop plans describing a treatment strategy, its purpose, and its anticipated outcome. Physical therapist assistants, under the direction and supervision of a physical therapist, may be involved in implementing treatment plans with patients. Physical therapist aides perform routine support tasks, as directed by the therapist.

Where Are Physical Therapists Employed?

Physical therapists work in hospitals, private physical therapy clinics, rehabilitations centers, nursing homes, schools, and other settings. The job of a physical therapist is to provide services aimed at preventing the onset of physical ailments and disabilities, assisting patients with care for sustained injuries and illnesses, and improving quality of life for anyone experiencing an ailment, illness, injury, or disability. The PT attempts to prevent pain or further damage and may train different muscles to compensate for damaged ones. Physical therapists are valuable members of the healthcare team who work with physicians, dentists, podiatrists, occupational therapists, nurses, speech and hearing professionals, psychologists, and social workers. Physical therapists may practice by referral from physicians, podiatrists, or dentists or have direct access to patients depending upon the jurisdiction.

Specialty Areas of Physical Therapy

Physical therapy encompasses practitioners who either generalize in all aspects of physical therapy or maintain specialization credentials in specific areas. Some physical therapists treat a wide range of ailments; others specialize in areas such as pediatrics, geriatrics, orthopedics, sports medicine, neurology, and cardiopulmonary physical therapy (*Guide to Physical Therapist Practice*, 2003). Physical therapists adhere to evidence-based practice whereby the administration and intervention of treatment and care is based upon proven and effective scientific and clinical studies. Patients with whom physical therapists work may include those who have osteoarthritis, fractures, head injuries, coronary artery disease, neurological disorders, low back pain, ankle sprains, amputations, and many other conditions. Though the actual percentage of physical therapists of minority background is small, the profession as a whole strongly embraces diversity because physical therapists treat patients of all ethnic and cultural backgrounds, races, and religions.

Physical therapy is a people-oriented profession. Physical therapists have many opportunities to improve the quality of their clients' lives as individuals or in small groups. Physical therapists educate patients in health promotion and conduct research to improve patient care. Physical therapists must have excellent observational and psychomotor skills.

History of the Physical Therapy Profession

The profession of physical therapy essentially began in the early 1900s. Primarily in the New England region of the United States, individuals were being treated for what is now referred to as "acute anterior poliomyelitis," called "infantile paralysis" at the time. The need for care directed toward those with locomotor functional deficits was growing. The first title used for physical therapists was actually termed "reconstruction aides." Those individuals who had experience using physical therapeutics in their civilian lives were recruited during the World Wars to assist with military healthcare needs. Reconstruction aides had some background in anatomy and human movement, as well as some psychosocial skills used commonly with those returning from the wars and facing emotional challenges resulting from disabilities. Assisting these individuals in returning to mainstream society was a major role of the reconstruction aide.

The American Women's Physical Therapeutic Association, established in 1921, was the first physical therapy association. In 1930, the association changed its name to the American Physiotherapy Association, at which time men were admitted as members and the overall membership grew to nearly 1,000 people. In the 1940s and 1950s during World War II and after, a nationwide polio epidemic served as the impetus for a greater demand of physical therapists to serve the nation. The need to learn and become more united and organized in the fight against physical ailments facilitated the membership of the association to nearly 8,000 people. At this time, educational preparation took on a greater level of importance as formal academic programs grew to nearly 40 across the country.

The association underwent yet another name change in the late 1940s, to the American Physical Therapy Association (APTA), the name it maintains to date. Membership continues to grow, with nearly 80,000 members throughout the United States. Physical therapists now serve the community as general practitioners, with some possessing specialized clinical credentials in a single area, such as pediatrics or cardiopulmonary.

Some of the major influential factors in the growth of the physical therapy profession occurred in the 1960s when public policy, driven by the federal government, established expanded opportunities for all Americans to receive healthcare benefits. The Medicare system and federal Social Security Act opened doors for the elderly and those with disabilities to receive physical therapy services, regardless of financial status, through government-funded initiatives. In 1973, legislation specifically pertaining to rehabilitation was enacted in an effort to reduce discrimination in the society against those with disabilities, yet again leading to a greater need for physical therapy services. In 1974, members of the APTA adopted the first draft of the *Essentials of an Accredited Educational Program for Physical Therapists*, serving as the standard for entry-level education (Swisher and Page, 2005).

The demand for those receiving physical therapy services began to exceed the number of professionally educated physical therapists in the United States in the mid-1980s. This then led to a large increase in the number of accredited physical therapy programs in addition to the more formal recognition of the physical therapist assistant as a member of the physical therapy team. The physical therapist assistant, working under the direction of the physical therapist, is able to perform certain administrative and clinical functions that assist in the delivery of physical therapy services to the public.

Physical Therapy Today

Today, there are approximately 120,000 licensed physical therapists and 20,000 physical therapist assistants in the United States. The practice of physical therapy has changed significantly, ranging from the clinical skills one needs to possess to the educational preparation delivered. *A Guide to Physical Therapy Practice* (2003) has been written and revised to better define the scope of physical therapy practice. The emphasis on evidence-based practice is a hallmark of the quality of care provided by physical therapists and physical therapist assistants today.

Physical therapists utilize a variety of treatment techniques to assist in the care of patients. Manual skills, physical agents, and assistive devices are all components of intervention planned and implemented by a physical therapist. The educational preparation to become a physical therapist is extensive and demanding to meet the needs of providing quality care to patients. Physical therapy educational programs have a competitive admissions process and demand discipline, perseverance, and hard work throughout the approximately three-year curriculum that combines classroom and clinical learning opportunities (Curtis, 2002).

A Day in the Life of the PT

A typical day for a physical therapist might begin with a review of the history and medical background of a specific patient. This may involve a consultation with other members of the medical and allied health teams, including but not limited to, physicians, occupational therapists, case study managers, nurses, and social workers. Physical therapists often consult with family members to have a total appreciation of a patient's home environment.

A physical therapist would then perform an evaluation to determine the patient's current functional and cognitive status. Subjective and objective measurements are recorded to help identify baseline ability and to monitor a patient's progress over time. An example of a subjective measurement would be asking a patient to rate his or her pain on a scale of one to ten, or to describe the type of pain that exists in terms of a descriptive word, such as sharp or dull. These are subjective measurements because they can't be proven and are taken upon the word of a patient. The PT also documents objective measurements in terms of degrees of range of motion that a joint possesses, temperature or blood pressure, the amount of swelling that exists, or the strength of a muscle.

A physical therapist may use any number of treatment interventions, including ultrasound, electrical stimulation, manual therapy, physical agents, thermal agents, and therapeutic exercise. A main component of intervention for a physical therapist includes patient education. Physical therapists educate patients on posture and body mechanics, proper walking and running mechanics, exercise techniques, and the use of assistive devices such as crutches, walkers, and canes.

A large part of the work for any healthcare provider pertains to documentation. There are legal and ethical guidelines outlining how and what needs to be documented in a patient's medical record. Documentation may be done in handwritten notes or via electronic methods, so long as thorough and complete recordings of a patient's interventions are recorded in an accurate and timely manner. Progress notes, billing statements, letters to physicians, and other forms of communication are all considered types of documentation that a physical therapist will routinely provide.

Not all physical therapists are full-time clinicians. Physical therapists serve as educators, researchers, administrators, and business owners. Most physical therapists are multidimensional professionals and are active in more than a single facet of physical therapy. A typical work week for a full-time physical therapist is a minimum of 40 hours and may include weekends and nights depending upon the setting.

Minimum Educational and Legal Requirements

Physical Therapist

All physical therapists have an undergraduate degree prior to enrolling in a graduate physical therapy program. Prerequisites for admission to physical therapy school often include courses in anatomy, biology, chemistry, physics, psychology, statistics, English, and humanities. Achieving good grades in these prerequisite classes as well as a good overall grade point average are important if one wishes to be viewed as a qualified applicant for physical therapy school.

Physical therapy education consists of basic and clinical sciences, biomechanics, neuroscience, orthopedics, physical therapy professional issues classes, differential diagnosis, pharmacology, pathology, and others. A large portion of the educational program consists of clinical internships so that students can gain supervised hands-on experience working with patients. Most doctoral physical therapy programs are approximately three years in length.

There are currently over 200 accredited physical therapy educational programs. Of these, just more than one half of them award degrees at the doctoral level, with the remaining programs offering a degree at the master's level.

Physical Therapist Assistant

A physical therapist assistant is supervised by a physical therapist and performs physical therapy interventions under the direction of a physical therapist. Physical therapist assistants are technically trained and graduate from an accredited physical therapist assistant program. This program may exist as a two-year degree at a community college or as a baccalaureate degree within a four-year college. The curriculum to complete a degree in physical therapy assisting includes classes related to anatomy, physiology, biomechanics, and technical courses related to physical therapy. Clinical affiliations/internships are included as part of the required learning experience. There are currently over 200 physical therapist assistant programs in the United States. Upon completion of a physical therapist assistant program, physical therapists must pass a national licensure examination. Over 40 states have some form of regulation for physical therapists to practice, either in the form of licensure, registration, or certification. Academic programs established to prepare individuals to enter the physical therapy profession are considered to be professional degree programs offered at the graduate level (BLS, 2006).

What Do Schools Look for in Physical Therapy Applicants?

Physical therapy programs do not look at any one specific element that determines a candidate's ability to succeed academically and enter the profession as a competent physical therapist. Rather, a combination of attributes and accomplishments are considered representative of a well-rounded and well-prepared individual.

One's overall grade point average is a key component in a candidate's application. While schools vary in what they consider to be a competitive grade point average, most look for a 3.0 to 4.0 or better. There are exceptions, in that being slightly under a 3.0 to 4.0 with other outstanding qualities or having a grade point average well above a 3.0 to 4.0 with deficits in other qualities may change the way schools view an applicant. Grades earned in the prerequisite classes, specifically science-related courses, are also looked at closely when comparing candidates. Oftentimes this serves as a better measure for comparison amongst applicants because applicants can have different majors and take very different courses. Comparing commonly required courses assists admissions committees in evaluating students' abilities more evenly. It is important to understand that most physical therapy schools do not specify that a student major in anything in particular for an undergraduate degree.

Historically, graduate record exams (GRE's) are an evaluative tool for admission criteria in physical therapy programs, though some schools have moved away from requiring GREs as part of the admissions process. Professional debate exists as to whether GREs are a predictor of success in physical therapy education. Schools that continue to require GREs as part of the application process primarily evaluate the quantitative and analytical components and look for an average score of approximately 1000, with neither section being lower than a 400. In some instances, these numbers are inflexible because they might be a part of the overall graduate school policy at an institution. In others, a school might choose to allow a student a sliding scale of evaluation whereby the GRE is a sole determinant of non-acceptance (Curtis, 2002).

A very important component of one's application is the formation of letters of recommendation. Schools typically request three letters of recommendation from an applicant. It is preferred that letters of recommendation come from a) educators who can speak to a student's academic performance and potential, and b) physical therapists who have supervised a student in some capacity that allows for a character judgment to be made. Information in these letters should speak directly to attributes that each individual program is asking for as well as what characteristics an individual possesses that would separate him or her from other applicants and serve as a predictor of success in the field. Letters of recommendation from family members and friends, or individuals who hold elected office or high-ranking positions but do not necessarily know the applicant well, are discouraged.

Physical therapy school applicants are required to spend time either volunteering or working as a paid aide in a physical therapy environment under the supervision of a physical therapist. Schools vary tremendously in the number of hours required to observe: some are as low as 20 hours, while some are as high as 200. The purpose of these supervised hours is not merely quantitative, but rather to ensure that a student has a total understanding of the role of a physical therapist prior to applying to graduate level physical therapy school. Students without experience in various physical therapy settings prior to admission will likely experience greater episodes of uncertainty and/or apprehension in unfamiliar environments during the clinical education component of school.

Formal physical therapy applications usually include a component of essay writing. Topics vary from asking one to describe significant life-altering events in one's life to discussing a trend or concern related to the profession of physical therapy. The intent with the essay portion of the application is to view how a student can organize thoughts and express them in written form with ample time for preparation and proofreading.

Some physical therapy schools conduct interviews as part of the application process. Consensus amongst programs does not exist as to whether or not an interview can predict the success of an applicant. However, during interviews, attire, mannerisms, communication skills, and sometimes impromptu writing samples are assessed. Preparing for an interview involves learning about the institution and its program, as well as asking appropriate questions regarding one's concerns about physical therapy school.

What a student should look for in a physical therapy school varies depending on the needs of each potential PT student. It is difficult to accurately rank physical therapy schools. Some sources, like the *US News and World Report*, provide such rankings based upon information the schools themselves submit to the magazine. Regardless of how a school is ranked, the key to finding a good physical therapy school is researching what school is the best match for an individual. The following is a list of some considerations that should be taken into account when choosing a physical therapy school:

- Cost of tuition
- Geographical location
- Licensure passing rate
- Graduation and attrition rate
- Length of program
- Clinical education opportunities and assignments
- Experience of faculty
- Entrance requirements/standards
- Cultural atmosphere
- Graduate placement outcomes.

Role of the National Professional Organization/Association

The American Physical Therapy Association (APTA) is the national professional organization for physical therapists and physical therapist assistants, representing over 70,000 members. The APTA provides information about the profession and accredited educational programs. The association strives to promote advancements in physical therapy practice, research, and education. With its national headquarters located in Alexandria, Virginia, the APTA is actively involved with political and legislative issues in Washington, DC in support of its members.

As an association, the APTA has adopted the following mission statement (APTA, 2006):

> The mission of the American Physical Therapy Association (APTA), the principle membership organization representing and promoting the profession of physical therapy, is to further the profession's role in the prevention, diagnosis, and treatment of movement dysfunctions and the enhancement of physical health and functional abilities of members of the public.

The APTA has also established a clear vision for its members' future and in doing so has outlined both a vision sentence and a vision statement. The vision sentence reads as follows (APTA, 2006):

> By 2020, physical therapy will be provided by physical therapists who are doctors of physical therapy, recognized by consumers and other health care professionals as practitioners of choice to whom consumers have direct access for the diagnosis of, interventions for, and prevention of impairments, functional limitations, and disabilities related to movement, function, and health.

Estimated Salary/Earnings/Work Environment

As of 2004, physical therapists earn a median salary of $60,180. This salary figure varies depending upon the work setting, number of years of experience, geographic location, and additional educational background or skills that one possesses (BLS, 2006). From 1999 to 2002 salary increases ranged from 12-19% on the average throughout the country, with the largest average increases reported for those working in acute care hospital settings. Though the profession consists of predominantly females, surveys reveal that male physical therapists earn a higher annual income. This has been attributed to a number of reasons, including the notion that females tend to place a greater emphasis on family responsibilities versus career success. This ultimately has an effect of interrupting professional growth opportunities of female counterparts. Unemployment rates for physical therapists have been reported to be extremely low, ranging between 1% to 3% on the average. Job satisfaction ratings have been favorable, and it appears as though with the trends in health care that the salaries, demand for employment, and quality of job satisfaction will continue to demonstrate positive findings.

As of 2004, physical therapist assistants earned a median income of $37,890. This salary figure also varies depending upon the work setting, number of years of experience, geographic location, and additional educational background or skills that the individual possesses (BLS, 2006).

Future Trends for the PT Profession

A proliferation of physical therapy programs produced many physical therapists entering the profession at a quick rate in the last decade. This is very different from just a decade ago when the profession saw fewer schools with larger class sizes and applicant pools. Efforts to slow the proliferation of newly accredited physical therapy programs so that the market for physical therapy jobs does not destabilize and leave graduates unemployed are topics of professional discussion. Concerns of decreasing availability of student clinical placements, increased demands on physical therapist clinician productivity, and greater demands to hire doctoral-trained qualified faculty for teaching and research purposes have contributed to the concerns. The APTA projects a 20% to 30% surplus of physical therapists between the years 2005 to 2007. Others believe there will remain a shortage of physical therapists needed to meet the growing demands of the general public (APTA, 2005).

Employment opportunities for physical therapist assistants have been steadily on the rise. Unemployment rates have been identified as below 4% as of 1991 by the American Physical Therapy Association (APTA, 2005). Advanced certifications and qualifications are also being developed to assure professional growth opportunities for physical therapist assistants. Employment for physical therapists is expected to grow faster than the average rate of most occupations through the year 2008 (BLS, 2006). Many factors contribute to this projection. Increased technology and clinical skills used to detect illness and disability will bring forth new approaches to rehabilitation; advances in surgical procedures to the elderly population will require physical therapy services; and the aging baby boomer generation will soon be faced with middle-aged and older health-related concerns. The emphasis of the government and society in general on health promotion and preventive care will open new areas of intervention for physical therapists. Specializations of physical-therapy-related care will expand, and consumers will seek individuals with greater levels of expertise in a given area of practice as is currently seen with physicians.

Issues Facing PT Today

Guided by the national association, the physical therapy profession has identified a number of critical issues facing its future. The ability to be reimbursed in an equitable manner for services still remains a challenge. Physical therapists have obtained what is referred to as "direct access" in most states, yet not in all. This simply means that a patient or client does not need to see a physician first to receive a medical diagnosis prior to seeing a physical therapist for a treatment. Furthermore, some insurance companies will not reimburse a physical therapist for services under a direct access treatment intervention without the referral of a physician. Receiving appropriate and equitable reimbursement for services rendered is a high priority for physical therapists. This is obtained through federal- and state-wide lobbying and legislative efforts.

Physical therapists are also strongly enforcing the notion that only physical therapists, and physical therapist assistants with appropriate supervision, are qualified to provide and bill for physical therapy services. This too requires initiatives at the state and federal levels in the form of legislation that recognizes such delivery and billing for services.

The federal government, and specifically the Centers for Medicare and Medicaid Services (CMS), have placed payment limitations on services provided by physical therapists to patients who are recipients of federally funded health insurance plans. This means that a patient in need of continued physical therapy services will be denied such services as a result of the federal guidelines regarding pre-established limits on reimbursements. In such a case, the patient will suffer from not receiving needed and appropriate care in a timely manner. Physical therapists, and other healthcare providers, are leading efforts to repeal this reimbursement cap imposed by the federal government.

The Physical Therapist Helping Patients: A Case Study

Rehabilitation Following a Total Hip Joint Replacement

Mr. Jones is a 68-year-old male who has recently undergone a successful total hip joint replacement after years of dealing with pain and activity limitations from degenerative joint arthritis. It is now the day after surgery, and the healthcare team is already working collaboratively to prepare Mr. Jones for a safe transition home. His orthopedic surgeon, floor nurse, social worker, occupational therapist, and physical therapist are meeting today to discuss how the surgical procedure went and the prognosis for his recovery. The status of his tissue and its healing properties are identified, as is his presurgical status. These factors will determine the rate at which he can progress through his rehabilitation. Each healthcare team member has a role in his recovery. The level of family support at home and the type of household that Mr. Jones lives in are discussed. The physical therapist notes that his wife is fairly healthy and will assist with basic activities of daily living. He will need some assistance with his transfers from the bed to standing up and with all of his furniture. He lives in a one-level home, so there are no stairs that need to be negotiated. He will need non-skid surfaces placed in his bathrooms, because they have tile floors, and handrails will need to be built in his shower stall. Mr. Jones had a cemented total hip joint replacement, and the physical therapist will work closely with his doctor as to the lessening of weight-bearing restrictions and his therapeutic exercise progression according to evidence-based outcomes supported in the medical literature for this surgical intervention and the associated rehabilitation phases. The discussion during this meeting will be documented and the physical therapist will educate the patient and his caregivers on the plan, including limitations, expectations, and guidelines for rehabilitation.

SUMMARY

According to the Bureau of Labor Statistics (2006), employment of physical therapists will grow much faster than the average through 2014. Over the long run, the demand for physical therapists should continue to rise as growth in the number of individuals with disabilities or limited function spurs demand for therapy services. Job opportunities should be particularly good in acute hospital, rehabilitation, and orthopedic settings, because the elderly receive the most treatment in these settings. The growing elderly population is particularly vulnerable to chronic and debilitating conditions that require therapeutic services. In addition, the baby-boom generation is entering the prime age for heart attacks and strokes, increasing the demand for cardiac and physical rehabilitation. Further, young people will need physical therapy as technological advances save the lives of a larger proportion of newborns with severe birth defects.

Future medical developments also should permit a higher percentage of trauma victims to survive, creating additional demand for rehabilitative care. In addition, growth may result from advances in medical technology that could permit the treatment of more disabling conditions. Widespread interest in health promotion also should increase demand for physical therapy services. A growing number of employers are using physical therapists to evaluate worksites, develop exercise programs, and teach safe work habits to employees in the hope of reducing injuries in the workplace. When illness, injury, or disability threatens individuals from birth through old age, the physical therapist is a vital part of the healthcare team, improving the quality and quantity of life.

ADDITIONAL RESOURCES

American Physical Therapy Association
1111 North Fairfax Street
Alexandria, VA 22314-1488
Phone: 703/684-APTA (2782) or 800/999-APTA (2782)
TDD: 703/683-6748
Fax: 703/684-7343
Internet: www.apta.org

REFERENCES

American Physical Therapy Association (APTA). (2005). APTA physical therapist employment survey fall 2001—Executive summary. Retrieved May 15, 2005 from http://www.apta.org.

Bureau of Labor Statistics, US Department of Labor (BLM). (2006). *Occupational outlook handbook, 2006–07 edition.* Physical therapists. Retrieved April 11, 2006 from http://www.bls.gov/oco/ocos080.htm.

Curtis, K. A. (2002). *Physical therapy professional foundations: Keys to success in school and career.* Thorofare, NJ: Slack.

Guide to Physical Therapist Practice (2nd ed.). (2003). Alexandria, VA: American Physical Therapy Association.

Purtilo R. (1999). *Ethical dimensions in the health professions* (3rd ed.). Philadelphia, PA: Saunders.

Rozier, C. K., Raymond, M. J., Goldstein, M. S., & Hamilton, B. L. (1998). Gender and physical therapy career success factors. *Physical Therapy, 78,* 690–703.

Swisher, L. & Page, C. (2005). *Professionalism in physical therapy: History, practice, & development* (3rd ed.). Philadelphia, PA: Saunders.

Chapter 14

Occupational Therapy

S. Margaret Maloney

OBJECTIVES

After studying this chapter, the student should be able to

1. Explain the role of the registered occupational therapist (OTR) in the healthcare system.
2. Describe the historical development of the profession of occupational therapy.
3. Describe the educational preparation and certification required for OTRs.
4. Identify the various healthcare environments employing OTRs.
5. Identify resources for additional information on the role of the OT.

INTRODUCTION

Monotony is the law of nature. Look at the monotonous manner in which the sun rises. The monotony of necessary occupation is exhilarating and life giving.
Mahatma Gandhi (1869–1948)

It is neither wealth nor splendor; but tranquility and occupation which give you happiness.
Thomas Jefferson (1743–1826)

People engage in occupations throughout their day as they care for themselves and others, drive, work or attend school, engage in play/leisure pursuits and social interaction, and perhaps express their spirituality (AOTA, 2002). Occupational therapy (OT) is a health and human services profession that assists clients across the lifespan to achieve independence and satisfaction in all dimensions of their lives by empowering them to engage in chosen "occupations." For occupational therapy clinicians, the interactions of mind, body, spirit, and environment, which foster the "doing" of an occupation, are central to the domain of the profession. Occupational therapy professionals have long viewed health and wellness from a holistic viewpoint.

What Does the Occupational Therapist Do?

According to the American Occupational Therapy Association (AOTA), occupational therapy is skilled treatment that helps individuals achieve independence in all facets of their lives. It gives people the "skills for the job of living" necessary for independent and satisfying lives. OT also gives people the skills for the *joy* of living. Services typically include (AOTA, 2005):

- Customized treatment programs to improve one's ability to perform daily activities
- Comprehensive home and job site evaluations with adaptation recommendations
- Performance skills assessments and treatment
- Adaptive equipment recommendations and usage training
- Guidance to family members and caregivers.

Any understanding of the OT profession requires comprehension of the word "occupation." Contrary to our current social usage of the word "occupation" as a method to describe our employment or vocational roles, the original definition of "occupation" encompassed a broader sense of an individual's engagement in relevant tasks or activities, which *take hold of,* or occupy, a person's time. Such occupations have both a purpose and a meaning for the person who chooses to engage in them (Kielhofner, 2002; Nelson, 1994, 1997). Occupations may be of an objective (physical) or a subjective (emotional or cognitive) nature (AOTA, 2002). For example, an individual may spend time reading books about knitting and studying patterns prior to actually engaging in the physical production of a woolen scarf.

Occupations are "clusters of activities and tasks in which a person engages in order to meet his/her intrinsic needs for self-maintenance, expression, and fulfillment carried out within the context of individual roles" (Law et al., 1996). Occupations occur within the conditions of individuals' roles and their cultural, physical, social, personal, temporal, and virtual environmental contexts (AOTA, 2002). Occupations will vary in their importance, purpose, and meaningfulness across a person's lifespan. Anne Wilcock (1998) takes the connection between occupational engagement and health a step further, and proposes an occupational theory of human nature built upon the premise that there is a link between health and occupation which not only allows man to survive, but ultimately to flourish. Whether occupational therapy practitioners utilize the terms *occupation* or *activity*, they are guided by the central tenet "that man, through the use of his hands as they are energized by mind and will, can influence the state of his health" (Reilly, 1962).

Clients of all ages may be referred to an occupational therapy professional related to developmental delays, onset or exacerbation of an illness, or an injury. Occupational therapy is available across the continuum of health care and human service settings and is provided in varied settings such as neonatal intensive care units, hospital acute care, long-term physical or behavioral health rehabilitation, school-based and community agencies, prisons, work-related injury centers, long-term nursing facilities, substance disorder clinics, private practice offices, or even an individual's home. Whatever the site of treatment, occupational therapy practitioners call upon the power of man's engagement in daily occupations as both the means to engage a client and the therapeutic end product of the intervention.

OTs help people improve their ability to perform tasks in their daily living and working environments. They help clients not only to improve their basic sensorimotor functions and reasoning abilities, but also to compensate for permanent loss of function. Their goal is to help clients have independent, productive, and satisfying lives. The OT assists clients in performing activities of all types, ranging from using a computer to caring for their own or others' daily needs such as dressing, personal hygiene, cooking, and eating. An OT might incorporate physical activity to assess or treat deficits in a client's endurance level, strength, and dexterity. Other therapeutic activities may improve visual acuity and the ability to discern patterns. A client with short-term memory loss might be encouraged to make lists or utilize a day-planner to aid recall. A person with neuromuscular deficits might participate in therapeutic crafts to improve eye-hand or fine motor coordination. Occupational therapists also use computer programs to help clients improve decision making, abstract reasoning, problem solving, and perceptual skills, as well as memory, sequencing, and coordination—all of which are important for independent living.

Therapists instruct those with permanent disabilities, such as spinal cord injuries, cerebral palsy, or muscular dystrophy in the use of adaptive equipment, including wheelchairs, splints, and assistive devices for eating and dressing. OTs must demonstrate creativity and ingenuity when called upon to construct special equipment to enhance a client's ability to manipulate and interact with typical objects in his or her home or work environment. Therapists develop computer-aided assistive devices and teach clients with severe limitations how to use that equipment in order to communicate better and control various aspects of their environment.

Some occupational therapists treat individuals whose ability to function in a work environment has been impaired. These practitioners arrange employment, evaluate the work environment, plan work activities, and assess the client's progress. Therapists also may collaborate with the client and the employer to modify the work environment so that the work can be successfully completed.

OTs may work exclusively with individuals in a particular age group or with particular disabilities. In schools, for example, they help children participate as fully as possible in school learning programs and social activities such as play. OTs evaluate children's abilities to engage in activities related to the learning process, such as impulse control or handwriting skills, and then recommend and provide therapy, modify classroom equipment, and consult with teachers and other team members such as a school psychologist.

Occupational therapy also is beneficial to the geriatric population. Therapists help the elderly lead more productive, active, and independent lives through a variety of methods, including the use of assistive devices, modification to their homes, education in techniques to conserve their energy, and driving assessment. In mental health settings, OTs treat individuals who have a major psychiatric disorder, such as schizophrenia, or are mentally retarded or developmentally delayed. To treat these conditions, therapists choose activities that help people learn to engage in and cope with daily life. Treatment might focus upon increasing coping and time management skills, creating a system to organize prescription medicines, assertiveness training, socialization and leisure pursuits, budgeting, shopping, homemaking, and the use of public transportation. Occupational therapists also may work with individuals who are dealing with alcoholism, drug abuse, depression, eating disorders, or stress-related disorders.

Assessing and documenting a client's activities and progress is an important part of an occupational therapist's job. Accurate records are essential for evaluating clients, for billing purposes, and for reporting to physicians and other healthcare providers. Thus, OTs must possess strong skills for both verbal and written communication to interact effectively with their clients, family members, and other team members such as physicians, nurses, social workers, teachers, case managers, physical therapists, psychologists and psychiatrists, and insurance providers.

A wide variety of people can benefit from occupational therapy, including those with the following issues or concerns (AOTA, 2005):

- work-related injuries, including lower back problems or repetitive stress injuries
- limitations following a stroke or heart attack

- arthritis, multiple sclerosis, or other serious chronic conditions
- birth injuries, learning problems, or developmental disabilities
- mental health or behavioral problems, including Alzheimer's, schizophrenia, and post-traumatic stress
- problems with substance use or eating disorders
- burns, spinal cord injuries, or amputations
- broken bones or other injuries from falls, sports injuries, or accidents
- vision or cognitive problems that threaten their ability to drive
- traumatic brain injury
- deficits associated with the natural aging process

History of Occupational Therapy

The profession of occupational therapy formally began in 1917 when the charter members of the newly formed National Society for the Promotion of Occupational Therapy (NSPOT) convened in Clifton Spring, New York to solidify their belief in the therapeutic power of naturalistic occupations and crafts. Their goal was to formalize the creation of the new discipline. As they assembled, George Barton, William Dunton, Jr., Susan Cox Johnson, Thomas Kidner, Isabel Newton, and Eleanor Clarke Slagle represented a variety of professions—psychiatry, arts and crafts, physical medicine, curative occupations, and architecture—which joined to create the strength and diversity of the newly created profession. Three other individuals, nurse Susan Tracy, Herbert Hall, MD, and neurobiologist Adolph Meyer, also influenced the early path of occupational therapy, although they did not attend the initial NSPOT meeting (Peloquin, 1991).

The profession traces its roots not only to these individuals but to the values and philosophy of humanitarianism, the moral treatment movement, the arts and crafts movement, and the personal anecdotal evidence of psychiatric and physical medicine practitioners regarding recovery from illness following engagement in occupation. Dunton (1919) believed occupational engagement to be as necessary for man as food and drink. Meyer elaborated his position that an individual's fundamental ability to organize "self" and time was a learned trait established by "doing" things (1922). Slagle felt that clients were able to overcome, modify, or construct new "habit reactions" while performing occupations, which allowed them to restore their health. Barton had experienced a year of institutionalization to treat tuberculosis and subsequently developed an unrelated left-side paralysis. In both cases, he rehabilitated himself using burgeoning occupational therapy treatment techniques based upon his belief that a patient would recuperate more quickly if engaged in "doing" (Barton, 1920).

Several factors are linked to the initial growth and acceptance of the new profession. First, World War I played an important role. The demand for occupation therapists (who were initially termed rehabilitation or reconstruction aides) grew as the public asserted an expectation that the approximately 148,000 returning injured soldiers were entitled to return to their social and economic usefulness regardless of whether their disability was from a physical or psychological condition (Ambrosi & Schwartz, 1995). Early entrants to the profession often cited patriotic duty and service to their country as being important aspects of their decision to do so (Quiroga, 1995). By 1918, rehabilitation aides were providing therapy to soldiers both in the United States and in the war zone. Walter Reed Hospital established one of the early OT programs where wounded soldiers were treated utilizing such occupations as chair caning, woodworking, printing, and weaving. In addition, over 200 reconstruction aides served in field hospitals in France.

Secondly, the onset of increased industrial mechanization in the early 20th century and the resultant increase in the number of work-related injuries can be traced to the growth in the early profession (Ambrosi & Schwartz, 1995). Third, because protracted institutionalization was the usual course of treatment for persons with tuberculosis treatment or with mental illness, the sanatoria became particularly ripe sites for implementing occupational therapy treatment programming.

Finally, social expectations had created both the need and the opportunity for women, particularly from the upper classes, to engage in employment or philanthropic duties outside of the home. This novice profession presented an acceptable alternative to two other female-dominated vocations, nursing and teaching (Quiroga, 1995), and women flocked to the OT training programs in large numbers. One early program, The War Service Classes for Training Reconstruction Aides for Military Hospitals, experienced a dramatic increase in the number of applicants from about 100 applicants for the first class in 1918, to over 1,000 applicants for the second class in 1919 (Quiroga, 1995).

The OTR and the COTA

The profession is divided into two levels of credentialed practitioners. At the professional level are registered occupational therapists (OTR). Certified occupational therapy assistants (COTA), who may only practice under the supervision of an OTR, have been serving clients at the technical level since the late 1950s. The level of supervision required depends upon the individual COTA's competency with complex interventions and general experience level. The *Standards of Practice for Occupational Therapy* (AOTA, 1999) delineates that COTAs require supervision as they collaborate with the OTR during the screening, evaluation, and intervention process (AOTA, 1999).

Education and Certification

Occupational therapists need patience and strong interpersonal skills to inspire trust and respect in their clients. Ingenuity and imagination in adapting activities to individual needs are assets. Those working in home healthcare services must be able to adapt to a variety of settings.

The pathway to employment for both occupational therapists and occupational therapy assistants consists of achieving three key milestones: (a) acceptance into and completion of an approved occupational therapy educational program; (b) securing credentialing through a national entry-level certification examination; and (c) obtaining licensure within the state(s) where employment is desired as required.

Prior to achieving official status, the curriculum of an occupational therapy or an occupational therapy assistant program is highly scrutinized by the profession through the Accreditation Council for Occupational Therapy Education (ACOTE). Developing and existing programs are monitored via annual written reports and formal on-site visits. ACOTE in turn complies with the criteria established by the United States Department of Education. ACOTE establishes rigorous standards for occupational therapy education in order to ensure the preparation of competent occupational therapy practitioners. In addition, ACOTE encourages the enhancement and improvement of existing educational programs through subsequent accreditation evaluations, which typically occur every five years.

Occupational therapists were previously able to enter the profession via either a bachelor's or an entry-level master's educational program. However, effective in 2007, all new therapists must be graduates of a master's level program in occupational therapy prior to taking the national certification exam. Therapists who were credentialed prior to 2007 will continue to be grandfathered into the profession at the bachelor's level. Many therapists who were graduates of bachelor's level occupational therapy programs prior to 2007 voluntarily sought additional educational training at the master's level, but it is not a requirement for them to do so in order to continue to practice.

There are currently over 150 master's level occupational therapy educational programs in the United States that have been approved by the Accreditation Council for Occupational Therapy Education (ACOTE). A listing of the programs is available through the American Occupational Therapy Association Web site (www.aota.org). Each educational institution establishes the prerequisites for acceptance into their program. In general, prerequisite education focuses upon guiding prospective students to develop a well-rounded liberal arts foundation with emphasis upon the biological, behavioral, and health sciences, as well as sociocultural and socioeconomic topics. In addition, many programs require documentation of observation or volunteer work within an occupational therapy setting, as well as a writing sample such as an autobiographical statement or essay concerning a topic relevant to health care. Some programs may also require an application interview in an individual or group format, as well as documentation of Graduate Record Exam or Miller Analogies Test scores. An interested student should contact the individual OT Program in order to learn specific application requirements.

There are two types of entry-level master's programs. One type is a combined bachelor's/master's program that typically takes approximately five years to complete. The other type is an entry-level master's program for students who already have acquired a bachelor's degree prior to seeking a master's degree. This type of program generally takes a student two to three years to complete following completion of the bachelor's degree. Students with a wide variety of undergraduate bachelor's degrees may apply to a master's program, provided that they have met the individual school's prerequisite requirements.

Course work within a master's program must comply with the *Standards for an Accredited Educational Program for the Occupational Therapist* (ACOTE, 1998a). Typical OT curricula cover

- the profession's history and ethics code;
- an understanding of occupations and activity analysis;
- human development across the lifespan; human anatomy, neuroanatomy, and physiology; etiology and management of medical and psychiatric conditions;
- the theoretical constructs guiding the professional in the occupational therapy process, including screening, evaluation, intervention planning, and documentation of services;
- research skills and research utilization; management and supervision; and leadership and advocacy for the profession.

All students complete a minimum of six months (480 hours) of fieldwork education under the direct supervision of an occupational therapist. The fieldwork experience consists of two separate three-month-long experiences, which occur within different types of practice settings. Some programs require three fieldwork experiences.

Occupational therapy assistant (OTA) programs are also required to comply with the ACOTE standards (ACOTE, 1998b). OTA programs receive accreditation at an associate degree level, although some are certificate-issuing programs. Because OTAs must work under the supervision of an occupational therapist, their training is similar, although there is less emphasis upon management, research skills, and anatomy/physiology. OTA students must complete only one three-month-long fieldwork experience.

Following the completion of all educational coursework and the fieldwork experience, new graduates must achieve certification to practice. Certification requires successfully passing either the occupational therapist or the occupational therapy assistant national exam administered by the National Board for Certification in Occupational Therapy, Inc. (NBCOT). The exam, created in conjunction with practicing clinicians, reflects the current standards of competency and scope of practice. After achieving initial certification, practitioners must demonstrate ongoing competence through training activities. NBCOT requires documentation to show completion of 36 continuing education units for professional development activities every three years in order to renew certification (NBCOT, 2005).

The final step prior to full practice is to secure credentialing in any state where the OT intends to practice. All 50 states have enacted some form of regulation to practice, usually in the form of licensure. Typically, the responsible state board will require proof of completion of an ACOTE-accredited program, successful completion of the NBCOT exam, a criminal background check, proof of knowledge of the state laws and code of ethics, a recent photograph, and a fee. Information on each particular state's requirements and a link to the regulatory agencies may be found on the AOTA Web page (www.aota.org). Most state agencies also require a practitioner to provide documentation of ongoing continuing education in order to maintain licensure, although the amount varies from state to state. For further information regarding the specific rules and regulations of each state, please consult the relevant regulatory agency.

In addition to the previously noted entry-level occupational therapy programs, approximately 50 programs exist to provide post-professional masters education in occupational therapy. This type of program requires a student to possess an occupational therapy degree prior to application. Doctoral-level education is available directly in the field of occupational therapy or in related disciplines. Degrees are available as a doctorate of philosophy (PhD), a doctorate of science (ScD), or an occupational therapy clinical doctorate (OTD). Over 15 universities offer doctoral-level education, and the number of such programs continues to increase. An up-to-date listing may be found on the AOTA Web page (www.aota.org).

Occupational science is new related academic discipline that has been evolving globally since the 1980s with the aim to support the work of occupational therapists. Elizabeth Yerxa (1993, p. 3) describes occupational sciences as the "study of the human as an occupational being." Through scholarly inquiry, occupational scientists strive to explore and understand the very nature and meaning of occupation from a social science perspective (Zemke & Clark, 1996). Occupational science has been described as being similar to anthropology, sociology, and psychology (Larson, Wood, & Clark, 2003). The first doctoral program in occupational science was established at the University of Southern California in the late 1980s and other programs at both the undergraduate and graduate degree level have been implemented since then. For an up-to-date listing of undergraduate and professional programs in occupational science, please consult the listing of education programs found at www.aota.org.

The American Occupational Therapy Association

The American Occupational Therapy Association, Inc. (AOTA) is the national-level organization charged with advancing the quality, availability, and support of occupational therapy. The organization is administered through a small number of paid staff along with extensive membership involvement. Membership in the association is voluntary, and the volunteer sector is composed of two groups: the Executive Board and the Representative Assembly. Within the Representative Assembly, several committees exist to administer specific duties, such as the Commission on Education, Commission on Standards and Ethics, Commission on Practice, Commission on Continuing Competence and Professional Development, Special Interest Section Steering Committee, and the Assembly of Student Delegates. An elected delegate represents each state.

The organization provides services such as development of standards of practice; political advocacy and public relations services; monitoring of educational programs; publication of research and practice articles; and monitoring the *Occupational Therapy Code*. In 1965, AOTA created The American Occupational Therapy Foundation (AOTF) as an independent 501(c)3 organization in order to create avenues to fund research endeavors designed to add to the knowledge base of the profession and to disseminate research in professional literature. In 2002, AOTA created a second independent 501(c)3 organization, The Fund to Promote Awareness of Occupation Therapy, in an effort to promote the general public's awareness of and demand for the profession through targeted education strategies, research, and professional development opportunities.

Work Settings and Estimated Salary for OTRs and COTAs

There were approximately 82,000 OTRs in the United States in 2002, and they earned an average salary of $51,900 (BLS, 2004). COTAs earn an average salary of $30,132 (AOTA, 2000). Women dominate the profession and compose 94% of the OTR professionals and 96% of COTAs (AOTA, 2000). The median age is 39-years-old for an OTR and is 40-years-old for COTAs, and both groups report practicing OT for an average of 12 years (AOTA, 2000). The largest portion of clinicians (over 50%) report working within a medical facility, with freestanding skilled nursing facilities being the largest single type of medical employer (AOTA, 2000). The second most common work setting (nearly 25%) is a school-based setting (AOTA, 2000). A typical OT practitioner works 35 hours per week (AOTA, 2000) but nearly 25% voluntarily work part-time (BLS, 2004).

Occupational therapists in hospitals and other health care and community settings usually worked a 40-hour week. Those in schools may participate in meetings and other activities during and after the school day. In large rehabilitation centers, therapists may work in spacious rooms equipped with machines, tools, and other devices generating noise. The work can be tiring, because therapists are on their feet much of the time. Those providing home healthcare services may spend time driving from appointment to appointment. Therapists also face hazards such as back strain from lifting and moving clients and equipment. Therapists increasingly are taking on supervisory roles. Due to rising healthcare costs, third-party payers are beginning to encourage occupational therapist assistants and aides to take more hands-on responsibility. By having assistants and aides work more closely with clients under the guidance of a therapist, the cost of therapy should decline (BLS, 2004).

Trends for Future Employment

Employment for occupational therapists is projected to increase faster than average through 2012 (BLS, 2004) as the country faces an aging population. In addition, medical and healthcare technological advancements have allowed more people to survive serious injury or illness and thus will also create a demand for more occupational therapists to assist them to regain independence as they return to home or community.

In addition to the typical employment settings where practitioners have historically worked, many occupational therapists have begun to create new opportunities in emergent practice arenas such as ergonomics consulting, lifestyle coaching, driver rehabilitation and training, and low vision services. They also work with technology and assistive device development and consulting, community mental health and welfare services, health and wellness programs, and programs aimed at violence prevention and addressing the psychosocial needs of school-aged children. Occupational therapists are involved with disaster relief services to help individuals strive to address their emotional stress and disruption of their occupational identity after experiencing a natural catastrophe or terrorism. In all settings, occupational therapy practitioners are dedicated to empowering clients to fully utilize their unique skills for the *joy* of living.

A Day in the Life of an OT

Jane, an occupational therapist, pulls into the parking lot of the mid-sized community hospital just as the street lights turn off. She hurries into the occupational therapy department and settles herself at her desk with a cup of tea, a bagel, and the morning referral orders in her hand. She notes that there have been five new admissions to the acute care floor and schedules time to review their charts and complete their evaluations this afternoon. The first part of her morning will be spent on the physical rehabilitation floor assisting two of her current patients as they complete their morning bathing and dressing routines. Later in the morning, she will participate in the weekly team meeting rounds with the social worker, physical therapist, nurse, and physician to discuss the progress of her patients on the unit.

She notes that her OT manager has scheduled a guest speaker from a local wheelchair manufacturer during the lunch hour for an in-house education session. She always enjoys the intellectual stimulation of their weekly "professional development lunch hour," which sometimes involves discussing pertinent research journal articles, presentations on unique medical or psychiatric conditions, or discussions of new treatment ideas.

Jane quickly gathers her clipboard, pen, and "treatment bag" and heads upstairs to see her first patient of the day. The bedside clock glows 7:00 AM as she enters the darkened private room, but the occupant is already awake and lies in her bed with the curtains drawn. Mrs. Anderson, or "Lilly" as she has instructed Jane to address her, is a 71-year-old, married, white woman who lives with her 80-year-old husband, Travis, in a self-contained home within a religious-affiliated retirement center. She looks up at Jane expectantly and nods a silent greeting.

Lilly was admitted to the emergency room two weeks ago after a fall down the stairs in her home during which she suffered a traumatic brain injury (TBI). Three days ago she was transferred to the rehabilitation unit. Jane's review of her chart revealed that six months ago, Lilly underwent a coronary-artery bypass. After she returned home, she developed pneumonia, which required further hospitalization. Jane's evaluation of Lilly indicated residual visual-perception deficits, short-term memory impairment, slight vertigo, generalized weakness, poor balance, and poor endurance to complete a typical daily self-care routine. She used a wheeled-walker for the last two months, and according to her husband usually only went up or downstairs to their bedroom once or twice a day with his assistance. Their home has a first floor bathroom and three steps which lead to the front door. Lilly stated that she was coming down the stairs alone the day of the fall because she didn't want to "bother" her husband. During Jane's first visit, Lilly was tearful and blamed herself for "being stupid and clumsy." She wondered how she was going to be able "to ever get better—it's too hard for Travis to care for me."

Prior to the bypass surgery, Lilly had been independent with self-care, drove her car to visit friends and family, swam once a week, and enjoyed cooking, tending to her small flower garden, and singing in the church choral group. Lilly and Jane have developed goals for her to return to these important roles of homemaker, grandmother, wife, and church member. Jane has educated Lilly and Travis about available safety and assistive equipment, which they have already purchased for installation at their home, such as a tub transfer bench in the bathroom and front-step handrails.

Today Jane works with Lilly bedside and in the bathroom to problem-solve ways to conserve her energy and simplify her routine of toileting, bathing, and dressing. Lilly completes her bathing using a tub bench and remarks how much easier it is to take a shower while seated. She exhibits visual deficits when she finds it difficult to see her white socks against the white sheet of the bed, but she laughingly says, "I guess I'll have to buy darker socks." She dresses and brushes her teeth and hair with moderate assistance from Jane. At one point she forgets for a moment what the next step in dressing is. As Jane prepares to leave, Lilly smiles broadly from her seat in a chair by the open window as she awaits her breakfast tray and says "Look, I did it! I'm dressed!"

In another wing of the hospital, another OT, Abby, has also arrived at her OT department on the behavioral health unit. She has scheduled her day between a mixture of individual and group patient treatment sessions on the in-patient unit, and one out-patient group for women experiencing eating disorders. She updates herself by reading the chart of a new referral to the unit. Dr. Winston Smith is a 75-year-old, married white male, who is a retired dentist. He reluctantly admitted himself into the substance abuse program three days ago after a visit to his general practitioner physician for what he thought was a routine physical. Mrs. Smith made the appointment because she was concerned that he was becoming increasingly "forgetful, unmotivated, tired—just not like himself." She revealed to the physician that she suspected her husband was consuming at least 25 Vicodin pills per day. Dr. Smith minimized the problem when he met with the physician and stated, "This is just a little problem; I only take three–five pills a day." Abby learns that the admitting psychiatrist noted acute opiate dependence, atypical depression, a history of alcohol dependence, and a history of low back pain secondary to a back injury in his youth. His blood pressure (157/90), respiration rate (20) and pulse (87) were high yesterday. Dr. Smith has received small dosages of methadone during the detoxification process in the last two days and had reported signs and symptoms of withdrawal from the opiates such as anxiety, sweating, nausea, vomiting, and diarrhea. Yesterday, Abby researched Vicodin and learned that it is a narcotic composed of hydrocodone bitartrate and acetaminophen, and is usually prescribed for short-term pain relief at a dose of a maximum of eight pills per day. She knows that Dr. Smith had self-prescribed the medication and has subsequently surrendered his dental license. Legal issues are still pending. She had introduced herself to him on his second day on the unit, but delayed the initial interview until he was through his detox phase.

Today Abby finds Dr. Smith sitting erectly in a chair at an empty table in his room. She notices that his knuckles are white as he firmly grasps the arms of his chair. He is attired in casual but crisp short-sleeved shirt and trousers, and his grooming is immaculate; even his shoes look buffed. The few personal items (including a framed photograph of himself with his family) are neatly arranged on his dresser. She introduces herself again and explains the role of an OT on the unit, and asks him what he would like her to call him. "Dr. Smith is fine," he replies without meeting her gaze.

Abby interviews him in an open-ended manner guided by the OT assessment instrument. She learns that he has a wife and a grown son from whom he is estranged following a disagreement about the son's career choice (to be an architect and not a physician as Dr. White would have liked). He retired from a thriving dental practice six years ago after almost 35 years of work. He was also busy as a guest lecturer at the local dental school, on call at three emergency rooms, and provided weekly pro bono pediatric dental care at a low-income clinic. He now spends some of his time volunteering at a local natural history museum and says, "I thought I'd be doing much more once I retired, but I just seem to stay at home." He used to enjoy fly-fishing and sometimes travels with his wife when she plans it and "drags me along." He appears irritated when questioned about his drug use and minimizes his actions: "I took the pain pills for pain; I did it responsibly and it did not interfere with my daily life—I am not a druggie."

Abby slowly draws more information out of Dr. Smith by asking reflective questions and observing his body posture, eye contact, tone of voice, and rate of speech. She notes that he tears up while discussing his wish to reestablish a relationship with his son, and shame in his awareness that he has caused his wife unhappiness. When asked what is most difficult for him, he replies, "with all this free time, I feel like a failure because I'm not succeeding at retirement. What kind of future is this?" Abby reflects that he did have a very busy schedule before and many more opportunities to interact with other people, and that professionals often have difficulty transitioning to the role of retiree. He nods his head and looks wistful.

Together they develop a plan of treatment to include attending occupational therapy group sessions three times a week to focus upon time utilization/management, socialization, pain-management techniques, and pursuing more leisure opportunities. Abby thinks about his need to be "a success" and wonders to herself if it would be beneficial to reestablish his role as a teacher. She says aloud that she was always interested in fly-fishing and asks if he would consider teaching her more about fly-tying. He looks startled for a second and then says "You'd listen to an old guy like me?"

"Of course," she laughs. "Just tell me what I should buy and I'll bring the stuff in tomorrow! Maybe we could get the group to try it, too." He eagerly writes her a list of a things to buy, and makes a suggestion of a shop to go to. "Tell them I sent you and they'll give you a deal."

Abby stands up to signal the end of the session and says "Thank you, Dr. Smith, for sharing your time with me."

He smiles slightly and says, "Please, call me Winston."

SUMMARY

The occupational therapist and certified occupational therapy assistant work across all domains of health. These professionals help patients live their lives to their best abilities. By providing guidance, support, and sometimes even devices to help patients from birth to grave, the OT strives to improve the quality of patients' lives, thus meeting the objectives of Healthy People 2010.

ADDITIONAL RESOURCES

Accreditation Council for Occupational Therapy Education
Education Division
c/o American Occupational Therapy Association
P.O. Box 31220
Bethesda, MD 20824-1220
Phone: (301) 652-2682
Internet: www.aota.org

American Occupational Therapy Association
4720 Montgomery Lane, PO Box 31220
Bethesda, MD 20824-1220
Phone: 301-652-2682—TDD: 1-800-377-8555
Fax: 301-652-7711
Internet: www.aota.org

American Occupational Therapy Foundation
4720 Montgomery Lane, P.O. Box 31220
Bethesda, MD 20824-1220
Phone: 301-652-2682 – TDD 1-800-377-8555
Fax: 301-656-3620
Internet: www.aotf.org

National Board for Certification in Occupational Therapy (NBCOT)
800 South Fredrick Avenue, Suite 200
Gaithersburg, MD 20877-4150
Phone: (301) 990-7979
Internet: www.nbcot.org/

Society for the Study of Occupation: USA
Internet: www.sso-usa.org

World Federation of Occupational Therapists
Internet: www.wfot.org

REFERENCES

Accreditation Council for Occupational Therapy Education (ACOTE). (1998a). *Standards for an accredited educational program for the occupational therapist*. Bethesda, MD: ACOTE.

Accreditation Council for Occupational Therapy Education (ACOTE). (1998b). *Standards for an accredited educational program for the occupational therapist assistant*. Bethesda, MD: ACOTE.

Ambrosi, E. & Schwartz, K. (1995). The profession's image, 1917–1925, Part II: Occupational therapy as represented by the profession. *American Journal of Occupational Therapy, 49*, 828–832.

American Occupational Therapy Association (AOTA). (1995). What is occupational therapy? Retrieved on September 25, 2005, from http://www.aota.org/featured/area6/index.asp.

American Occupational Therapy Association (AOTA). (1999). Standards of practice for occupational therapy. *American Journal of Occupational Therapy, 53,* 294–295.

American Occupational Therapy Association (AOTA). (2000). *AOTA 2000 member compensation survey.* Bethesda, MD: AOTA.

American Occupational Therapy Association (AOTA). (2002). Occupational therapy practice framework: Domain and process. *American Journal of Occupational Therapy, 56,* 609–639.

American Occupational Therapy Association (AOTA). (2005). *About occupational therapy.* Retrieved September 25, 2005, from http://www.aota.org.

Barton, G. E. (1920). What occupational therapy may mean to nursing. *Trained Nurse and Hospital Review, 64,* 304–310.

Bureau of Labor Statistics, US Department of Labor (BLM). (2004). Occupational outlook handbook. Retrieved July 30, 2005, from www.bls.gov/oco/ocos078.htm.

Dunton, W. R. (1919). *Reconstruction therapy.* Philadelphia, PA: Saunders.

Kielhofner, G. (2002). *A model of human occupation: Theory and application* (3rd ed.). Baltimore, MD: Lippincott Williams & Wilkins.

Larson, E., Wood, W., & Clark, C. (2003). Occupational science: Building the science and practice of occupation through an academic discipline. In E. Crepeau, E. Cohn, & B. Schell (Eds.), *Willard & Spackman's occupational therapy* (10th ed., pp. 15–26). Philadelphia, PA: Lippincott Williams & Wilkins.

Law, M., Cooper, B., Strong, S., Stewart, D., Rigby, P., & Letts, L. (1996). The Person-Environment-Occupational Model: A transactive approach to occupational performance. *Canadian Journal of Occupational Therapy, 63,* 9–23.

Meyer, A. (1922). The philosophy of occupational therapy. *Archives of Occupational Therapy, 1,* 1–10.

National Board for Certification in Occupational Therapy (NBCOT). (2005). *NBCOT Certification Renewal Handbook.*

Nelson, D. L. (1994). Occupational form, occupational performance, and therapeutic occupation. Lesson 2. In C. B. Royeen (Ed.). *AOTA Self-study series: The practice of the future: Putting occupation back into therapy* (pp. 9–48). Rockville, MD: American Occupational Therapy Association.

Nelson, D. L. (1997). Why the profession of occupational therapy will flourish in the 21st century. 1996 Eleanor Clarke Slagle lecture. *American Journal of Occupational Therapy, 51,* 11–24.

Peloquin, S. M. (1991). Occupational therapy services: Individual and collective understanding of the founders. Part 1. *American Journal of Occupational Therapy, 45,* 352–360.

Quiroga, V. A. (1995). Occupational therapy: The first 30 years: 1900–1930. Bethesda, MD: American Occupational Therapy Association.

Reilly, M. (1962). Occupational therapy can be one of the great ideas of 20th century medicine. 1962 Eleanor Clarke Slagle lecture. *American Journal of Occupational Therapy, 16,* 2–9.

Wilcock, A. A. (1998). *An occupational perspective of health.* Thorofare, NJ: Slack.

Yerxa, E. (1993). Occupational science: A new source of power for participants in occupational therapy. *Occupational Science: Australia. 1,* 3–10.

Zemke, R. & Clark, F. (1996). Occupational science: The evolving discipline. Philadelphia, PA: F.A. Davis.

Chapter 15

Athletic Training

Connie L. Peterson

OBJECTIVES

After studying this chapter, the student should be able to

1. Explain the role and function of the certified athletic trainer.
2. Explain the historical development of athletic training as a profession.
3. Describe the educational preparation and certification required for athletic trainers.
4. Summarize the estimated earning and career potential of certified athletic trainers.
5. Identify resources for additional information on the role of athletic trainers.

INTRODUCTION

> *An athlete who tells you the training is always easy and always fun simply hasn't been there. Goals can be elusive, which makes the difficult journey all the more rewarding.*
>
> Alberto Salazar, American sprinter, (1958–)

Sports medicine is a generic term that encompasses multiple disciplines. Among these disciplines, you can find physicians, athletic trainers, physical therapists, exercise physiologists, emergency medical technicians, biomechanists, nutritionists, podiatrists, massage therapists, and sport psychologists. While each of these professions has a specific role to play within the sports medicine team, collectively, these individuals will be more successful working together to provide an optimal environment for safe, healthy, maximal sport performance. The sports medicine healthcare team helps both sports teams and individual athletes to prevent injuries (primary prevention), detect injuries (secondary prevention), and provide rehabilitation of sports injuries (tertiary prevention). Athletic trainers function within all three levels of prevention, and of all these professionals, frequently having the most regular contact with the athlete. The role of the athletic trainer is expanding beyond the sports arena to provide skills to physically active individuals of all ages.

What Is a Certified Athletic Trainer?

Certified athletic trainers (ATCs) are medical experts who specialize in the prevention, assessment, emergency care, treatment, and rehabilitation of injuries and illnesses that occur to athletes and the physically active. The American Medical Association recognizes Athletic Training as an allied healthcare profession. As part of a complete healthcare team, the ATC works under the direction of a licensed physician and in cooperation with other healthcare providers, athletic administrators, coaches, and parents. They provide a critical link between school-based sports programs and the medical community in implementing healthcare programs. In addition, athletic trainers are a valuable resource to educate and counsel athletes in the prevention of chronic diseases and degenerative injuries through life-long activity-related fitness and health education. The ATC specializes in six professional practice areas or domains: prevention; clinical evaluation and diagnosis; immediate care; treatment, rehabilitation, and reconditioning; organization and administration; and professional responsibility. A typical day for an athletic trainer may include the following tasks:

- Preparing an athlete for practices or competition, including taping, bracing, and bandaging
- Evaluating injuries to determine management and possible referral to other healthcare providers
- Developing and implementing treatment, rehabilitation, and reconditioning programs
- Completing administrative tasks such as injury and treatment documentation, ordering supplies, submitting insurance reimbursement forms, and communicating with coaches, parents, and other healthcare providers.

The Beginning of Athletic Training

Athletic training has roots dating back to ancient Greece where athletics was an important part of Greek culture. Individuals called Paidotribes (boy-rubber) and Aleittes (anointer) suggest that massage played an important role in athletic performance. The medical gymnastae (trainers) were said to possess ideas of the effect of diet, rest, and exercise on the development of the body. Hippocrates, the "father of modern medicine," and his student Claudius Galen often advised their patients to exercise in the gymnasia as a means of recovering from their ills.

As sport began to reemerge in society during the late 19th century, few individuals recognized the need for medical care for injured athletes. Athletes, their coaches, teammates, and spectators often managed their own injuries and the injuries of team members. In 1869, Rutgers and Princeton introduced the sport of football to the American scene. As a result of 18 deaths and 159 serious injuries in 1905, President Roosevelt was threatening to abolish football as an intercollegiate sport. This spurred a few educational institutions to hire individuals whose duties included those of athletic trainer (although usually not exclusively).

The early "trainers" were mainly responsible for carrying water jugs, acting as team managers, and providing an occasional massage. These trainers typically worked independently and rarely shared ideas with others. Upon graduating from the University of Illinois in 1914 with a degree in physical education, Samuel E. Bilik enrolled in medical school. The Illini hired Bilik to serve as a part-time athletic trainer, thus changing the norm. Bilik published his first book, *Athletic Training*, two years later and soon began teaching intensive summer courses for athletic trainers that supported using sound, logical, physiological, and scientific facts to practice medicine with athletes. Other progress during this time must be credited to the Cramer brothers, Charles ("Chuck") and Frank, who founded the Cramer Chemical Company, which furnished supplies to training rooms throughout the country. After traveling with the US Olympic team in 1932, the brothers wanted to share what they had learned, so they set up a series of traveling workshops and began publishing The *First Aider*, a newsletter with practical practice tips for the fledgling Athletic Training profession. The *First Aider* gave athletic trainers insight into the latest athletic training methods, provided a forum for the exchange of ideas regarding the conditioning and training of athletes, the discussion of training room problems, and the care and treatment of minor injuries in athletics.

A few prominent individuals realized that if they started working together, sharing ideas, and supporting each other, perhaps the profession would have an opportunity to grow and develop. Organization on the national level could provide a collective voice on matters of mutual concern, set minimum standards of practice, and serve as a forum for the exchange of ideas. The first attempt to organize an association for athletic trainers occurred at the Drake Relays in Des Moines, Iowa during the spring of 1938. Unfortunately, only those athletic trainers with teams participating in the competition were able to attend. Just as the first National Athletic Trainers' Association (NATA) was beginning to take shape, the United States began mobilizing its forces for

World War II. Athletic trainers went from preparing boys for athletic competition to conditioning men for armed service. As the war evolved, the organization struggled with financial and logistical challenges. Regional bickering and accusations of athletic trainers "keeping" their best secrets to themselves abounded. By the end of the war, the first NATA was no longer around.

Despite the failure of the first attempts at organizing the profession, those earlier attempts set the foundation for what would become one of the fastest growing professional organizations in the country. During the late 1940s, unity began to reemerge in the form of regional and conference-based athletic training organizations. It was quickly identified that if athletic training was to develop into a full-fledged profession, a national association must be established to set and enforce recognizable and respectable standards of practice and care. On June 24 and 25, 1950, The Cramer Chemical Company sponsored what is considered the first National Athletic Trainers Clinic in Kansas City, Missouri. From this meeting emerged the foundation of the National Athletic Trainers' Association in the form of an elected a board of directors, a purpose for the association, and classes of membership. Generously, the Cramer Chemical Company continued to underwrite the expenses of the NATA, allowing for growth without concern of financial support.

William E. "Pinky" Newell's appointment as executive secretary of NATA in 1956 coincided with numerous milestones. Under Newell's tenure, the profession established a journal of scholarly research and discourse (1956), adopted a code of ethics (1957), aligned itself with numerous organizations including the National Collegiate Athletic Association (1957), and approved a model curriculum for athletic training of students (1959). Advocating education, Newell helped elevate the profession to a level of competence and effectiveness such that in 1967 the AMA recognized the NATA as a professional organization worthy of the "support" of the medical community.

In 1956, Arthur Dickinson colorfully described the evolution of the athletic trainer. In a speech to the American Association of Health, Physical Education, and Recreation, he said:

> the word "trainer" has stuck like a bloody tick from the time racehorses demanded a valet, who slept in the stables and probably shared part of the horse's menus. Following this, the boxing profession broke out with a rash of handlers—men who appeared at the ringside with a bucket and sponge and hurled meaningless advice to the toiling gladiators, and later slapped them when they got on the rubbing table after the bout. These also were called trainers. Universities and colleges . . . figured that if racehorses and boxers could stand up under the treatment meted out by these characters, why wouldn't it be good for the football team? So, they lowered

themselves socially and hired these chaps who left the ringside and stables in droves. So much chewing tobacco was sprayed on the dressing room walls of our institutions that Congress nearly went into an extra session to pass laws preventing such things. . . . Soon, college presidents, tiring of having men on the staff who signed the payroll with an X, demanded at least an 8th grade diploma. Thus, education took a gigantic step forward. (Ebel, 1999).

The proposed curriculum model of 1959 was to have accelerated the development of athletic training education programs by colleges and universities. By 1970, four schools had submitted their curricula for approval by the NATA. The 1970s also saw the emergence of licensing of athletic trainers by states in which they practiced, and the demise of the "men only" profession as women's sports and interest in the profession grew. Accelerating the development of athletic training programs coincided with the implementation of a national certifying exam in 1971. While this exam created controversy among its relatively "trade" trained members, it was a necessary step for the association to achieve its goal of respected credentials consistent with other allied healthcare providers. To sit for this exam, candidates had to complete required course work, gain practical experience under the direct supervision of a NATA athletic trainer, and complete requirements for a bachelor's degree. The certification examination and ATC credential remained the responsibility of the NATA Board of Certification committee until 1989. At that time, the Board of Certification (BOC) became an independent, nonprofit organization. This independence assures the public that athletic trainers have achieved a minimal level of competency through the certification exam and have continued to meet requirements for certification through continuing education courses. From humble beginnings, the association has expanded to encompass a global membership totaling nearly 30,000, plus a full-time executive director and staff. Today, members serve as leaders for the association, which has more than 30 committees working together to help advance the profession.

Where Do Athletic Trainers Work?

Athletic Trainers can be found working almost anywhere people are physically active. Some of these work environments are described in the following.

Secondary Schools

Administrators and parents recognize the value of qualified medical professionals in keeping today's young athletes safe. Many athletic trainers are able to find yment in both private and public secondary schools. In 1998, the American Medical Association recommended, "those high schools with athletic programs provide the services of a certified athletic trainer for their athletes" (NATA, 2006). High school athletic trainers may also teach classes at the school or may be employed through a clinic or hospital to provide outreach care.

Colleges and Universities

There is tremendous variability in the different positions available at colleges and universities. Smaller institutions may hire athletic trainers with the expectation that they wear many different hats, including part-time teacher, athletic trainer, and administrator. Larger institutions typically hire many athletic trainers who are employed clinically by the athletic department and may or may not have any teaching responsibilities. These athletic trainers work daily with athletic teams and athletes. Institutions with accredited athletic training education programs may hire ATCs to teach athletic training classes, supervise athletic training students, and/or conduct research related to athletic training areas of interest. These athletic trainers may or may not have clinical responsibilities.

Professional Sports

While employment in this setting is often desired, there are very few opportunities available. The growth of professional sport opportunities for women is creating parallel growth opportunities within the athletic training profession. Athletic trainers working in professional sports work year-round conducting off-season rehabilitation, conditioning, and prevention programs.

Sports Medicine Clinics

Athletic trainers working in sports medicine clinics have the opportunity to work with different healthcare providers and a diverse patient population. Roles may vary from acting as a physician extender provider, providing rehabilitation care, doing outreach care at a local high school, developing marketing and promotional tools, working in community outreach and education, and providing possible special event medical coverage.

Military

The US Military is one of the fastest growing employment markets within athletic training. Athletic trainers may provide health care for one of the military school sports teams, work in on- and off-base fitness and wellness centers, be a part of the healthcare team for active duty service people, and/ or work with new recruit readiness preparation programs.

Industrial and Corporate

Athletic trainers are often hired by large corporations to work with physicians and other healthcare providers in delivering employee fitness programs, performing ergonomic assessments, serving as first responders to emergencies, and overseeing rehabilitation and return to work reconditioning programs for injured employees.

Hospitals

Athletic trainers may work directly with occupational health physicians, performing ergonomic assessments, conducting employee wellness programs, providing in- and out-patient rehabilitation, or managing/operating hospital-based fitness centers.

Health Clubs

Using their knowledge in nutrition, injury prevention, and rehabilitation, athletic trainers may design fitness and wellness programs for clients or work in the areas of risk management and performance enhancement.

Performing Arts

Athletic trainers work with performing artists to ensure proper conditioning, flexibility, and rehabilitation following injury. The Radio City Rockettes, Blue Man Group, and Cirque du Soleil™ all employ ATCs.

Olympic Sports

The US Olympic Committee employs approximately 25 full-time athletic trainers at its various Olympic training centers throughout the United States. In addition, athletic trainers are selected through a competitive process to provide care to teams in various international competitions. Individual national governing bodies may also have short-term positions available for special competitions. These positions are largely volunteer, but provide memorable experiences.

Additional work settings may include youth, recreational, and amateur sports teams, government, and law enforcement. While these settings do not employ a lot of athletic trainers, they are certainly areas of potential growth and represent the diversity into which athletic trainers are employable. New areas of employment continue to emerge as athletic trainers educate the public about their diversity of expertise.

Minimum Education/Certification Requirements for Athletic Trainers

To become a certified athletic trainer, students must complete degree requirements from an accredited athletic training education program and pass a national certification exam and/or meet state accrediting agency requirements. After completing certification requirements, many students continue to pursue an advanced degree. In fact, 70% of athletic trainers have earned graduate degrees in athletic training and related fields.

Athletic training education programs, an academic major or the equivalent, are accredited by the Commission on the Accreditation of Allied Health Education Programs (CAAHEP) via the Joint Review Committee-Athletic Training (JRC-AT) and lead to a bachelor's or master's degree. A list of CAAHEP Accredited Curriculum Programs can be found at http://www.caahep.org/programs.asp. However, athletic training certification programs transitioned to a new, independent accreditation process in July 2006. The Commission on the Accreditation of Athletic Training Education (CAATE) then became the certifying agency. Programs already granted accreditation under the old process will be honored until their re-accreditation date, at which time they must demonstrate requisite changes to meet the CAATE standards. Prospective athletic training students should ask questions about their school's program to assure the new standards are being met.

Educational content is based on cognitive (knowledge), psychomotor (skill), affective competencies (professional behaviors), and clinical proficiencies (professional, practice-oriented outcomes). Athletic training students receive formal instruction in the following specific subject matter areas:

Foundation Courses:
- Human physiology
- Human anatomy
- Exercise physiology
- Kinesiology/biomechanics
- Nutrition
- Therapeutic modalities
- Acute care of injury and illness

- Statistics and research design
- Strength training and reconditioning.

Professional Courses—Content Areas:
- Risk management and injury/illness prevention
- Pathology of injury/illness
- Assessment of injury/illness
- General medical conditions and disabilities
- Therapeutic exercise: rehabilitation techniques
- Healthcare administration
- Weight management and body composition
- Psychosocial intervention and referral
- Medical ethics and legal issues
- Pharmacology
- Professional development and responsibilities.

In addition, students are required to complete a minimum of two years of academic clinical education. Using a competency-based approach, students are instructed and evaluated by Approved Clinical Instructors. These clinical experiences should occur in a variety of settings to expose students to different work environments. Possible venues include

- College and university athletic training rooms or health centers
- Industrial settings
- Secondary schools
- Hospitals
- Professional sports
- Olympic sports
- Sports medicine and physical therapy clinics
- Any other setting employing a certified athletic trainer.

Typically, undergraduate students can expect to complete general education and prerequisite athletic training courses during their first one–two years in an accredited athletic training education program. Most programs requires a formal application into the athletic training program and are competitive based on grades, previous experiences, letters of recommendation, and a formal interview. Many upper-level athletic training classes combine traditional classroom learning with laboratory, clinical, and "hands on" learning opportunities. This is a good major for students who tend to learn not only from reading, but also from "doing."

Athletic training students, who have completed requirements for graduation from an accredited program, are then eligible to take a certification exam administered by the Board of Certification, Inc. (BOC). The certification exam covers a variety of topics within the six domains of practice listed earlier in this chapter. Most of today's practicing athletic trainers completed an exam which included a written portion with multiple choice questions, a practical exam where students demonstrated their psychomotor proficiency, and a written simulation test consisting of situations designed to approximate real-life decision making and the ability to resolve cases similar to those an athletic trainer might encounter in actual practice. Beginning in Spring 2006, the BOC certification exam will be delivered electronically and integrate all components of the exam—written, written simulation, and practical—into a single format. This exam will assess the candidate's knowledge with regard to the many skills and procedures required for higher-level critical thinking.

The Education Council serves as the NATA's voice in matters related to athletic training education. The council is specifically responsible for facilitating continuous quality improvement in entry-level, graduate, and continuing athletic training education. This committee has an ongoing responsibility for determining educational competencies (content) required of entry-level athletic training programs. A quick look at the history of athletic training education suggests that as the scope of practice has broadened over the years, so too has the number and type of competencies being taught to entry-level athletic trainers.

Another topic of interest regarding the future of athletic training education is the exploration of the development of Certificates of Advanced or Added Qualification (CAQs). This type of specialty education would result in an advanced preparation beyond that of an entry-level certified athletic trainer.

Athletic training educators are also debating whether to increase the entry level of education to that of a master's degree. Physician assistant, physical, and occupational therapy programs have all moved to this model. The question remains—should athletic training move to a similar model? A recent task force studied this question and unanimously recommended to leave the entry level as an undergraduate degree rather than raise it to a master's degree. However, research regarding this move continues to progress and the decision will most likely be revisited in the near future. As it stands, there are entry-level graduate programs that are similar to undergraduate athletic training education programs as well as accredited graduate athletic training education programs which emphasize advanced qualifications within athletic training.

Once athletic training students pass the certification examination demonstrating sufficient knowledge within each of the six domains, they use the designation "ATC." This credential is an entry-level credential which ensures high standards of professional practice and is required by most employers. In addition to the BOC credential, athletic trainers usually must also meet individual state licensing requirements. To determine if these added requirements apply, certified athletic trainers are encouraged to check with the states in which they practice (http://www.bocatc.org/atc/STATE/). Often, state accrediting agencies accept the ATC credential as sufficient.

Because athletic training is a constantly evolving profession, certified athletic trainers must complete continuing education requirements set by the Board of Certification in order to retain their certification. These requirements include

- Completion and reporting of 75 continuing education units, including recertification in CPR at least once in each three-year term. Continuing education units are awarded for various activities, such as attending educational meetings, publishing manuscripts in professional journals, giving an educational presentation to colleagues or the public, or the completion of course work relative to the field of athletic training. Additional information can be obtained by visiting the Board of Certification Web site: http://www.bocatc.org/atc/CE/REP0305/.
- Adherence to the BOC Standards of Professional Practice.

The purposes of these requirements are to ensure that ATCs continue to

- Obtain current professional development information
- Explore new knowledge in specific content areas
- Master new athletic training-related skills and techniques
- Expand approaches to effective athletic training
- Further develop professional judgment
- Conduct professional practice in an ethical and appropriate manner

While the technical requirements to become an athletic trainer are well defined, personality impacts professional success. Though not inclusive, the following personality traits (italicized) are traits a prospective athletic trainer should consider before pursuing a career in athletic training:

Athletic trainers need to have a *love of sports*. While professional athletes may make large salaries, the trickle-down effect to the support staff, including the athletic training staff, is not typically a reason athletic trainers cite as a reason to pursue the profession. Athletic trainers often find themselves assigned to work with sports for which they have no background, but because of their general love of sports, they are extremely satisfied with their jobs. A love of sports is also necessary under different work conditions, for example, when the climate isn't so pleasant. Athletes and athletic trainers are outside or inside in all types of weather competing and practicing. If you don't love what you are doing, you probably won't stay in the profession very long.

A typical day in the athletic training clinical setting may also be physically demanding. Often times, athletic trainers must carry coolers of ice and water, remove an injured athlete from the playing field, work nontraditional hours (long days), or assist athletes performing functional sport activities through a rehabilitation program. *Good physical conditioning and stamina* assure that the athletic trainer is not fatigued and capable of performing their job responsibilities despite being tired.

Both *written and oral communication skills* are critical for success in athletic training. A review of athletic trainers' daily activities brings this to life. In a typical day, an athletic trainer may have to talk with a salesperson about supplies and equipment for their facility, submit a daily injury report to the coaching staff so they are aware of athletes available for practice, document daily treatment and rehabilitation activities in patient charts, educate athletes about their injuries, provide treatment or rehabilitation exercises, refer an athlete to a physician (phone referral), and perhaps teach a new skill to a student. And this is only a brief example of the role communication skills play in the daily life of an ATC.

Athletic Trainers are also bound by a "code of ethics." *Ethical behavior* assures high-quality health care; protects the rights, welfare, and dignity of the public; and presents a standard of behavior that all members should strive to achieve. The NATA Code of Ethics can be found at http://www.nata.org/about/codeofethics.htm.

Intellectual curiosity helps athletic trainers achieve success by allowing them to be open and receptive to learning new ideas and techniques. It is impossible to expect all athletic trainers to practice in the exact same fashion. Many times, the actual practice of athletic training is an art based on sound scientific principles. Injuries present and respond differently from what textbooks teach and guidelines suggest. Having the curiosity to pursue different treatment options, and the realization that it is impossible to know everything, helps keep the profession of athletic training exciting. Closely paralleling intellectual curiosity is the ability to adapt to a situation. Not all athletic trainers work in the perfect environment with every possible piece of equipment available to them. High school athletic trainers often provide excellent care on small budgets simply because they are able to adapt to their situation by using a creative approach to problem solving. By simply asking the question, "How can I do this?" rather than stating "I cannot do this," athletic trainers achieve tremendous results.

The *ability to empathize* with an injured athlete as they struggle through physical pain and often psychological depression is critical. Understanding that injury may mean the end of a season, the loss of a game, a change in personal identity, or perhaps the end of a career, goes a long way in developing an athlete's trust. Often times, this requires digging deep into psychological healing skills to help the athlete to see that it is not the end, but rather a bump in the road. A *sense of humor* is one tool which may be valuable in successfully treating injured athletes. Humor can also help athletic trainers survive long days at work, often in challenging environments.

Roles of the National Professional Organization/Association

The National Athletic Trainers' Association (NATA) is a not-for-profit organization dedicated to advancing, encouraging, and improving the athletic training profession. It accomplishes this by supporting and representing the profession through public awareness, education, and research. The National Athletic Trainers' Association's roles within the profession closely follow the purposes outlined in the bylaws.

1. **To enhance the quality of health care for the physically active.** The credential of ATC assures the public that the individual has met minimal standards to provide quality care to the physically active.

2. **To advance the profession of athletic training through education and research in the prevention, evaluation, management, and rehabilitation of injuries.** Some of the activities that help the association achieve this goal include:
   - Publishing the *Journal of Athletic Training*. This journal features peer-reviewed scientific articles written by experts in the field.
   - Sponsoring regional and national educational seminars.
   - Supporting the NATA Research and Education Foundation in awarding scholarships, research grants, and continuing education opportunities.
   - Initiation of the development of the World Federation of Athletic Trainers and Therapists. This group is a coalition of national organizations of healthcare professionals in the fields of sport, exercise, injury/illness prevention, and treatment.

3. **To safeguard and advance the interests of its members by presenting the professions' viewpoints, concerns, and other important information to the media and to appropriate legislative, administrative, regulatory, and private sector bodies, and by developing a working relationship with appropriate governmental and private sector not-for-profit and for-profit entities.** This role is accomplished by some of the following activities:
   - Writing and publishing position statements. While not binding documents, these statements serve as a guideline for appropriate professional practice. These can be found at http://www.nata.org/publicinformation/position.htm.

- Hiring legal consultants and legislative lobbyists to protect the interests of the profession and professional organization in state and national laws.
- Sponsoring, encouraging, and assisting members with opportunities to meet local politicians and representatives.
- Monitoring the news for stories, both positive and negative, to promote and protect the interests of its members.
- Developing, distributing, and encouraging activities to promote the profession. (March is NATA month.)

4. **To advance members' levels of knowledge through the collection, interpretation, and dissemination of information on subjects appropriate to the profession.** In addition to the *Journal of Athletic Training*, the NATA publishes

- The *NATA News* (monthly) to communicate mainly key administrative issues to members in a timely fashion.
- An e-Blast newsletter to communicate time-sensitive information and alert members to new developments that may require their immediate action or can increase the credibility and awareness of the profession, and to remind members of upcoming events and deadlines.
- A salary survey of its members. The membership is surveyed yearly and the results are made available in an electronic database.

In addition, the national association offers members NATA-sponsored group liability, disability, medical, and life insurance, as well as discounted auto insurance, financial planning, and travel-related services. An online database for job searching is available as is an online membership directory and access to professional book and literature review services.

Estimated Salary/Earnings by Work Environment

The NATA surveys its membership on a regular basis to identify trends within the profession. The most recent NATA salary survey (conducted in 2004) indicated that athletic trainers work in very diverse settings. The average number of hours worked per week is 54. In addition to the salaries listed, most respondents list that their employer offered and paid part of their health insurance, dental insurance, and retirement plan costs. The salary of an athletic trainer depends on experience and job responsibilities. The median annual earnings of athletic trainers were $33,940 in 2004 (BLS, 2006).

Years of experience, level of education (BS, MS, PhD), and geographic regions may impact potential salary. Also, some positions may only be 9- or 10-month positions, allowing the athletic trainer to earn additional income in other positions should they desire.

The Future of Athletic Training

Athletic training has been on a moderate to fast growth rate since tracking began in 1974. Membership has grown from about 4,500 members in 1974 to over 31,000 in 2005, an increase of over 600%. Taking a conservative estimate of a 30% growth rate, athletic training should see an increase of about 7,000 new positions by 2012. However, because of the flexibility of athletic trainers to work within other healthcare positions, job growth within healthcare services must also be considered. An aging population and longer life expectancies are factors driving up the demand for qualified healthcare providers. Further, this aging population and medical community recognize the impact physical activity has on living longer, healthier, more independent, and productive lives. One thing to be certain about is that as long as people are participating in sports, injuries will occur, and the demand for qualified healthcare providers to evaluate, treat, and manage these injuries will continue to be necessary. Athletic trainers are the ideal professionals to deliver high-quality health care to a wide range of individuals.

Challenges Facing the Profession

In contrast to the early athletic trainers who kept their trade secrets to themselves, the profession of athletic training has expanded into a well-educated, international network, with individuals working together to achieve quality health care for physically active individuals. What started as a profession in athletics has grown to a profession in health care that is expanding to a global frontier. Despite this growth, the profession continues to face an identity crisis. Athletic trainers are often misperceived as "personal trainers" or "coaches" or "massage therapists." A change in name has been explored as one possible solution to the dilemma, yet a change in name is likely to create more confusion and undo much of the hard work of the leaders in the profession to date.

Reimbursement for services provided continues to be an ongoing struggle within the profession. Currently, the insurance industry and legislative bodies often consider athletic trainers as second-tier service providers. That is, they don't often recognize that athletic trainers are capable healthcare providers and fail to reimburse companies using athletic trainers to provide health care. Until this issue is resolved, growth and professional respect will continue to be stifled. Numerous other governmental affairs issues also provide a challenge to the profession of athletic training. However, the leadership of the NATA is working hard to protect the interests of its members and keep the profession on a path of growth and development.

A Day in the Life of an Athletic Trainer

During a college football game, a wide receiver took a lateral blow to the head by an oncoming defensive tackle. The injury occurred in the middle of the field immediately after the wide receiver caught a 27-yard pass. He was soundly hit on the left side of the head by the opponent's helmet, forcing a whiplash mechanism to occur before he fell to the ground. The player was lying on the ground in an unconscious state as the head athletic trainer came to the field. The head athletic trainer had responsibility for the primary management of the athlete on the field and focused on stabilizing the head. The assistant athletic trainer performed the primary survey and summoned the emergency medical technicians (EMTs) to the field with the spine board. The primary survey found that the athlete was regaining consciousness and that airway, breathing, and circulatory status were all satisfactory. The EMTs assisted the athletic training staff in log rolling the athlete on the spine board, paying careful attention to stabilization of the head, spine, torso, and pelvis at all times because the presence or absence of a cervical fracture or dislocation had not been confirmed. Once secured on the spine board, the athlete was loaded on the ambulance and taken to the emergency room by the EMTs, accompanied by the assistant athletic trainer.

Immediately upon arrival to the emergency room, radiographs of the cervical spine, magnetic resonance imaging (MRI) of the brain and spinal cord, and a computed axial tomography (CAT) scan of the cervical spine were obtained by the radiologist. The results of each of these were negative. The emergency room doctor examined the athlete after being briefed by the assistant athletic trainer on the mechanism of injury, history, and the initial assessment. The athlete remained in the hospital for the rest of the night for periodic neurological evaluations, conducted by registered nurses and emergency room doctors to assess changes in the athlete's sensory and motor function.

The athletic trainer scheduled an appointment with the team neurosurgeon and neuropsychological team, who conducted a complete history, physical, and neurological examination. The athlete was diagnosed with a cerebral concussion. As a part of the team's concussion program, the athletic trainer and neuropsychologist administered a concussion screening to compare the results with the baseline screening that had been administered five months prior.

After 48 hours, the athlete's sensory, motor, and cognitive tests were within normal limits and his chief complaint was muscular soreness in the neck and shoulders from the whiplash mechanism. The athletic trainer developed a treatment and rehabilitation program to assist this athlete in regaining cervical range of motion and strength. An appointment with the team's massage therapist was also scheduled for the next day.

Once the athlete was asymptomatic at rest, the team doctor gave clearance for a heavily monitored functional progression program to begin. The athletic trainer designed a light exercise program consisting of non-sport-specific aerobic activity (stationary bike) and sport-specific activities (throwing a football). The athletic trainer and doctor monitored the athlete carefully during this stage of progression. Gradually the level of intensity and perceived exertion was increased. As he advanced and continued to be symptom free, communication about return to competition increased between the athlete, coaches, parents, athletic trainer, and doctor. Once the athlete felt confident and comfortable with his level of function and was asymptomatic at rest, exertion, and with contact, he was able to return to play for the remainder of the season.

SUMMARY

Athletic training has evolved from a male-only profession without well-defined standards of practice or educational requirements, to a diverse profession, recognized by the American Medical Association, with rigorous academic preparation, national certification, and state practice requirements. The knowledge and skills possessed by athletic trainers proves their skills as healthcare providers in a wide variety of practice settings, not just in athletics. It is anticipated that the profession will continue to grow in numbers and opportunities as more people are exposed to the advantages and capabilities of these providers.

ADDITIONAL RESOURCES

National Athletic Trainers Association	http://www.nata.org
NATA Foundation (research and scholarships)	http://www.natafoundation.org
Board of Certification (how to become and stay certified)	http://www.bocatc.org

Joint Review Committee— Education programs	http://www.jrc-at.org/index.html
Education Council (initial and continuing education)	http://www.nataec.org/
World Federation of Athletic Trainers and Therapists	http://www.wfatt.org/
Employment (jobs, salaries)	http://www.nata.org/employment/index.htm
State accrediting agencies	http://www.bocatc.org/atc/STATE/
NATA Code of Ethics	http://www.nata.org/about/codeofethics.htm
Journal of Athletic Training	http://www.nata.org/jat/
American College of Sports Medicine	http://www.acsm.org/

DISCUSSION QUESTIONS

The following section contains study questions to stimulate student thinking/comprehension of the profession.

1. List and describe three specific activities an athletic trainer would perform within each of the six practice domains.

2. Select five different work settings for athletic trainers. Then list three reasons you would like working in these settings and two reasons you would *not* like working in this setting.

3. How does the profession of athletic training differ from personal training?

4. What role does sharing knowledge play in the development of a profession?

5. What role(s) did the Cramer Company play in the development of athletic training?

6. Why was a certification exam developed for athletic trainers?

7. Use the NATA Web site to find out who, in addition to Gatorade®, are current major sponsors of the NATA.

8. What general type of courses should high school students take to prepare them for an athletic training major program?

9. To sit for the Board of Certification Exam, what criteria must an applicant complete?

10. Examine your own personal skill set. Explain why you feel athletic training would or would not be a good fit for you.

11. March is National Athletic Training month. Describe three public relations activities you could implement to promote the profession of athletic training in your school community.

12. The World Federation of Athletic Trainers and Therapists (WFATT) is a coalition of national organizations of health professionals in sport, exercise, injury/illness prevention, and treatment. In addition to the United States (through the NATA), what other countries are represented in the coalition?

13. If a law were to be enacted stating that only physical therapists could provide rehabilitation services in doctors' offices, how would the practice of athletic training be impacted? What role(s) does the NATA play in protecting against such legislation?

14. Once an athletic training student has completed degree requirements for a bachelor's degree, describe steps they can take to increase their employment prospects.

15. Discuss the pros and cons of changing the entry-level requirements for certification to a master's degree.

16. In what year was the first national certification examination given?

17. In what year was the current NATA founded?

REFERENCES

Bureau of Labor Statistics, US Department of Labor, Occupational Outlook Handbook, 2006–2007 Edition, Athletic Trainers, on the Internet at http://www.bls.gov/oco/ocos294.htm (visited Nov. 28, 2006).

Ebel, R. G. (1999). *Far beyond the shoe box—Fifty years of the National Athletic Trainers' Association*. New York: Forbes Publishing.

Chapter 16

Communication Disorders: Speech–Language Pathology and Audiology

Stephanie Chisolm

OBJECTIVES

After studying this chapter, the student should be able to

1. Explain the role of communication sciences in the healthcare system.
2. Explain the difference between the speech-language pathologist and audiologist.
3. Describe the educational preparation and certification required for speech-language pathology and audiology.
4. Identify resources for additional information pertaining to the role of and training for a career in the communication sciences.

INTRODUCTION

> *Good communication is as stimulating as black coffee*
> *and just as hard to sleep after.*
> Anne Morrow Lindbergh, *Gift From the Sea*

C ommunication, whether as stimulating as a cup of black coffee or bland as boiled water, is the exchange of information, the sending and receiving of messages. Speech includes vocal communication or conversations.

It is the production of sounds in meaningful combinations by the lips, tongue, teeth, palate, vocal cords, and lungs for communication. Communication is essentially the art and technique of using words effectively to impart information or ideas. Communication is a two-way interaction requiring interpersonal rapport and the participation of a sender and a receiver. The sender encodes and transmits a message that the receiver then decodes. Communication breakdowns can occur if either party has difficulty performing his or her role. If the sender does not speak clearly or intelligibly, or does not use language appropriately, in a meaningful way, the receiver may not understand the message. If the receiver has a hearing impairment, an oral/spoken message may not be received.

Communication Is a Speech and Hearing Health Concern

Speak properly, and in as few words as you can,
but always plainly; for the end of speech
is not ostentation, but to be understood.
William Penn (1644–1718)

Two of the professions concerned with human communication and disorders associated with speaking and hearing are *speech-language pathology*, and *audiology*. Speech-Language Pathology is the study of human communication disorders. This includes disorders of speech, language, and swallowing. Audiologists evaluate and treat people who have hearing, balance, and related ear problems. Communication disorders can be congenital or acquired, and can affect individuals of any age.

American Speech-Language-Hearing Association (ASHA), the professional, scientific, and credentialing association, summarizes the role of the speech-language pathologist and audiologist in the following statement:

Of all the gifts bestowed upon humanity, the ability to communicate is one of the most important. Any impairment of this ability can have far-reaching consequences, affecting every aspect of a person's life, from learning, to work, to interactions with family, friends, and community. Audiologists and speech-language pathologists provide services to prevent, diagnose, evaluate, and treat communication disorders.

Speech-Language Pathologists

Speech-language pathologists (SLPs), sometimes called *speech therapists*, assess, diagnose, treat, and help to prevent speech, language, cognitive, communication, voice, swallowing, fluency, and other related disorders. They work with people who cannot make speech sounds, or cannot make them clearly. The SLP also works with individuals with speech rhythm and fluency problems, such as stuttering; people with voice quality problems, such as inappropriate pitch or harsh voice; and those with problems understanding and producing language. Some SLPs may help those who wish to improve their communication skills by modifying an accent; those with cognitive communication impairments, such as attention, memory, and problem-solving disorders; and those with hearing loss who use hearing aids or cochlear implants in order to develop auditory skills and improve communication. They also work with people who have swallowing difficulties. An SLP may work with individuals with oral motor problems that cause eating and swallowing difficulties. This may apply to clients of all ages, from infant feeding to the elderly, where the SLP evaluates aerodigestive functions and refers those clients to appropriate medical professionals. In addition, speech-language pathologists may

- Prepare future professionals in colleges and universities.
- Manage agencies, clinics, organizations, or private practices.
- Engage in research to enhance knowledge about human communication processes.
- Develop new methods and equipment to test and evaluate problems.
- Establish treatments that are more effective.
- Investigate behavioral patterns associated with communication disorders.

Speech-language pathologists often work as part of a team, which may include teachers, physicians/nurses, audiologists, psychologists, social workers, rehabilitation counselors, occupational therapists, and others. Corporate speech-language pathologists also work with employees to improve communication with their customers.

Speech and language problems can result from a variety of problems including hearing loss, brain injury or deterioration, cerebral palsy, stroke, cleft palate, voice pathology, mental retardation, or emotional problems. Problems can be congenital, developmental, or acquired. Speech-language pathologists use written and oral tests, as well as special instruments, to diagnose the nature and extent of impairment and to record and analyze speech, language, and swallowing irregularities.

The speech-language pathologist develops an individualized plan of care, tailored to each patient's needs. For individuals with little or no speech capability, speech-language pathologists may select augmentative or alternative communication methods, including automated devices and sign language, and teach their use. They teach these individuals how to make sounds, improve their voices, or increase their language skills to communicate more effectively. Speech-language pathologists help patients develop or recover reliable communication skills so patients can fulfill their educational, vocational, and social roles, thus improving their quality of life.

Training and Certification for Speech Language Pathology

About 233 colleges and universities offer graduate programs in speech-language pathology. Courses cover anatomy and physiology of the areas of the body involved in speech, language, swallowing, and hearing; the development of normal speech, language, swallowing, and hearing; the nature of communication disorders; acoustics; and psychological aspects of communication. Graduate students also learn to evaluate and treat speech, language, swallowing, and hearing disorders and receive supervised clinical training in communication disorders.

Speech-language pathologists can acquire the Certificate of Clinical Competence in Speech-Language Pathology (CCC-SLP) offered by the American Speech-Language-Hearing Association. To earn a CCC, a person must have a graduate degree and 400 hours of supervised clinical experience, complete a 36-week postgraduate clinical fellowship, and pass the Praxis Series examination in speech-language pathology administered by the Educational Testing Service (ETS).

In 2005, 47 states required licensure for speech-language pathologists if they worked in a healthcare setting, and all states required a master's degree or equivalent and a passing score on the national examination on speech-language pathology. Other requirements typically are 300 to 375 hours of supervised clinical experience and 9 months of postgraduate professional clinical experience. Forty-one states have continuing education requirements for licensure renewal. Medicaid, Medicare, and private health insurers generally require an SLP practitioner to have a license to qualify for reimbursement (SLP, 2006).

Only 11 states require this same license to practice in the public schools. The other states issue a teaching license or certificate that typically requires a master's degree from an approved college or university. Some states will grant a temporary teaching license or certificate to bachelor's degree applicants, but the speech pathologist must earn a master's degree within three to five years. A few states grant a full teacher's certificate or license to bachelor's degree applicants.

The Employment Environment for SLPs

According to the Bureau of Labor Statistics (SLP, 2006), speech-language pathologists held about 96,000 jobs in 2004. About half of jobs were in educational services, including preschools, elementary and secondary schools, and colleges and universities. Others were in hospitals; offices of other health practitioners, including speech-language pathologists; nursing care facilities; home healthcare services; individual and family services; outpatient care centers; child day care services; or other facilities. A few speech-language pathologists are self-employed in private practice. They contract to provide services in schools, offices of physicians, hospitals, or nursing care facilities, or work as consultants to industry.

Speech-language pathologists provide direct clinical services to individuals with communication or swallowing disorders. In speech and language clinics, they may independently develop and carry out treatment programs. In medical facilities, they may work with physicians, social workers, psychologists, and other therapists. Speech-language pathologists in schools develop individual or group programs, counsel parents, and may assist teachers with classroom activities. A growing number of speech pathologists have begun catering to clients whose needs are professional rather than medical. Speech pathologists may help business people communicate more effectively by reducing their regional and foreign accents.

Speech-language pathologists keep records to track patient progress and justify the cost of treatment when applying for reimbursement. They counsel individuals and their families concerning communication disorders as well as how to cope with the stress and misunderstanding that often accompany them. Some speech-language pathologists conduct research on how people communicate. Others design and develop equipment or techniques for diagnosing and treating speech problems. In school settings, the speech pathologist may participate in classroom activities.

Employment Trends for Speech-Language Pathologists

The Bureau of Labor Statistics expects employment of speech-language pathologists to grow faster than the average through the year 2012. Members of the baby boom generation are now entering middle age, when the possibility of neurological disorders and associated speech, language, swallowing, and hearing impairments increases. Medical advances are also improving the survival rate of premature infants and trauma and stroke victims, who then need assessment and possible treatment. Many states now require that all newborns receive screening for hearing loss and receive appropriate early intervention services.

In health services facilities, the impact of proposed federal legislation imposing limits on reimbursement for therapy services may adversely affect the short-term job outlook for therapy providers. However, over the long run, the demand for therapists should continue to rise as growth in the number of individuals with disabilities or limited function spurs demand for therapy services.

Employment in educational services will increase along with growth in elementary and secondary school enrollments, including the enrollment of special education students. Federal law guarantees special education and related services to all eligible children with disabilities. Greater awareness of the importance of early identification and diagnosis of speech, language, swallowing, and hearing disorders will also increase employment.

Median annual earnings of speech-language pathologists were $52,410 in May 2004. Median annual earnings in the industries employing the largest numbers of speech-language pathologists in May 2004 were (SLP, BLS, 2006):

Offices of other health practitioners	$57,240
General medical and surgical hospitals	$55,900
Elementary and secondary schools	$48,320

Entry Requirements for Speech-Language Pathology

To enter this career, one must have a sincere interest in helping people, an above-average intellectual aptitude, and the sensitivity, personal warmth, and perspective to be able to interact with a person who has a communication problem. Scientific aptitude, patience, emotional stability, tolerance, and persistence are necessary, as well as resourcefulness and imagination. Other essential traits include a commitment to work cooperatively with others and the ability to communicate effectively orally and in writing.

Prospective speech-language pathologists should consider a program with courses in biology, physics, social sciences, English, and mathematics, as well as in public speaking, language, and psychology. On the undergraduate level, a strong liberal arts focus is recommended, with course work in linguistics, phonetics, anatomy, psychology, human development, biology, physiology, and semantics. A program of study in communication sciences and disorders is available at the undergraduate level. The work of speech-language pathologists is further enhanced by graduate education, which is mandated by ASHA. Speech-language pathologists and audiologists are also required by ASHA to obtain the ASHA Certificate of Clinical Competence (CCC) which involves the completion of a master's degree, a supervised Clinical Fellowship (CF), and a passing score on a national examination. In some areas, such as college teaching, research, and private practice, a PhD degree is desirable. In most states, speech-language pathologists and audiologists also must comply with state regulatory (licensure) standards to practice and/or have state education certification. The requirements are very similar or identical to ASHA's CCC requirements.

Future Outlook for SLPs

The future of the speech-language pathology profession appears excellent. More frequent recognition of problems in preschool and school-age children by teachers and parents, combined with the increased numbers of older citizens and medical advances have created a growing need for speech and language services. In addition, opportunities in research and higher education are expected to increase as baby boomers currently in these positions retire. Clinical opportunities will be especially strong for those with bilingual and multicultural expertise. There are shortages of qualified personnel in some areas of the country, especially in the inner city, rural, and less populated areas. Job opportunities in medically related areas are expected to grow at an above-average rate. Although competition for positions in some areas is keen, the potential for private practice and contract work is increasing rapidly.

Audiologists

Hearing is one of our most vital senses, and audiologists are experts in the non-medical management of the auditory and balance systems. They specialize in the study of

- Normal and impaired hearing.
- Prevention of hearing loss.
- Identification and assessment of hearing and balance problems.
- Rehabilitation of persons with hearing and balance disorders.

More than 28 million Americans have some type of hearing problem. Hearing difficulties are often unrecognized by the person involved. Children and teenagers seldom complain about the symptoms of hearing loss, and adults may lose their hearing so gradually they do not realize it is happening.

The first step in treatment of a hearing problem is a hearing evaluation by an audiologist. The audiologist works with people who have hearing, balance, and related ear problems. They examine individuals of all ages and identify those with the symptoms of hearing loss and other auditory, balance, and related neural problems. They then assess the nature and extent of the problems and help the individuals manage them. Using audiometers, computers, and other testing devices, they measure the loudness at which a person begins to hear sounds, the ability to distinguish between sounds, and the impact of hearing loss or balance problems on an individual's daily life. Audiologists interpret these results and may coordinate them with medical, educational, and psychological information to make a diagnosis and determine a course of treatment.

Hearing disorders can result from a variety of causes, including trauma at birth, viral infections, genetic disorders, exposure to loud noise, certain medications, or aging. Treatment may include examining and cleaning the ear canal, fitting and dispensing hearing aids, fitting and tuning cochlear implants, and audiologic rehabilitation.

Audiologic rehabilitation emphasizes counseling on adjusting to hearing loss, training on the use of hearing instruments, and teaching communication strategies for use in a variety of listening environments. For example, audiologists may provide instruction in lip reading. They also may recommend, fit, and dispense personal or large area amplification systems and alerting devices.

In audiology (hearing) clinics, they may independently develop and carry out treatment programs. Audiologists, in a variety of settings, work with other health professionals as a team in planning and implementing services for children and adults, from birth to old age. Audiologists also keep records on patient/client progress, which helps pinpoint problems, and justify the cost of treatment when applying for reimbursement.

Some audiologists specialize by working in a particular setting or with a specific population, such as the elderly, children, or hearing-impaired individuals who need special therapy programs. Others develop and implement ways to protect workers' ears from on-the-job injuries. They measure noise levels in workplaces and conduct hearing protection programs in factories, as well as in schools and communities. Audiologists may conduct research on types of—and treatment for—hearing, balance, and related disorders. Others design and develop equipment or techniques for diagnosing and treating these disorders.

What Do Audiologists Do?

Hearing testing. Audiologists use specialized equipment to obtain accurate results about hearing loss. These tests are typically conducted in sound-treated rooms with calibrated equipment. The audiologist is trained to inspect the eardrum with an otoscope, perform limited earwax removal, conduct diagnostic audiologic tests, and check for medically related hearing problems. Hearing loss is caused by medical problems about 10% of the time. Audiologists are educated to recognize these medical problems and refer patients to ear, nose, and throat physicians (known as otolaryngologists). Most persons with hearing impairment can benefit from the use of hearing aids, and audiologists are knowledgeable about the latest applications of hearing aid technology.

Hearing services for infants and children. Good hearing is essential to the social and intellectual development of infants and young children. Audiologists test hearing and identify hearing loss in children of all ages. This includes conducting newborn and infant hearing screening and diagnostic hearing tests with young children. Audiologists provide hearing therapy and fit hearing aids on babies and young children with hearing loss.

Services for school children. Audiologists provide a full range of hearing and rehabilitative hearing services in private and public schools for students in all grades. Such services are essential to the development of speech, language, and learning skills in children with hearing problems.

Hearing services and counseling. Audiologists are vitally concerned that every person, regardless of age, benefit from good hearing. Audiologists provide individual counseling to help those with hearing loss function more effectively in social, educational, and occupational environments. It is a fact that we lose hearing acuity as we grow older, and that hearing problems are commonly associated with the elderly. Audiologists are committed to helping senior citizens hear better.

Hearing aids and assistive listening devices. Audiologists provide complete hearing aid services to clients with hearing problems. Audiologists are also experts with assistive listening equipment and personal alerting devices. Audiologists provide education and training so that persons with hearing impairment can benefit from amplification and communication devices. Audiologists dispense the majority of hearing aids in the United States. Audiologists use the most advanced computerized procedures to individualize the fitting of hearing aids. Hearing aid options are thoroughly discussed with each potential user based on the results of a complete hearing aid test battery and the individual needs of each patient. Follow-up care and hearing aid accessories are routinely available from dispensing audiologists.

Hearing conservation programs. Prolonged exposure to loud noise causes permanent hearing loss. Because audiologists are concerned with the prevention of hearing loss, they are often involved in implementing programs to protect the hearing of individuals exposed to noisy industrial and recreational situations.

Hearing research. Audiologists engage in a wide variety of research activities to develop new hearing assessment techniques and new rehabilitative technologies, particularly in the area of hearing aids. Research reports of audiologists can be found in the professional literature of medical and scientific journals. Audiologists write textbooks on hearing evaluation, hearing aids, and the management of people with hearing loss. Audiologists help develop professional standards and are represented on the boards of national and government agencies.

Training and Certification for Audiology

Of the 48 states that require a license to practice audiology, almost all require that individuals have a master's degree in audiology or the equivalent; however, a clinical doctoral degree is becoming the new standard, along with a passing score on a national examination on audiology offered through the Praxis Series of the Educational Testing Service. Other requirements are 300 to 375 hours of supervised clinical experience and 9 months of postgraduate professional clinical experience. An additional examination may be required in order to dispense hearing aids. Forty states have continuing education requirements for licensure renewal. Medicaid, Medicare, and private health insurers generally require licensure for practitioners to qualify for reimbursement.

About 107 colleges and universities offer graduate programs in audiology in the United States. About 39 of these offer a Doctor of Audiology (AuD) degree. Requirements for admission to programs in audiology include courses in English, mathematics, physics, chemistry, biology, psychology, and communication sciences. Graduate course work in audiology includes anatomy; physiology; physics; genetics; normal and abnormal communication development; auditory, balance, and neural systems assessment and treatment; diagnosis and treatment; pharmacology; and ethics.

Audiologists can acquire the Certificate of Clinical Competence in Audiology (CCC-A) offered by the American Speech-Language-Hearing Association. To earn a CCC, a person must have a graduate degree and 375 hours of supervised clinical experience, complete a 36-week postgraduate clinical fellowship, and pass the Praxis Series examination in audiology, administered by the Educational Testing Service. According to the American Speech-Language-Hearing Association, as of 2007, audiologists will need to have a bachelor's degree and complete 75 hours of credit toward a doctoral degree in order to seek certification. As of 2012, audiologists will have to earn a doctoral degree in order to be certified.

The American Board of Audiology certifies audiologists. Applicants must earn a master's or doctoral degree in audiology from a regionally accredited college or university, achieve a passing score on a national examination in audiology, and demonstrate that they have completed a minimum of 2,000 hours of mentored professional practice in a two-year period with a qualified audiologist. Renewing certification every three years requires the audiologists earns 45 hours of approved continuing education within the three-year period. Beginning in the year 2007, all applicants must earn a doctoral degree in audiology.

The audiologist must effectively communicate diagnostic test results, diagnoses, and proposed treatments in a manner easily understood by their clients. They must be able to approach problems objectively and provide support to clients and their families. Because a client's progress may be slow, patience, compassion, and good listening skills are necessary.

Employment of Audiologists

Audiologists held about 12,899 jobs in 2004. About one half provided services in non-residential healthcare facilities, including private physician offices, private practices, and speech and hearing centers. More than 72% were employed in hospitals, 17% in school settings, and 8% in colleges and universities. Some audiologists contract to provide services in schools, hospitals, nursing homes, or work as consultants to the industry. The majority of audiologists provide direct clinical services but others serve as program administrators, university professors, scientists, consultants, and expert witnesses. Some provide consultation about community noise.

The Working Environment for Audiologists

Audiologists work in private practice offices, hospitals and medical centers, clinics, public and private schools, universities, rehabilitation or speech and hearing centers, health maintenance organizations, and nursing homes. Audiologists work closely with government agencies such as state and local health departments, practicing physicians, and hearing aid manufacturers. Audiologists conduct clinical activities with patients, are involved in hearing research, dispense hearing aids and assistive listening devices, and teach at universities and medical schools.

In industrial audiology, the audiologist plans and executes programs of hearing conservation for workers. Audiologists frequently work with other medical specialists, speech-language pathologists, educators, engineers, scientists, and allied health professionals and technicians.

Future Employment and Earnings of Audiologists

According to the Bureau of Labor Statistics, employment of audiologists will grow as fast as the average for all occupations through the year 2014. Because hearing loss is strongly associated with aging, rapid growth in older population groups will cause the number of persons with hearing and balance impairments to increase markedly. Medical advances are also improving the survival rate of premature infants and trauma victims, who then need assessment and possible treatment. Greater awareness of the importance of early identification and diagnosis of hearing disorders in infants also will increase employment. Most states now require that all newborns receive screening for hearing loss and receive appropriate early intervention services.

Employment in educational services will increase along with growth in elementary and secondary school enrollments, including the enrollment of special education students. The number of audiologists in private practice will rise due to the increasing demand for direct services to individuals as well as the increasing use of contract services by hospitals, schools, and nursing care facilities.

While there does not appear to be a shortage of demand for services, growth in employment of audiologists will be moderated by limitations on insurance reimbursements for the services they provide. In addition, increased educational requirements may limit the pool of workers entering the profession and any resulting higher salaries may cause doctors to hire more lower paid ear technicians to perform the functions that audiologists provide in doctors' offices. The number of audiologists in private practice will rise due to the increasing demand for direct services to individuals as well as increasing use of contract services by hospitals, schools, and nursing care facilities. Only a few job openings for audiologists will arise from the need to replace those who leave the occupation, because the occupation is small.

Median annual earnings of audiologists were $51,470 in May 2004. According to a 2004 survey by the American Speech-Language-Hearing Association, the median annual salary for full-time certified audiologists who worked on a calendar-year basis, generally 11 or 12 months annually, was $56,000. For those who worked on an academic-year basis, usually 9 or 10 months annually, the median annual salary was $53,000. The median starting salary for certified audiologists with one to three years of experience was $45,000 on a calendar-year basis (BLM, 2006).

Entry Requirements for Audiology

To enter this career, one must have the ability to relate to patients/clients and their families/caregivers about the diagnosis of disability and audiologic rehabilitation plans and explain technology developments and devices that assist children and adults with hearing loss. Audiologists must effectively communicate diagnostic test results and interpret and propose treatment in a manner easily understood by their clients and professionals. They must be able to approach problems objectively and provide support to clients and their families. A client' s progress may be slow, so patience, compassion, and good listening skills are necessary.

Prospective audiologists should consider a program with courses in biology, physics, mathematics, and psychology. On the undergraduate level, a strong liberal arts focus is recommended, with course work in linguistics, phonetics, psychology, speech and hearing, and/or the biological and physical sciences. A program of study in audiology is not available at the undergraduate level. Typically, students obtain an undergraduate degree in communication sciences, which provides introductory course work in audiology.

About 95 colleges and universities offer graduate programs in audiology in the United States. Course work includes anatomy and physiology, basic science, math, auditory, balance, and normal and abnormal communication development. The American Speech-Language-Hearing Association requires those with a graduate degree to obtain the ASHA Certificate of Clinical Competence (CCC). To earn the CCC, a person must have a graduate degree and 375 hours of supervised clinical experience, complete a 36-week postgraduate clinical fellowship, and pass a written examination. In most states, speech-language pathologists and audiologists also must comply with state regulatory (licensure) standards to practice and/or have state education certification. These requirements are very similar or identical to ASHA's CCC requirements (BLM, 2006).

Speech, Language, and Hearing Scientists

Providing the research on which SLP and audiology clinicians base their methodology requires that speech, language and hearing scientists

- Explore trends in communication sciences.
- Develop strategies for expanding the knowledge base in their field.
- Investigate the biological, physical, and physiological processes of communication.
- Explore the impact of psychological, social, and other factors on communication disorders.
- Develop evidence-based methods for diagnosing and treating individuals with speech, language, and hearing problems.
- Collaborate with related professionals (such as engineers, physicians, dentists, educators) to develop a comprehensive approach to diagnosing and treating individuals with speech, voice, language, and hearing problems.

In addition, researchers may

- Prepare future professionals and scientists in colleges and universities.
- Conduct research at, or consult with, universities, hospitals, government health agencies, and industries.

As with audiologists and speech-language pathologists, research scientists are educated in their specific area of interest. However, while clinicians can practice with a master's degree or clinical doctorate, scientists must earn a research doctorate. Some researchers do not hold the American Speech-Language-Hearing Association's (ASHA) Certificate of Clinical Competence (CCC) because the credential usually is not required to conduct scientific research within a laboratory setting. However, scientists conducting data-based research in some employment settings (for example, colleges and universities) do become ASHA certified. The speech, hearing, and language scientists work in research laboratories and institutes, colleges and universities, and state and federal government agencies, as well as within private industry.

Entry Requirements for Speech, Language, and Hearing Scientists

To become a speech, language, and hearing scientist, you must have a sincere interest in the development of the field of human communication sciences and disorders. You should also select undergraduate courses from a variety of scientific disciplines including physics, biology, chemistry, mathematics, linguistics, psychology, as well as a program of study in the speech, language, and hearing sciences. The next step is to obtain a master's degree. This will begin to direct you into a particular area of interest—an area that you believe deserves further exploration. Give careful thought to the doctoral programs to which you apply, because your chosen program will act as a vehicle for making contact with other professionals in the field, and those with whom you will work on your doctoral dissertation. This work will be the basis of future research pursuits in the communication sciences and disorders.

Future Outlook for Speech, Language, and Hearing Scientists

With genetics and hereditary research being the driving force of the future, research scientists have much to look forward to. Not only will there be opportunity to examine causality and progression issues, there will also be time to explore new techniques to prevent, identify, assess, and rehabilitate speech, language, and hearing impairments. In addition, researchers will continue to investigate the neurobiological, neurophysiological, and physical processes underlying normal communication. Furthermore, the future holds great opportunity for research scientists to investigate and examine cultural diversity in human communication. In addition, there will be more opportunities for scientists and clinical practitioners to collaborate as they design and implement multicenter randomized behavioral and medical treatment protocols for disorders of speech, voice/swallowing, language, hearing, and balance. There are extreme shortages of speech, language, and hearing scientists and teacher-scholars in all areas of the country, especially in inner-city, rural, and less populated areas (BLS, 2006).

The Professional Organizations for Speech-Language Pathology and Audiology

The American Speech-Language-Hearing Association (ASHA) is the professional, scientific, and credentialing association for more than 120,000 members and affiliates who are audiologists, speech-language pathologists, and speech, language, and hearing scientists in the United States and internationally. The mission of the American Speech-Language-Hearing Association is to promote the interests of and provide the highest quality services for professionals in audiology, speech-language pathology, and speech and hearing science, and to advocate for people with communication disabilities (About ASHA, 2006 http://www.asha.org, retrieved 9/20/06).

The American Academy of Audiology is the world's largest professional organization of, for, and by audiologists. The active membership of more than 9,600 audiologists joins together to provide the highest quality of hearing healthcare service to children and adults described by their national slogan "Caring for America's Hearing." The American Academy of Audiology promotes quality hearing and balance care by advancing the profession of audiology through leadership, advocacy, education, public awareness, and support of research (About ASHA, 2006 http://www.audiology.org/, retrieved 9/20/06).

SUMMARY

Without speech, there is nothing to hear, and speaking without being understood can be frustrating. The complementary professionals described in this chapter often function within similar working environments, with the same clients. For instance, within the school system, a speech-language pathologist may

- Provide speech-language services to a number of schools on an itinerant basis.
- Provide services to infants, toddlers, preschoolers, school-age children, and adolescents.
- Teach full-time in a special education classroom setting with students who have language-learning disorders.
- Work with children with severe and/or multiple disorders.
- Teach listening and communication skills in a regular classroom.
- Collaborate with other professionals and parents to facilitate a student's communication and learning in an educational environment.
- Conduct screenings and diagnostic evaluations.

- Write reports and participate in annual review conferences.
- Serve on program planning and teacher assistance teams.
- Develop Individualized Education Plans (IEP) and Individualized Family Service Plans (IFSPs).

Audiologists working in the schools may

- Identify children with hearing loss.
- Provide habilitation activities, such as language habilitation, auditory training, or speech reading.
- Create and administer programs for the prevention of hearing loss.
- Develop and supervise a hearing screening program for preschool and school-age children.
- Identify and evaluate children with hearing loss and assess central auditory function.
- Make recommendations and ensure proper fit and functioning of hearing aids, cochlear implants, group and classroom amplification, and assistive listening devices.
- Provide services in the areas of speech reading, listening, communication strategies, use and care of amplification devices such as cochlear implants, and the self-management of hearing needs.
- Serve as a member of the educational team in the evaluation, planning, and placement process for students with hearing loss or other auditory disorders.
- Provide in-service training on hearing and hearing loss and their implications for school personnel, children, and parents.
- Educate parents, children, and school personnel about hearing loss prevention.
- Collaborate with the school, parents, teachers, special support personnel, and relevant community agencies and professionals to ensure delivery of appropriate services.

Acute care, rehabilitation, and psychiatric hospitals and health maintenance organizations (HMOs) may offer audiology, speech, and language services on an in- or out-patient basis. Hospitals may provide services for patients of all ages, and some, such as children's hospitals or hospitals for military or veteran personnel, may house specialized populations. The speech-language pathologist may (SLP, BLM, 2006)

- Diagnose and treat a wide range of communication disorders.
- Diagnose and treat swallowing problems.
- Function as part of a multidisciplinary treatment team.
- Provide counseling to patients and their families.

The audiologist in this medical setting may

- Measure hearing ability of individuals of all ages, including infants.
- Administer and interpret screening, assessment, and diagnostic procedures, such as air conduction, bone conduction, speech audiometry, acoustic emmittance (impedance) tests, evoked potential tests, and electronystagmography.
- Identify the presence and severity of hearing loss.
- Provide aural rehabilitation counseling about handling communication situations at home, work, and school to reduce the effects of hearing loss.
- Assess the benefit of amplification devices, such as hearing aids.
- Instruct in the use of hearing aids or other assistive listening devices in a variety of contexts.
- Instruct in the care and maintenance of amplification and other assistive devices.
- Design rehabilitation programs to help persons learn to identify sound heard.
- Collaborate with teams of professionals, individuals, and families of caregivers on strategies to meet the communication needs of children or adults with hearing loss.
- Conduct Auditory Brainstem Response/Evoked Potentials.

There arc increasing opportunities for the speech-language pathologist and audiologist to work with older persons in nursing homes and geriatric centers. In addition to providing traditional services, speech-language pathologists may work with other disciplines in developing programs to help inpatients with dementia, such as Alzheimer's disease, maintain communication function. The cliché from the cell phone ad, "Can you hear me now?", nicely sums up the complementary role of the speech-language pathologist and audiologist.

CAREER INFORMATION

ASHA has many resources to help members and people interested in a career in audiology; speech-language pathology; or speech, language, and hearing science to meet their educational and professional goals.

General information on careers in speech-language pathology and audiology is available from

American Speech-Language-Hearing Association
10801 Rockville Pike
Rockville, MD 20852
Internet: http://www.asha.org

American Academy of Audiology
11730 Plaza America Dr., Suite 300
Reston, VA 20190
Internet: http://www.audiology.org

REFERENCES

About the American Speech-Language-Hearing Association (ASHA). Retrieved 11/22/06 from http://asha.org/about_asha.htm.

Bureau of Labor Statistics, US Department of Labor (BLM). (2005). *Occupational outlook handbook, 2004–05 edition*. Audiologists. Retrieved November 03, 2005, from http://www.bls.gov/oco/ocos085.htm.

Bureau of Labor Statistics, US Department of Labor (BLM). (2006). *Occupational outlook handbook, 2006–07 edition*. Speech-language pathologists. Retrieved September 20, 2006, from http://www.bls.gov/oco/ocos099.htm.

Chapter 17

Mental Health Professions

Stephanie Chisolm

OBJECTIVES

After studying this chapter, the student should be able to

1. Explain the role of the mental health professionals in the healthcare system.
2. Describe the difference between psychiatrists, social workers, counselors, and psychologists.
3. Describe the educational preparation and certification required for each of the mental health professions.
4. Identify the various healthcare, business, and academic environments that employ mental health professionals.
5. Identify resources for additional information on the role of mental health professionals.

INTRODUCTION

Anguish of mind has driven thousands to suicide; anguish of body, none. This proves that the health of the mind is of far more consequence to our happiness, than the health of the body, although both are deserving of much more attention than either of them receive.
C. C. Colton, English writer

The first few years of the 21st century have seen dramatic events in this country and around the world that have brought issues of mental health to the forefront of public health. The September 11, 2001 terrorist attack; wars in the Middle East; and natural disasters such as hurricanes, tornados, tsunamis, and fires, all broadcast in the media, leave images of physical and mental suffering that impact us all. There are as many responses to crisis as there are people affected. Most have intense feelings after a traumatic event but completely recover from the trauma; others are more vulnerable—especially those who have had previous traumatic experiences—and will need additional help. Considering health and illness as points along a continuum helps us appreciate that neither state exists in pure isolation from the other. In years past, the mental health field often focused principally on mental illness in order to serve those individuals most severely affected. However, individuals may fall on either extreme of the mental health continuum or somewhere in the middle. Even those without a clinical diagnosis of mental illness may sometimes benefit from a wide range of mental health therapies.

Mental Health Today and Yesterday

Mental health refers to the successful performance of mental functions in terms of thought, mood, and behavior. Mental disorders are those health conditions in which alterations in mental functions are paramount. Mental illness is a disorder of the brain that results in a disruption in a person's thinking, feeling, moods, and ability to relate to others. Mental illness is distinct from the legal concepts of sanity and insanity. Mental health, mental hygiene, behavioral health, and mental wellness are terms that describe the state or absence of mental illness. However, mental health is not defined simply as the absence of mental illness, because it infers the ability to enjoy life, resilience, balance, flexibility, and self-actualization.

A 1999 Surgeon General's report highlights the stigmatization of people with mental disorders that has persisted throughout history. Manifested by bias, distrust, stereotyping, fear, embarrassment, anger, and/or avoidance, this stigma leads others to avoid living, socializing, or working with, renting to, or employing people with mental disorders, especially severe disorders such as schizophrenia. This stigmatization reduces patients' access to resources and opportunities (for example, housing, jobs) and leads to low self-esteem, isolation, and hopelessness. Its milder manifestation deters the public from seeking, and wanting to pay for, mental health care. In its most overt and egregious form, stigma results in outright discrimination and abuse. More tragically, it deprives people of their dignity and interferes with their full participation in society (Surgeon General, 1999).

In colonial times in the United States, people with mental illness were described as "lunatics" and were largely cared for by families. There was no concerted effort to treat mental illness until urbanization in the early 19th century created a societal problem previously relegated to families scattered among small rural communities. Social policy assumed the form of isolated asylums where persons with mental illness were administered the reigning treatments of the era. Throughout the history of institutionalization in asylums (later renamed mental hospitals), reformers strove to improve treatment and curtail abuse. Several waves of reform culminated in the deinstitutionalization movement that began in the 1950s with the goal of shifting patients and care to the community (Surgeon General, 1999).

According to the National Institute of Mental Health (2001), mental disorders are common in the United States and internationally. An estimated 22.1% of Americans ages 18 and older—about one in five adults—suffer from a diagnosable mental disorder in a given year. In addition, 4 of the 10 leading causes of disability in the United States and other developed countries are mental disorders—major depression, bipolar disorder, schizophrenia, and obsessive-compulsive disorder. In 2000, more than 90% of the 29,350 people who died by suicide in the United States had a diagnosable mental disorder, commonly a depressive disorder or a substance abuse disorder. Approximately 9.5% of the US population age 18 and older has a depressive disorder. Women are more likely than men to have an anxiety disorder. Approximately twice as many women as men suffer from panic disorder, post-traumatic stress disorder, generalized anxiety disorder, agoraphobia, and specific phobia, though about equal numbers of women and men have obsessive-compulsive disorder and social phobia. Autism and related disorders (also called autism spectrum disorders or pervasive developmental disorders) develop in childhood and generally are apparent by age three (NIMH, 2001). These are a few of the wide array of mental health and mental illness issues known today. Fortunately, we have better means of treating individuals with mental illness today than the institutional methods of the early 20th century. This chapter will highlight psychiatrists, psychologists, social workers, and counselors who serve as mental health professional in the healthcare system.

Diagnosing Mental Disorders

Many people suffer from more than one mental disorder at a given time. In the United States, mental disorders are diagnosed based on the *Diagnostic and Statistical Manual of Mental Disorders, fourth edition (DSM-IV)*. Mental Health Professionals use this manual when working with patients in order to better understand their illness and potential treatment and to help third-party payers (for example, insurance) understand the needs of the patient. The book is an invaluable resource for any professional who makes psychiatric diagnoses in the United States and many other countries.

You know I think that going into therapy is a very positive thing,
and talking about it is really helpful, because the more you
talk the more your fears fade, because you get it out.

Fran Drescher, Actor

Psychiatrists

Psychiatrists are primary caregivers (physicians) in the area of mental health. They assess and treat mental illnesses through a combination of psychotherapy, psychoanalysis, hospitalization, and medication. Psychotherapy involves regular discussions with patients about their problems; the psychiatrist helps them find solutions through changes in their behavioral patterns, the exploration of their past experiences, and group and family therapy sessions. Psychotherapy does not include physiological interventions, such as drug therapy or electroconvulsive therapy, although it may be used in combination with such methods. Behavior therapy aims to help the patient eliminate undesirable habits or irrational fears through conditioning. Techniques include systematic desensitization, particularly for the treatment of clients with irrational anxieties or fears, and aversive conditioning, which uses negative stimuli to end bad habits. Humanistic therapy tends to be more optimistic, basing its treatment on the theory that individuals have a natural inclination to strive toward self-fulfillment. Psychoanalysis involves long-term psychotherapy and counseling for patients. In many cases, medications are administered to correct chemical imbalances that may be causing emotional problems. Psychiatrists may also administer electroconvulsive therapy to those of their patients who do not respond to, or who cannot take, medications. For more details about the professional preparation of psychiatrists, physicians who specialize in mental health, please look in Chapter 7.

Social Workers

Social work is a profession for those with a strong desire to help improve people's lives. Social workers help people function the best way they can in their environment, deal with their relationships, and solve personal and family problems. Social workers often see clients who face a life-threatening disease or a social problem. These problems may include inadequate housing, unemployment, serious illness, disability, or substance abuse. Social workers also assist families that have serious domestic conflicts, including those involving child or spousal abuse. They often provide social services in health-related settings governed by managed care organizations. To contain costs, these organizations are emphasizing short-term intervention, ambulatory and community-based care, and greater decentralization of services. Most social workers specialize in a particular area. Although some conduct research or are involved in planning or policy development, most social workers prefer an area of practice in which they interact with clients.

Child, family, and school social workers provide social services and assistance to improve the social and psychological functioning of children and their families and to maximize the family well-being and academic functioning of children. Some social workers assist single parents; arrange adoptions; and help find foster homes for neglected, abandoned, or abused children. In schools, they address such problems as teenage pregnancy, misbehavior, and truancy. They also advise teachers on how to cope with problem students. Some social workers may specialize in services for senior citizens. They run support groups for family caregivers or for the adult children of aging parents. Some advise elderly people or family members about choices in areas such as housing, transportation, and long-term care; they also coordinate and monitor services. Through employee assistance programs, they may help workers cope with job-related pressures or with personal problems that affect the quality of their work. Child, family, and school social workers typically work in individual and family services agencies, schools, or state or local governments. These social workers may be known as child welfare social workers, family services social workers, child protective services social workers, occupational social workers, or gerontology social workers.

Many of us want to imagine that we will live forever—young and pain-free. *Medical and public health social workers* are among those rare beings willing to look at illness and death as part of life's experiences. They do all they can to help people get well—but when illness is terminal (deadly), they turn their attention to helping their clients die peacefully. Medical and public health social workers provide persons, families, or vulnerable populations with the psychosocial support needed to cope with chronic, acute, or terminal illnesses, such as Alzheimer's disease, cancer, or AIDS. They also advise family caregivers, counsel patients, and help plan for patients' needs after discharge by arranging for at-home services—from meals-on-wheels to oxygen equipment. Some work on interdisciplinary teams that evaluate certain kinds of patients—geriatric or organ transplant patients, for example. Medical and public health social workers may work for hospitals, nursing and personal care facilities, individual and family services agencies, or local governments. Government economists expect job growth for medical and public health social workers to be faster than the average for all careers through 2012. One reason has to do with the fact that hospital stays are shorter than they used to be. People often need attention after they leave the hospital, and social workers can provide it.

Mental health and substance abuse social workers assess and treat individuals with mental illness or substance abuse problems, including abuse of alcohol, tobacco, or other drugs. Mental health social workers provide services for persons with mental or emotional problems. Such services include individual and group therapy, outreach, crisis intervention, social rehabilitation, and training in skills of everyday living. They may also help plan for supportive services to ease patients' return to the community. Substance abuse social workers counsel drug and alcohol abusers as they recover from their dependencies. They also arrange for other services that may help clients find employment or get training. They generally are employed in substance abuse treatment and prevention programs. Mental health and substance abuse social workers are likely to work in hospitals, substance abuse treatment centers, individual and family services agencies, or local governments. These social workers may be known as clinical social workers.

Other types of social workers include social work planners and policy makers, who develop programs to address such issues as child abuse, homelessness, substance abuse, poverty, and violence. These workers research and analyze policies, programs, and regulations. They identify social problems and suggest legislative and other solutions. They may help raise funds or write grants to support these programs.

Education and Employment for Social Workers

A bachelor's degree in social work (BSW) is the most common minimum requirement to qualify for a job as a social worker; however, majors in psychology, sociology, and related fields may be adequate to qualify for some entry-level jobs, especially in small community agencies. Although a bachelor's degree is sufficient for entry into the field, an advanced degree has become the standard for many positions. A master's degree in social work (MSW) is typically required for positions in health settings and is required for clinical work. Some jobs in public and private agencies also may require an advanced degree, such as a master's degree in social services policy or administration. Supervisory, administrative, and staff training positions usually require an advanced degree. College and university teaching positions and most research appointments normally require a doctorate in social work (DSW or PhD).

As of 2004, the Council on Social Work Education (www.CSWE.org) accredited 442 BSW programs and 168 MSW programs. BSW programs prepare graduates for direct service positions such as caseworker. They include courses in social work values and ethics, dealing with a culturally diverse clientele, at-risk-populations, promotion of social and economic justice, human behavior and the social environment, social welfare policy and services, social work practice, social research methods, and field education. Accredited BSW programs require a minimum of 400 hours of supervised field experience.

Master's degree programs prepare graduates for work in their chosen field of concentration and continue to develop the skills required to perform clinical assessments, manage large caseloads, and explore new ways of drawing upon social services to meet the needs of clients. A full-time master's program lasts two years and includes a minimum of 900 hours of supervised field instruction, or internship. Entry into a master's program does not require a bachelor's in social work, but courses in psychology, biology, sociology, economics, political science, and social work are recommended. In addition, a second language can be very helpful. Most master's programs offer advanced standing for those with a bachelor's degree from an accredited social work program.

All states and the District of Columbia have licensing, certification, or registration requirements regarding social work practice and the use of professional titles. Although standards for licensing vary by state, a growing number of states are placing greater emphasis on communications skills, professional ethics, and sensitivity to cultural diversity issues. In addition, the National Association of Social Workers (NASW) offers voluntary credentials. Social workers with an MSW may be eligible for the Academy of Certified Social Workers (ACSW), the Qualified Clinical Social Worker (QCSW), or the Diplomate in Clinical Social Work (DCSW) credential based on their professional experience. Credentials are particularly important for those in private practice; some health insurance providers require social workers to have them in order to be reimbursed for services.

Social workers should be emotionally mature, objective, and sensitive to people and their problems. They must be able to handle responsibility, work independently, and maintain good working relationships with clients and coworkers. Volunteer or paid jobs as a social work aide offer ways of testing one's interest in this field.

Full-time social workers usually work a standard 40-hour week; however, some occasionally work evenings and weekends to meet with clients, attend community meetings, and handle emergencies. Some, particularly in voluntary nonprofit agencies, work part-time. Social workers usually spend most of their time in an office or residential facility, but also may travel locally to visit clients, meet with service providers, or attend meetings. Some may use one of several offices within a local area in which to meet with clients. The work, while satisfying, can be emotionally draining. Understaffing and large caseloads add to the pressure in some agencies. To tend to patient care or client needs, many hospitals and long-term care facilities are employing social workers on teams with a broad mix of occupations—including clinical specialists, registered nurses, and health aides. Advancement to supervisor, program manager, assistant director, or executive director of a social service agency or department is possible, but usually requires an advanced degree and related work experience. Other career options for social workers include teaching, research, and consulting. Some of these workers also help formulate government policies by analyzing and advocating policy positions in government agencies, in research institutions, and on legislators' staffs.

Some social workers go into private practice. Most private practitioners are clinical social workers who provide psychotherapy, usually paid for through health insurance or by the clients themselves. Private practitioners must have at least a master's degree and a period of supervised work experience. A network of contacts for referrals also is essential. Many private practitioners work part-time while they work full-time elsewhere. Competition for social worker jobs is stronger in cities, where demand for services often is highest and training programs for social workers are prevalent. However, opportunities should be good in rural areas, which often find it difficult to attract and retain qualified staff. By specialty, job prospects may be best for those social workers with a background in gerontology and substance abuse treatment.

The Bureau of Labor Statistics expects employment of social workers to grow faster than the average for all occupations through 2012 (BLS, 2006c). The rapidly growing elderly population and the aging baby boom generation will create greater demand for health and social services, resulting in particularly rapid job growth among gerontology social workers. Many job openings also will stem from the need to replace social workers who leave the occupation. As hospitals continue to limit the length of patient stays, the demand for social workers in hospitals will grow more slowly than in other areas. Because hospitals are releasing patients earlier than in the past, social worker employment in home healthcare services is growing. However, the expanding senior population is an even larger factor. Employment opportunities for social workers with backgrounds in gerontology should be good in the growing numbers of assisted-living and senior-living communities. The expanding senior population will also spur demand for social workers in nursing homes, long-term care facilities, and hospices.

Employment of substance abuse social workers will grow rapidly over the 2002 to 2012 projection period (BLS, 2006c). Substance abusers are increasingly placed into treatment programs instead of being sentenced to prison. As this trend grows, demand will increase for treatment programs and social workers to assist abusers on the road to recovery. Employment of school social workers also is expected to steadily grow. Expanded efforts to respond to rising student enrollments and continued emphasis on integrating disabled children into the general school population may lead to more jobs. Availability of state and local funding will be a major factor in determining the actual job growth in schools.

Opportunities for social workers in private practice will expand but growth may be somewhat hindered by restrictions that managed care organizations put on mental health services. The growing popularity of employee assistance programs is expected to spur some demand for private practitioners, some of whom provide social work services to corporations on a contractual basis. However, the popularity of employee assistance programs will fluctuate with the business cycle, as businesses are not likely to offer these services during recessions.

The Bureau of Labor Statistics (2006c) reports median annual earnings of child, family, and school social workers of $34,820 in 2004. Median annual earnings in the industries employing the largest numbers of child, family, and school social workers in 2004 were

Elementary and secondary schools	$44,300
Local government	$40,620
State government	$35,070
Individual and family services	$30,680
Other residential care facilities	$30,550

Median annual earnings of medical and public health social workers were $40,080 in 2004. Median annual earnings in the industries employing the largest numbers of medical and public health social workers in 2004 were

General medical and surgical hospitals	$44,920
Local government	$39,390
Nursing care facilities	$35,680
Individual and family services	$32,100

Median annual earnings of mental health and substance abuse social workers were $33,920 in 2004. Median annual earnings in the industries employing the largest numbers of mental health and substance abuse social workers in 2004 were

Local government	$35,720
Psychiatric and substance abuse hospitals	$36,170
Outpatient care centers	$33,220
Individual and family services	$32,810

For information about career opportunities in social work and voluntary credentials for social workers, contact

- National Association of Social Workers, 750 First St. NE., Suite 700, Washington, DC 20002-4241. Internet: http://www.socialworkers.org.

For a listing of accredited social work programs, contact

- Council on Social Work Education, 1725 Duke St., Suite 500, Alexandria, VA 22314-3457. Internet: http://www.cswe.org.

Information on licensing requirements and testing procedures for each state may be obtained from state licensing authorities, or from

- Association of Social Work Boards, 400 South Ridge Pkwy., Suite B, Culpeper, VA 22701. Internet: http://www.aswb.org.

Counselors

The practice of professional *counseling* is the application of mental health, psychological, or human development principles, through cognitive, affective, behavioral, or systemic intervention strategies that address wellness, personal growth, or career development, as well as pathology. Counselors assist people with personal, family, educational, mental health, and career decisions and problems. Their duties depend on the individuals they serve and on the settings in which they work. A professional counseling specialty is narrowly focused on one particular area (for example, substance abuse), requiring advanced knowledge in the field founded on the premise that all counselors must first meet the requirements for the general practice of professional counseling.

Educational, vocational, and school counselors provide individuals and groups with career and educational counseling. In school settings—elementary through postsecondary—they are usually called school counselors and they work with students, including those considered to be at risk and those with special needs. They advocate for students and work with other individuals and organizations to promote the academic, career, and personal and social development of children and youths. School counselors help students evaluate their abilities, interests, talents, and personality characteristics in order to develop realistic academic and career goals. Counselors use interviews, counseling sessions, tests, or other methods in evaluating and advising students. They also operate career information centers and career education programs. High school counselors advise students regarding college majors, admission requirements, entrance exams, financial aid, trade or technical schools, and apprenticeship programs. They help students develop job search skills such as resume writing and interviewing techniques. College career planning and placement counselors assist alumni or students with career development and job-hunting techniques.

Elementary school counselors observe younger children during classroom and play activities and confer with their teachers and parents to evaluate the children's strengths, problems, or special needs. They also help students develop good study habits. Elementary school counselors do less vocational and academic counseling than do secondary school counselors.

School counselors at all levels help students understand and deal with social, behavioral, and personal problems. These counselors emphasize preventive and developmental counseling to provide students with the life skills needed to deal with problems before they occur and to enhance the student's personal, social, and academic growth. Counselors provide special services, including alcohol and drug prevention programs and conflict resolution classes. Counselors also try to identify cases of domestic abuse and other family problems that can affect a student's development. Counselors work with students individually, with small groups, or with entire classes. They consult and collaborate with parents, teachers, school administrators, school psychologists, medical professionals, and social workers in order to develop and implement strategies to help students be successful in the education system.

Vocational counselors who provide mainly career counseling outside the school setting are also referred to as *employment counselors* or *career counselors*. Their chief focus is helping individuals with their career decisions. Vocational counselors explore and evaluate the client's education, training, work history, interests, skills, and personality traits, and arrange for aptitude and achievement tests to assist in making career decisions. They also work with individuals to develop their job search skills, and they assist clients in locating and applying for jobs. In addition, career counselors provide support to persons experiencing job loss, job stress, or other career transition issues.

Rehabilitation counselors help people deal with the personal, social, and vocational effects of disabilities. They counsel people with disabilities resulting from birth defects, illness or disease, accidents, or the stress of daily life. They evaluate the strengths and limitations of individuals, provide personal and vocational counseling, and arrange for medical care, vocational training, and job placement. Rehabilitation counselors interview individuals with disabilities and their families, evaluate school and medical reports, and confer and plan with physicians, psychologists, occupational therapists, and employers to determine the capabilities and skills of the individual. Conferring with the client, they develop a rehabilitation program that often includes training to help the person develop job skills. Rehabilitation counselors also work toward increasing the client's capacity to live independently.

Mental health counselors work with individuals, families, and groups to address and treat mental and emotional disorders and to promote optimum mental health. They are trained in a variety of therapeutic techniques used to address a wide range of issues, including depression, addiction and substance abuse, suicidal impulses, stress management, problems with self-esteem, issues associated with aging, job and career concerns, educational decisions, issues related to mental and emotional health, and family, parenting, and marital or other relationship problems. Mental health counselors often work closely with other mental health specialists, such as psychiatrists, psychologists, clinical social workers, psychiatric nurses, and school counselors.

Substance abuse and behavioral disorder counselors help people who have problems with alcohol, drugs, gambling, and eating disorders. They counsel individuals who are addicted to drugs, helping them identify behaviors and problems related to their addiction. These counselors hold sessions for one person, for families, or for groups of people.

Marriage and family therapists apply principles, methods, and therapeutic techniques to individuals, family groups, couples, or organizations for the purpose of resolving emotional conflicts. In doing so, they modify people's perceptions and behaviors, enhance communication and understanding among all family members, and help to prevent family and individual crises. Marriage and family therapists also may engage in psychotherapy of a non-medical nature, with appropriate referrals to psychiatric resources, and in research and teaching in the overall field of human development and interpersonal relationships.

Other counseling specialties include gerontological, multicultural, and genetic counseling. A gerontological counselor provides services to elderly persons who face changing lifestyles because of health problems; the counselor helps families cope with the changes. A multicultural counselor helps employers adjust to an increasingly diverse workforce. Genetic counselors provide information and support to families who have members with birth defects or genetic disorders and to families who may be at risk for a variety of inherited conditions. These counselors identify families at risk, investigate the problem that is present in the family, interpret information about the disorder, analyze inheritance patterns and risks of recurrence, and review available options with the family.

Most school counselors work the traditional 9- to 10-month school year with a 2- to 3-month vacation, although increasing numbers are employed on 10.5- or 11-month contracts. They usually work the same hours that teachers do. College career planning and placement counselors work long and irregular hours during student recruiting periods. Rehabilitation counselors usually work a standard 40-hour week. Self-employed counselors and those working in mental health and community agencies, such as substance abuse and behavioral disorder counselors, frequently work evenings to counsel clients who work during the day. Both mental health counselors and marriage and family therapists also often work flexible hours, to accommodate families in crisis or working couples who must have evening or weekend appointments.

Counselors must possess high physical and emotional energy to handle the array of problems they address. Dealing daily with these problems can cause stress. Because privacy is essential for confidential and frank discussions with clients, counselors usually have private offices.

Counselors held about 601,000 jobs in 2004 (BLS, 2006a). Employment was distributed among the counseling specialties as follows:

Educational, vocational, and school counselors	248,000
Rehabilitation counselors	131,000
Mental health counselors	96,000
Substance abuse and behavioral disorder counselors	76,000
Marriage and family therapists	24,000

Educational, vocational, and school counselors work primarily in elementary and secondary schools and colleges and universities. Other types of counselors work in a wide variety of public and private establishments, including health care facilities; job training, career development, and vocational rehabilitation centers; social agencies; correctional institutions; and residential care facilities, such as halfway houses for criminal offenders and group homes for children, the elderly, and the disabled. Some substance abuse and behavioral disorder counselors work in therapeutic communities where addicts live while undergoing treatment. Counselors also work in organizations engaged in community improvement and social change and work in drug and alcohol rehabilitation programs and state and local government agencies. A growing number of counselors are self-employed and working in group practices or private practice. Laws allowing counselors to receive payments from insurance companies and the growing recognition that counselors are well-trained professionals fuel this growth in the profession.

All states require school counselors to hold state school counseling certification and to have completed at least some graduate course work; most require the completion of a master's degree. Some states require public school counselors to have both counseling and teaching certificates and to have had some teaching experience before receiving certification. For counselors based outside of schools, 47 states and the District of Columbia had some form of counselor credentialing, licensure, certification, or registration that governed their practice of counseling. Requirements typically include the completion of a master's degree in counseling, the accumulation of two years or 3,000 hours of supervised clinical experience beyond the master's degree level, the passage of a state-recognized exam, adherence to ethical codes and standards, and the satisfaction of annual continuing education requirements. Counselors must be aware of educational and training requirements that are often very detailed and that vary by area and by counseling specialty. Prospective counselors should check with state and local governments, employers, and national voluntary certification organizations in order to determine which requirements apply.

Licensed or certified counselors typically have a master's degree. A bachelor's degree often qualifies a person to work as a counseling aide, rehabilitation aide, or social service worker. Some states require counselors in public employment to have a master's degree; others accept a bachelor's degree with appropriate counseling courses. Counselor education programs in colleges and universities usually are in departments of education or psychology. Fields of study include college student affairs, elementary or secondary school counseling, education, gerontological counseling, marriage and family counseling, substance abuse counseling, rehabilitation counseling, agency or community counseling, clinical mental health counseling, counseling psychology, career counseling, and related fields. Courses are grouped into eight core areas: human growth and development, social and cultural diversity, relationships, group work, career development, assessment, research and program evaluation, and professional identity. In an accredited master's degree program, 48 to 60 semester hours of graduate study, including a period of supervised clinical experience in counseling, are required for a master's degree.

In 2003, 176 institutions offered programs in counselor education that were accredited by the Council for Accreditation of Counseling and Related Educational Programs (CACREP). CACREP also recognizes many counselor education programs, apart from those in the 176 accredited institutions that use alternative instruction methods, such as distance learning. Programs that use such alternative instruction methods meet evaluation criteria based on the same standards for accreditation that CACREP applies to programs that employ the more traditional methods. Another organization, the Council on Rehabilitation Education (CORE), accredits graduate programs in rehabilitation counseling. Accredited master's degree programs include a minimum of two years of full-time study, including 600 hours of supervised clinical internship experience.

Many counselors elect to earn national certification by the National Board for Certified Counselors, Inc. (NBCC), which grants the general practice credential "National Certified Counselor." To be certified, a counselor must hold a master's or higher degree, with a concentration in counseling, from a regionally accredited college or university; must have at least two years of supervised field experience in a counseling setting (graduates from counselor education programs accredited by CACREP are exempted). Certified counselors must provide two professional endorsements, one of which must be from a recent supervisor; and must have a passing score on the NBCC's National Counselor Examination for Licensure and Certification (NCE). This national certification is voluntary and is distinct from state certification. However, in some states, those who pass the national exam are exempted from taking a state certification exam. NBCC also offers specialty certification in school, clinical mental health, and addiction counseling. Beginning January 1, 2004, new candidates for NBCC's National Certified School counselor (NCSC) credential must pass a practical simulation examination in addition to fulfilling the current requirements. To maintain their certification, counselors retake and pass the NCE or complete 100 hours of acceptable continuing education credit every five years.

Another organization, the Commission on Rehabilitation Counselor Certification, offers voluntary national certification for rehabilitation counselors. Many employers require rehabilitation counselors to be nationally certified. To become certified, rehabilitation counselors usually must graduate from an accredited educational program, complete an internship, and pass a written examination. (Certification requirements vary according to an applicant's educational history. Employment experience, for example, is required for those with a counseling degree in a specialty other than rehabilitation.) After meeting these requirements, candidates are designated "Certified Rehabilitation Counselors." To maintain their certification, counselors must successfully retake the certification exam or complete 100 hours of acceptable continuing education credit every five years. Other counseling organizations also offer certification in particular counseling specialties. Usually these are voluntary, but having one may enhance one's job prospects. Counselors must participate in graduate studies, workshops, and personal studies to maintain their certificates and licenses.

Persons interested in counseling should have a strong interest in helping others and should possess the ability to inspire respect, trust, and confidence. They should be able to work independently or as part of a team. Counselors must follow the code of ethics associated with their respective certifications and licenses.

Prospects for advancement vary by counseling field. School counselors can move to a larger school; become directors or supervisors of counseling, guidance, or pupil personnel services; or, usually with further graduate education, become counselor educators, counseling psychologists, or school administrators. Some counselors choose to work for a state's department of education. For marriage and family therapists, doctoral education in family therapy emphasizes the training of supervisors, teachers, researchers, and clinicians in the discipline. Counselors can become supervisors or administrators in their agencies. Some counselors move into research, consulting, or college teaching, or go into private or group practice.

The Bureau of Labor Statistics (2006a) expects overall employment of counselors to grow faster than the average for all occupations through 2012, and job opportunities should be very good because there are usually more job openings than graduates of counseling programs. In addition, numerous job openings will occur as many counselors retire or leave the profession.

Employment of educational, vocational, and school counselors is expected to grow as fast as the average for all occupations due to increasing student enrollments, particularly in secondary and postsecondary schools; state legislation requiring counselors in elementary schools; and an expansion in the responsibilities of counselors. For example, counselors are becoming more involved in crisis and preventive counseling, helping students deal with issues ranging from drug and alcohol abuse to death and suicide. Although schools and governments realize the value of counselors in achieving academic success in their students, budget constraints at every school level will dampen job growth of school counselors. However, federal grants and subsidies may fill in the gaps and allow the current ongoing reduction in student-to-counselor ratios to continue.

Demand for vocational or career counselors should grow as the notion of staying in one job over a lifetime continues to be rejected and replaced by the concept of managing one's own career and taking responsibility for it. In addition, changes in welfare laws that require beneficiaries to work will continue to create demand for counselors by state and local governments. Other opportunities for employment counselors will arise in private job-training centers that provide training and other services to laid-off workers, as well as to those seeking a new or second career or wanting to upgrade their skills.

Demand continues to be strong for substance abuse and behavioral, mental health, and marriage and family therapists and for rehabilitation counselors, for a variety of reasons. For one, California and a few other states have recently passed laws requiring substance abuse treatment instead of jail for people caught possessing a drug. This shift will require more substance abuse counselors in those states. Second, the increasing availability of funds to build statewide networks to improve services for children and adolescents with serious emotional disturbances and for their family members should increase employment opportunities for counselors. Under managed care systems, insurance companies are increasingly providing for reimbursement of counselors as a less costly alternative to psychiatrists and psychologists. In addition, legislation is pending that may provide counseling services to Medicare recipients.

The number of people who will need rehabilitation counseling will grow as the population continues to age and as advances in medical technology continue to save lives that only a few years ago would have been lost. In addition, legislation requiring equal employment rights for people with disabilities will spur demand for counselors, who not only will help these people make a transition into the workforce, but also will help companies comply with the law.

Employment of mental health counselors and marriage and family therapists will grow, as the nation becomes more comfortable seeking professional help for a variety of health and personal and family problems. Employers increasingly offer employee assistance programs that provide mental health, alcohol, and drug abuse services. More people are expected to use these services as society focuses on ways of developing mental well-being, such as controlling stress associated with job and family responsibilities.

Median annual earnings of educational, vocational, and school counselors in 2004 were $45,570. School counselors can earn additional income working summers in the school system or in other jobs. Median annual earnings in the industries employing the largest numbers of educational, vocational, and school counselors in 2004 were as follows (BLS, 2006a):

Elementary and secondary schools	$51,160
Junior colleges	$45,730
Colleges, universities, and professional schools	$39,110
Individual and family services	$30,240

Median annual earnings of substance abuse and behavioral disorder counselors in 2004 were $32,130. Median annual earnings of mental health counselors in 2004 were $32,960. Median annual earnings of rehabilitation counselors in 2004 were $27,870. For substance abuse, mental health, and rehabilitation counselors, government employers generally pay the highest wages, followed by hospitals and social service agencies. Residential care facilities often pay the lowest wages (BLS, 2006a).

Median annual earnings of marriage and family therapists in 2004 were $38,980. Median annual earnings in 2004 were $33,620 in individual and family social services, the industry employing the largest numbers of marriage and family therapists. Self-employed counselors who have well-established practices, as well as counselors employed in group practices, usually have the highest earnings (BLS, 2006a).

For general information about counseling, as well as information on specialties such as school, college, mental health, rehabilitation, multicultural, career, marriage and family, and gerontological counseling, contact:

- American Counseling Association, 5999 Stevenson Ave., Alexandria, VA 22304-3300. Internet: http://www.counseling.org.

For information on accredited counseling and related training programs, contact:

- Council for Accreditation of Counseling and Related Educational Programs, American Counseling Association, 5999 Stevenson Ave., 4th floor, Alexandria, VA 22304. Internet: http://www.counseling.org/cacrep.

For information on national certification requirements for counselors, contact:

- National Board for Certified Counselors, Inc., 3 Terrace Way, Suite D, Greensboro, NC 27403-3660. Internet: http://www.nbcc.org.

State departments of education can supply information on those colleges and universities which offer guidance and counseling training that meets state certification and licensure requirements.

State employment service offices have information about job opportunities and about entrance requirements for counselors.

Psychologists

A magician pulls rabbits out of hats.
An experimental psychologist pulls habits out of rats.
Anonymous

Psychologists study the human mind and human behavior. Research psychologists investigate the physical, cognitive, emotional, or social aspects of human behavior. Psychologists in health service fields provide mental health care in hospitals, clinics, schools, or private settings. Psychologists employed in applied settings such as business, industry, government or nonprofit agencies provide training, conduct research, design systems, and act as advocates for the profession. Like other social scientists, psychologists formulate hypotheses and collect data to test their validity. Research methods vary depending on the topic under study. Psychologists sometimes gather information through controlled laboratory experiments or by administering personality, performance, aptitude, and intelligence tests. Other methods include observation, interviews, questionnaires, clinical studies, and surveys. Psychologists apply their knowledge to a wide range of endeavors, including health and human services, management, education, law, and sports. In addition to working in a variety of settings, psychologists usually specialize in one of a number of different areas.

Clinical psychologists—who constitute the largest specialty—most often work in counseling centers, independent or group practices, hospitals, or clinics. They help mentally and emotionally disturbed clients adjust to life and may help medical and surgical patients deal with illnesses or injuries. Some clinical psychologists work in physical rehabilitation settings, treating patients with spinal cord injuries, chronic pain or illness, stroke, arthritis, and neurological conditions. Others help people deal with times of personal crisis, such as divorce or the death of a loved one. Clinical psychologists often interview patients and give diagnostic tests. They may provide individual, family, or group psychotherapy, and design and implement behavior modification programs. Some clinical psychologists collaborate with physicians and other specialists to develop and implement treatment and intervention programs that patients can understand and comply with. Other clinical psychologists work in universities and medical schools, where they train graduate students in the delivery of mental health and behavioral medicine services. Some administer community mental health programs.

Areas of specialization within clinical psychology include health psychology, neuropsychology, and geropsychology. *Health psychologists* promote good health through health maintenance counseling programs designed to help people achieve goals, such as to stop smoking or lose weight. *Neuropsychologists* study the relation between the brain and behavior. They often work in stroke and head injury programs. *Geropsychologists* deal with the special problems faced by the elderly. The emergence and growth of these specialties reflects the increasing participation of psychologists in providing direct services to special patient populations. Often, clinical psychologists will consult with other medical personnel regarding the best treatment for patients, especially treatment that includes medications. Clinical psychologists generally are not permitted to prescribe medications to treat patients; only psychiatrists and other medical doctors may prescribe medications. However, one state, New Mexico, has passed legislation allowing clinical psychologists who undergo additional training to prescribe medication, and similar proposals have been made in additional states.

Counseling psychologists use various techniques, including interviewing and testing, to advise people on how to deal with problems of everyday living. They work in settings such as university counseling centers, hospitals, and individual or group practices.

School psychologists work in elementary and secondary schools or school district offices to resolve students' learning and behavior problems. They collaborate with teachers, parents, and school personnel to improve classroom management strategies or parenting skills, counter substance abuse, work with students with disabilities or gifted and talented students, and improve teaching and learning strategies. They may evaluate the effectiveness of academic programs, behavior management procedures, and other services provided in the school setting.

Industrial-organizational psychologists apply psychological principles and research methods to the workplace in the interest of improving productivity and the quality of work life. They also are involved in research on management and marketing problems. They conduct applicant screening, training and development, counseling, and organizational development and analysis. An industrial psychologist might work with management to reorganize the work setting to improve productivity or quality of life in the workplace. They frequently act as consultants, brought in by management in order to solve a particular problem.

Developmental psychologists study the physiological, cognitive, and social development that takes place throughout life. Some specialize in behavior during infancy, childhood, and adolescence, or changes that occur during maturity or old age. They also may study developmental disabilities and their effects. Increasingly, research is developing ways to help elderly people remain independent as long as possible.

Social psychologists examine people's interactions with others and with the social environment. They work in organizational consultation, marketing research, systems design, or other applied psychology fields. Prominent areas of study include group behavior, leadership, attitudes, and perception.

Experimental or *research psychologists* work in university and private research centers and in business, nonprofit, and governmental organizations. They study behavior processes using human beings and animals, such as rats, monkeys, and pigeons. Prominent areas of study in experimental research include motivation, thought, attention, learning and memory, sensory and perceptual processes, effects of substance abuse, and genetic and neurological factors affecting behavior.

A psychologist's subfield and place of employment determine working conditions. Clinical, school, and counseling psychologists in private practice have their own offices and set their own hours. However, they often offer evening and weekend hours to accommodate their clients. Those employed in hospitals, nursing homes, and other health facilities may work shifts including evenings and weekends, while those who work in schools and clinics generally work regular hours. Psychologists employed as faculty by colleges and universities divide their time between teaching and research and also may have administrative responsibilities. Many have part-time consulting practices. Most psychologists in government and industry have structured schedules.

Increasingly, many psychologists work as part of a team and consult with other psychologists and professionals. Many experience pressures due to deadlines, tight schedules, and overtime work. Travel usually is required, in order to attend conferences or conduct research.

Psychologists held about 179,000 jobs in 2004. Educational institutions employed about one out of four salaried psychologists in positions other than teaching, such as counseling, testing, research, and administration. Two out of 10 were employed in health care, primarily in offices of mental health practitioners and in outpatient care facilities, private hospitals, nursing and residential care facilities, and individual and family service organizations. Government agencies at the state and local levels employed 1 in 10 psychologists, primarily in public hospitals, clinics, correctional facilities, and other settings. Some psychologists work in research organizations, management consulting firms, marketing research firms, religious organizations, and other businesses. After several years of experience, some psychologists—usually those with doctoral degrees—enter private practice or set up private research or consulting firms. About 4 out of 10 psychologists were self-employed in 2004. In addition, many psychologists held faculty positions at colleges and universities, and as high school psychology teachers (BLS, 2006b).

A doctoral degree usually is required for employment as an independent licensed clinical or counseling psychologist. Psychologists with a PhD qualify for a wide range of teaching, research, clinical, and counseling positions in universities, healthcare services, elementary and secondary schools, private industry, and government. Psychologists with a Doctor of Psychology (PsyD) degree usually work in clinical positions or in private practices. A doctoral degree usually requires five to seven years of graduate study. The PhD degree culminates in a dissertation based on original research. Courses in quantitative research methods, which include the use of computer-based analysis, are an integral part of graduate study and are necessary to complete the dissertation. The PsyD may be based on practical work and examinations rather than a dissertation. In clinical or counseling psychology, the requirements for the doctoral degree usually include at least a one-year internship.

Persons with a master's degree in psychology may work as industrial-organizational psychologists or school psychologists. They also may work as psychological assistants, under the supervision of doctoral-level psychologists, and conduct research or psychological evaluations. A master's degree in psychology requires at least two years of full-time graduate study. Requirements usually include practical experience in an applied setting and a master's thesis based on an original research project. Competition for admission to graduate programs is keen. Some universities require applicants to have an undergraduate major in psychology. Others prefer only coursework in basic psychology with courses in the biological, physical, and social sciences; and statistics and mathematics.

A bachelor's degree in psychology qualifies a person to assist psychologists and other professionals in community mental health centers, vocational rehabilitation offices, and correctional programs. They may work as research or administrative assistants or become sales or management trainees in business. Some work as technicians in related fields, such as marketing research. In the federal government, candidates having at least 24 semester hours in psychology and one course in statistics qualify for entry-level positions. However, competition for these jobs is keen because this is one of the few areas of psychology that does not require an advanced degree.

The American Psychological Association (APA) presently accredits doctoral training programs in clinical, counseling, and school psychology. The National Council for Accreditation of Teacher Education, with the assistance of the National Association of School Psychologists, also is involved in the accreditation of advanced degree programs in school psychology. The APA also accredits institutions that provide internships for doctoral students in school, clinical, and counseling psychology.

Psychologists in independent practice or those who offer any type of patient care—including clinical, counseling, and school psychologists—must meet certification or licensing requirements in all states and the District of Columbia. Licensing laws vary by state and by type of position and require licensed or certified psychologists to limit their practice to areas in which they have developed professional competence through training and experience. Clinical and counseling psychologists usually require a doctorate in psychology, completion of an approved internship, and one to two years of professional experience. In addition, all states require that applicants pass an examination. Most state licensing boards administer a standardized test, and many supplement that with additional oral or essay questions. Most states certify those with a master's degree as school psychologists after completion of an internship. Some states require continuing education for license renewal.

The National Association of School Psychologists (NASP) awards the Nationally Certified School Psychologist (NCSP) designation, which recognizes professional competency in school psychology at a national level, rather than at a state level. Currently, 22 states recognize the NCSP and allow those with the certification to transfer credentials from one state to another without taking a new state certification exam. In those states that recognize the NCSP, the requirements for state licensure and the NCSP often are the same or similar. Requirements for the NCSP include completion of 60 graduate semester hours in school psychology; a 1,200-hour internship, 600 hours of which must be completed in a school setting; and a passing score on the National School Psychology Examination.

The American Board of Professional Psychology (ABPP) recognizes professional achievement by awarding specialty certification, primarily in clinical psychology, clinical neuropsychology, and counseling, forensic, industrial-organizational, and school psychology. Candidates for ABPP certification need a doctorate in psychology, postdoctoral training in their specialty, five years of experience, professional endorsements, and a passing grade on an examination.

Aspiring psychologists who are interested in direct patient care must be emotionally stable, mature, and able to deal effectively with people. Sensitivity, compassion, good communication skills, and the ability to lead and inspire others are particularly important qualities for persons wishing to do clinical work and counseling. Research psychologists should be able to do detailed work independently and as part of a team. Patience and perseverance are vital qualities because achieving results from psychological treatment of patients or from research usually takes a long time.

Overall employment of psychologists is expected to grow faster than the average for all occupations through 2012, due to increased demand for psychological services in schools, hospitals, social service agencies, mental health centers, substance abuse treatment clinics, consulting firms, and private companies (BLS, 2006b). Clinical, counseling, and school psychologists will grow faster than the average, while industrial-organizational psychologists will have average growth.

Among the specialties in this field, school psychologists may enjoy the best job opportunities. Growing awareness of how students' mental health and behavioral problems, such as bullying, affect learning is increasing demand for school psychologists to offer student counseling and mental health services. Clinical and counseling psychologists will be needed to help people deal with depression and other mental disorders, marriage and family problems, job stress, and addiction. The rise in healthcare costs associated with unhealthy lifestyles, such as smoking, alcoholism, and obesity, has made prevention and treatment more critical. The increase in the number of employee assistance programs, which help workers deal with personal problems, also should spur job growth in clinical and counseling specialties. Industrial-organizational psychologists will be in demand to help to boost worker productivity and retention rates in a wide range of businesses. Industrial-organizational psychologists will help companies deal with issues such as workplace diversity and antidiscrimination policies. Companies also will use psychologists' expertise in survey design, analysis, and research to develop tools for marketing evaluation and statistical analysis.

Demand should be particularly strong for persons holding doctorates from leading universities in applied specialties, such as counseling, health, and school psychology. Psychologists with extensive training in quantitative research methods and computer science may have a competitive edge over applicants without this background.

Master's degree holders in fields other than school or industrial-organizational psychology will face keen competition for jobs because of the limited number of positions that require only a master's degree. Master's degree holders may find jobs as psychological assistants or counselors, providing mental health services under the direct supervision of a licensed psychologist. Still others may find jobs involving research and data collection and analysis in universities, government, or private companies.

Opportunities directly related to psychology will be limited for bachelor's degree holders. Some may find jobs as assistants in rehabilitation centers, or in other jobs involving data collection and analysis. Those who meet state certification requirements may become high school psychology teachers.

Median annual earnings of wage and salary clinical, counseling, and school psychologists in 2004 were $54,950. Median annual earnings in the industries employing the largest numbers of clinical, counseling, and school psychologists in 2004 were as follows (BLS, 2006b):

Offices of other health practitioners	$64,460
Elementary and secondary schools	$58,360
Outpatient care centers	$46,850
Individual and family services	$42,640

Median annual earnings of wage and salary industrial-organizational psychologists in 2004 were $71,400.

For information on careers, educational requirements, financial assistance, and licensing in all fields of psychology, contact

- American Psychological Association, 750 1st St. NE., Washington, DC 20002. Internet: http://www.apa.org.

For information on careers, educational requirements, certification, and licensing of school psychologists, contact

- National Association of School Psychologists, 4340 East West Hwy., Suite 402, Bethesda, MD 20814. Internet: http://www.nasponline.org.

Information about State licensing requirements is available from

- Association of State and Provincial Psychology Boards, P.O. Box 241245, Montgomery, AL 36124-1245. Internet: http://www.asppb.org.

Information about psychology specialty certifications is available from

- American Board of Professional Psychology, Inc., 514 East Capitol Ave., Jefferson City, MO 65101. Internet: http://www.abpp.org.

SUMMARY

Remember that mental health is not defined simply as the absence of mental illness. Mental health infers the ability to enjoy life, resilience, balance, flexibility, and self-actualization. With as many as one in five American adults suffering from diagnosable mental disorders, the need for mental health professionals continues to grow. The diversity of employment settings makes mental health professions desirable for those individuals who want to help others through a variety of therapeutic modalities. While some can enter mental health professions with a bachelor's degree, many go on for advanced degrees to hone their professional skills at treating a wide array of mental illnesses. Many mental health workers are part of the healthcare teams striving to improve the quality of life for all Americans, a goal of Healthy People 2010.

ADDITIONAL RESOURCES

The National Mental Health Association is the country's oldest and largest nonprofit organization addressing all aspects of mental health and mental illness. With more than 340 affiliates nationwide, NMHA works to improve the mental health of all Americans, especially the 54 million people with mental disorders, through advocacy, education, research, and service.

National Mental Health Association
2001 N. Beauregard Street, 12th Floor
Alexandria, Virginia 22311
Internet: http://www.nmha.org/

National Institute of Mental Health (NIMH)
Public Information and Communications Branch
6001 Executive Boulevard, Room 8184, MSC 9663
Bethesda, MD 20892-9663
Phone: 301-443-4513 (local) 1-866-615-6464 (toll-free)

DISCUSSION QUESTIONS

1. What is the DSM-IV? How is it used in mental health care?
2. What social/demographic changes are supporting the growth of mental health professions for the next decade?
3. What areas can social workers specialize in?
4. What personality characteristics should mental health workers have?

REFERENCES

Bureau of Labor Statistics, US Department of Labor (BLM). (2006a). *Occupational outlook handbook, 2006–07 edition*. Counselors. Retrieved November 25, 2006, from http://www.bls.gov/oco/ocos067.htm.

Bureau of Labor Statistics, US Department of Labor (BLM). (2006b). *Occupational outlook handbook, 2006–07 edition*. Psychologists. Retrieved November 22, 2006, from http://www.bls.gov/oco/ocos056.htm.

Bureau of Labor Statistics, US Department of Labor (BLM). (2006c). *Occupational outlook handbook, 2006–07 edition*. Social Workers. Retrieved November 22, 2006, from http://www.bls.gov/oco/ocos060.htm.

National Institute of Mental Health (NIMH). (2001). The numbers count: Mental disorders in America. A summary of statistics describing the prevalence of mental disorders in America. Retrieved September 7, 2005 from, http://www.nimh.nih.gov/publicat/numbers.cfm.

Report of the Surgeon General, US Public Health Service (Surgeon General). (1999). Admiral David Satcher. Mental health and mental illness: A public health approach. Washington, DC: Health and Human Services Department.

Chapter 18

Public Health

Kristi L. Lewis and
Stephanie Chisolm

OBJECTIVES

After studying this chapter, the student should be able to

1. Define the field of public health.
2. Describe the difference between health education, epidemiology, and environmental health professionals.
3. Describe the educational preparation and certification required for careers in public health.
4. Identify the various government agencies' environments that make up the public health infrastructure.

INTRODUCTION

> *Health care matters to all of us some of the time;*
> *public health matters to all of us all of the time.*
> C. Everett Koop, former US Surgeon General

What do the tsunami in Asia, hurricane Katrina, avian flu, drinking water, HIV/AIDS, and bio-terrorism have in common? If you guessed that each could affect the health of large populations, you are correct. These and many other issues are examples of public health concerns emerging in the first decade of the new millennium. Public health consists of a variety of efforts organized by society to protect, promote, and restore the people's health. The Leading Health Indicators mentioned in earlier chapters are the ten high-priority public health issues in the United States. The indicators are intended to help everyone more easily understand how healthy we are as a nation. They reveal the most important changes we can make to improve our health as well as the health of our families and communities.

What Is Public Health?

Public health is the art and science dealing with the protection and improvement of community health by organized community effort, including preventive medicine, sanitation, and social science. Public health involves education, promotion of healthy lifestyles, and research for disease and injury prevention. Public health efforts involve the knowledge and application of many different disciplines in its research, teaching, service, and practice activities, including biology, sociology, mathematics, anthropology, public policy, medicine, education, psychology, information technology, epidemiology, and many other fields. What distinguishes public health from the rest of the healthcare system is the principal focus of public health efforts on entire populations rather than individuals. These populations can be as small as a local neighborhood, or as big as an entire country. Where clinical health professionals focus on a disease diagnosis and treatment, public health centers on prevention and health promotion.

Public health professionals try to prevent problems from happening or recurring through implementing educational programs, developing policies, administering services, and conducting research, in contrast to clinical professionals, such as doctors and nurses, who focus primarily on treating individuals after they become sick or injured. According to the Institute of Medicine's Committee for the Study of the Future of Public Health ("The Future of Public Health," 1988), the mission of public health is to "fulfill society's interest in assuring conditions in which people can be healthy."

In public health, a strong infrastructure provides the capacity to prepare for and respond to both acute and chronic threats to the nation's health, whether they are bioterrorism attacks, emerging infections, disparities in health status, or increases in chronic disease and injury rates. Such an infrastructure serves as the foundation for planning, delivering, and evaluating public health. The public health infrastructure comprises the workforce, data and information systems, and public health organizations. Research also is a key activity of the public health infrastructure in identifying opportunities to improve health, strengthen information systems and organizations, and make more effective and efficient use of resources.

What Areas Do Public Health Professionals Address in Their Careers?

Public health is an aspect of health services concerned with threats to the overall health of a community based on population health analysis. It generally includes surveillance and control of infectious disease and promotion of healthy behaviors among members of the community. Prevention is another important principle in the public health focus. Primary prevention through vaccination programs and free distribution of condoms are examples of public health measures. Public health promotes, not simply the absence of disease, but mental, physical, and emotional well-being. National bodies such as the Centers for Disease Control and Prevention in Atlanta, Georgia and the US Public Health Service are leaders in responding to public health threats domestically and even abroad. The domestic frontlines for public health initiatives are often state and local health departments. The Surgeon General, leader of the US Public Health Service (USPHS), is a national leader in public health activities.

Public health carries out its mission through organized, interdisciplinary efforts that address the physical, mental, and environmental health concerns of communities and populations at risk for disease and injury. Its mission is achieved through the application of health promotion and disease prevention technologies and interventions designed to improve and enhance quality of life, ultimately moving the nation toward the goals and objectives of Healthy People 2010. Health promotion and disease prevention technologies encompass a broad array of functions and expertise, including the three core public health functions:

- assessment and monitoring of the health of communities and populations at risk, to identify health problems and priorities;

- formulating public policies, in collaboration with community and government leaders, designed to solve identified local and national health problems and priorities;

- assuring that all populations have access to appropriate and cost-effective care, including health promotion and disease prevention services, and evaluation of the effectiveness of that care.

Public health agencies perform assessments of situations, assurance of quality and safety, as well as develop policies and regulations. According to the Public Health Functions Project (1995), public health also prevents epidemics and the spread of disease, protects against environmental hazards, prevents injuries, and encourages healthy behaviors. Public health professionals respond to disasters and assist communities in recovery efforts. They also assure the quality and accessibility of health services in communities.

Impact of Public Health

The dramatic achievements of Public Health in the 20th century have improved quality of life, increased life expectancy, reduced infant and child mortality worldwide, and eliminated or reduced many communicable diseases. Today, and into the 21st century, public health leaders must strengthen their roles as advocates for improved population-based health in an international, global community.

History and Health Departments

In order to understand the role and function of public health and the many organizations involved, including local, state and federal governments, one must have a good understanding of the history of public health. Public health began in 1798 with an act of Congress establishing health for merchant seaman. In 1870, the first Marine Hospital Services (MHS) began and in 1891, the MHS began taking on the role of screening immigrants as they arrived at Staten Island, New York. Today, immigrant health is still a public health concern. In 1887, after extensive studying of microbiology and the possible health consequences of microorganisms, a research laboratory opened at the Marine Hospital on Staten Island. This laboratory later became the National Institutes of Health (NIH). The National Institutes of Health is now located in Bethesda Maryland, a part of the US Department of Health and Human Services. The NIH is the primary federal agency for conducting and supporting medical research. Helping to lead the way toward important medical discoveries that improve people's health and save lives, NIH scientists investigate ways to prevent disease as well as the causes, treatments, and even cures for common and rare diseases.

In 1871, Dr. John Woodworth became the first "Supervising Surgeon" for the United States. This position later evolved into the post of the US Surgeon General, recognized today as one of the leading experts on prevention and health. Dr. C. Everett Koop brought attention to the position in the late 1980s with his campaign to reduce smoking by providing education to the public on the harmful effects of tobacco usage, especially among teenagers and young adults.

At the beginning of the 20th century, the population within the United States shifted from individuals living in rural areas of the country to more urban areas mostly due to industrialization and immigration. With this shift came the increase in outbreaks from communicable diseases such as cholera, tuberculosis, and malaria. It became clear that there needed to be a system to deal with such outbreaks and other health concerns that would plague the nation.

Long before the drafting of the United States Constitution, individual states had taken on the role of protecting the health of citizens (Stivers, 1991). By the early 1900s, most states had established state health departments to deal with public health issues related to communicable diseases.

1. *Vaccinations.* Vaccinations have resulted in the eradication of smallpox; elimination of poliomyelitis in the Americas; and control of measles, rubella, tetanus, diphtheria, Haemophilus influenzae type b, and other infectious diseases in the United States and other parts of the world.

2. *Motor-vehicle safety.* Improvements in motor-vehicle safety have resulted from engineering efforts to make both vehicles and highways safer and from successful efforts to change personal behavior (for example, increased use of safety belts, child safety seats, and motorcycle helmets and decreased drinking and driving). These efforts have contributed to large reductions in motor-vehicle-related deaths.

3. *Safer workplaces.* Work-related health problems, such as coal workers' pneumoconiosis (black lung), and silicosis—common at the beginning of the century—have come under better control. Severe injuries and deaths related to mining, manufacturing, construction, and transportation also have decreased; since 1980, safer workplaces have resulted in a reduction in the rate of fatal occupational injuries.

4. *Control of infectious diseases.* Control of infectious diseases has resulted from clean water and improved sanitation. Dramatic reductions in infections such as typhoid and cholera transmitted by contaminated water, a major cause of illness and death early in the 20th century, occur because of improved sanitation. In addition, the discovery of antimicrobial therapy has been critical to successful public health efforts to control infections such as tuberculosis and sexually transmitted diseases (STDs).

5. *Decline in deaths from coronary heart disease and stroke.* Decline in deaths from coronary heart disease and stroke have resulted from risk-factor modification, such as smoking cessation and blood pressure control coupled with improved access to early detection and better treatment.

6. *Safer and healthier foods.* Since 1900, safer and healthier foods have resulted from decreases in microbial contamination and increases in nutritional content. Identifying essential micronutrients and establishing food-fortification programs have almost eliminated major nutritional deficiency diseases such as rickets, goiter, and pellagra in the United States.

7. *Healthier mothers and babies.* Healthier mothers and babies have resulted from better hygiene and nutrition, availability of antibiotics, greater access to health care, and technologic advances in maternal and neonatal medicine. Since 1900, infant mortality has decreased 90%, and maternal mortality has decreased 99%.

8. *Family planning.* Access to family planning and contraceptive services has altered social and economic roles of women. Family planning has provided health benefits such as smaller family size and longer interval between the birth of children; increased opportunities for preconception counseling and screening; fewer infant, child, and maternal deaths; and the use of barrier contraceptives to prevent pregnancy and transmission of human immunodeficiency virus and other STDs.

9. *Fluoridation of drinking water.* Fluoridation of drinking water began in 1945 and in 1999 reaches an estimated 144 million persons in the United States. Fluoridation safely and inexpensively benefits both children and adults by effectively preventing tooth decay, regardless of socioeconomic status or access to care. Fluoridation has played an important role in the reductions in tooth decay (40%–70% in children) and of tooth loss in adults (40%–60%).

10. *Recognition of tobacco use as a health hazard.* Recognition of tobacco use as a health hazard and subsequent public health anti-smoking campaigns have resulted in changes in social norms to prevent initiation of tobacco use, promote cessation of use, and reduce exposure to environmental tobacco smoke. Since the 1964 Surgeon General's report on the health risks of smoking, the prevalence of smoking among adults has decreased, and millions of smoking-related deaths have been prevented.

Figure 18.1 *The 20th Century's Ten Great Public Health Achievements in the United States*
Source: (CDC, 1999)

Following the establishment of state health departments, by 1908, most counties and cities within the United States had established local health departments that could serve the local health needs of the community. By the mid 1900s, both state and local health departments had engaged in public health activities that would help to reduce the spread of communicable diseases. The development of a public health infrastructure led to sewage and waste disposal, chlorination and treatment of water supplies, and education for the general public on proper hygiene.

One of the most important milestones in public health was the development of antibiotics, specifically in the 1940s with the discovery of penicillin. With the development of antibiotics, the implementation of public health actions, and later the establishment of vaccination programs, mortality due to infectious or communicable diseases declined sharply in the United States.

The Communicable Disease Center (CDC), established in 1946 as a military program to control the spread of malaria (Warwick, 2002), worked closely with the state and local health departments to combat the existence and prevent the reemergence of newly infectious agents. The Communicable Disease Center became the Centers for Disease Control and Prevention and still today uses the acronym CDC. Even with the establishment of the CDC, public health experts were concerned about the possibility of disease outbreaks. The Epidemic Intelligence Service (EIS), established in 1951 to serve as a response team for health emergencies, led to the implementation of national surveillance systems.

The Public Health Infrastructure

Most counties and cities within the United States have local health departments that assist local constituents. Many people even today believe that health departments both at the local and state level provide only medical care for those lacking health insurance or for those unable to pay their medical expenses (medically uninsured or underserved). However, both local and state health departments provide a wide range of services and programs for the public at large. These services include environmental inspection and monitoring of soil and water for residential and business use and epidemiological surveillance and investigation. Other services include the development, implementation, and administrative oversight of federal public health programs including vaccination and public health clinics that provide primary care. Most health departments have divisions including Epidemiology, Environmental Health, Immunization, Tuberculosis, Water, Nutrition, and Maternal and Child Health, Injury prevention, and some have a Substance Abuse division.

Because health departments provide a wide range of services, they must have a wide range of program staff. The size of the city, county, or state often influences the number of health department programs and employees. Health departments at the local and state level employ a variety of health professionals, including public health nurses, epidemiologists, physicians, environmental health specialists, laboratory technicians, and nutritionists. All public health employees must be able to work with a diverse population and socioeconomic background. They must have a good understanding of the public health infrastructure and laws. Public health workers must also have good oral and written communication skills and be able to work with computers and computer software. Many of the health professionals described in this text can work in the public health field. The following highlights three additional public health professionals: environmental health specialists, epidemiologists, and health educators.

Environmental Health Specialists

The environment is everything that isn't me.
Albert Einstein (1879–1955)

According to Blumenthal and Rutterber (1995), environmental health can be defined as the relationship between the environment and human health. Many feel that the environment is one of the largest factors of human health. Most local, district, regional, and state health departments have an environmental health program staffed with environmental health specialists (formerly known as sanitarians). Environmental health specialists perform a variety of tasks to ensure the safety and well-being of the community. They focus on possible vectors and vehicles of disease transmission. For example, West Nile Virus, spread by mosquitoes, was first identified in the United States in 1999 through the diligent work of environmental health specialists trained to investigate possible environmental factors in disease transmission. In essence, environmental health involves the study of disease transmission via air, water, soil, and food. It also involves the identification of toxic substances that could pose a possible health hazard.

Specific tasks for environmental health specialists include inspection of restaurants and food establishments to ensure the safe preparation and consumption of food and the reduction of possible foodborne illnesses such as salmonella and E. coli. Environmental health staff will also often inspect hotels and resorts for public health issues, including their swimming pools and hot tubs. Environmental health specialists take soil and water samples for testing and evaluation purposes. The environmental health specialist investigates both domestic and wild animals to prevent the spread of rabies, a public health concern across the United States.

Since the position is not a desk job, environmental health specialists must be willing to work in the "field" and interact with the community. Individuals desiring a career in environmental health must obtain course work in science. Environmental health specialists often have degrees in the physical sciences such as biology or chemistry. An undergraduate or graduate-level degree in environmental health usually requires course work in toxicology, solid waste management, radiological health, and epidemiology.

Epidemiology and Epidemiologists

In addition to environmental health services, depending on the size of the community, some local, district, or regional health departments provide epidemiological services. Epidemiology is a branch of medical science that deals with the incidence, distribution, and control of disease in a population. Most state health departments have epidemiologists on staff to provide epidemiological assessment of health issues and concerns.

Some specific tasks of epidemiologists include investigating possible outbreaks, conducting surveillance activities, and disseminating information to healthcare providers and the public. For example, an epidemiologist may work closely with an environmental health specialist to investigate a possible foodborne illness associated with eating at a local restaurant. The epidemiologist would assist in identifying cases and interviewing individuals associated with the outbreak to find a common source. After identifying the source of the outbreak, an epidemiologist would set up specific control measures to eliminate the problem and prevent other similar outbreaks from occurring in the future.

Epidemiologists also provide assistance with surveillance activities to identify the amount and type of diseases present in the community. For example, during the late fall and winter months (October through April) an epidemiologist may track the number of influenza cases and identify characteristics of the individuals with the illness to have a better understanding of the disease and possible risk factors for those in the community. Trend analysis surveillance helps determine if the type and amount of disease present in the community is greater than expected and therefore becoming a possible public health concern. The field of epidemiology has become more visible since the events of September 11, 2001 with the concern of possible bioterrorism events. With additional threat concerns of newly emerging infectious or communicable diseases such as West Nile Virus, avian influenza, and Sudden Acute Respiratory Syndrome (SARS), epidemiology has received more publicity in recent years. There are many subspecialties within epidemiology, including chronic disease epidemiology, infectious disease epidemiology, genetic epidemiology, environmental epidemiology, and behavioral epidemiology.

Most epidemiologists have a background in the biological or chemical sciences. Almost all epidemiologists have an advanced degree in epidemiology or public health with a concentration in epidemiology. To pursue an advanced degree in public health with an emphasis in epidemiology it is recommended that individuals have a strong science and mathematical background. Many epidemiologists go on to pursue a doctoral degree in epidemiology or public health. This enables them to hold academic or upper-level managerial positions with public health agencies at the state or federal level.

Health Education and Health Educators

The importance of health education for the general public can not be dismissed. Providing accurate information on the prevention of both infectious and chronic conditions is extremely important to the health of the overall population. Health educators can work in a variety of locales, including public health departments, hospitals, and clinics. One major role for health educators includes applying public health strategies and principles in the development and dissemination of health information. Health educators may use social marking techniques to help them apply public health practices to the public. One important characteristic of health educators is that they must be willing to work with people in community settings. Most health educators have skills in conducting community assessments, developing and evaluating health programs, and writing grants. Health educators usually have a wide spectrum of educational backgrounds. Many have degrees in sociology, psychology, education, and health education.

The US Public Health Service

The US Public Health Service is the umbrella organization that oversees much of the public health efforts and organizations in this country. Founded first by President John Adams as a loose network of hospitals to support the health of American seamen, it is the uniformed service of the United States Department of Health and Human Services. The mission of the Public Health Service (PHS) Commissioned Corps is to provide highly trained and mobile health professionals who carry out programs to promote the health of the nation, understand and prevent disease and injury, assure safe and effective drugs and medical devices, deliver health services to federal beneficiaries, and furnish health expertise in time of war or other national or international emergencies. As one of the seven Uniformed Services of the United States, the PHS Commissioned Corps is a specialized career system designed to attract, develop, and retain a variety of health professionals who may be assigned to federal, state, or local agencies or international organizations to accomplish its mission.

To accomplish this mission, the agencies/programs are designed to

- Help provide health care and related services to medically underserved populations, such as American Indians and Alaska Natives, and to other population groups with special needs;
- Prevent and control disease, identify health hazards in the environment and help correct them, and promote healthy lifestyles for the nation's citizens;
- Improve the nation's mental health;
- Ensure that drugs and medical devices are safe and effective, food is safe and wholesome, cosmetics are harmless, and that electronic products do not expose users to dangerous amounts of radiation;
- Conduct and support biomedical, behavioral, and health services research and communicate research results to health professionals and the public; and
- Work with other nations and international agencies on global health problems and their solutions.

The PHS Commissioned Corps, led by the Surgeon General, consists of approximately 6,000 officers in the following professional categories: dentists, pharmacists, dietitians, physicians, engineers, scientists, environmental health, therapists, veterinarians, nurses, and other health service professionals.

The Surgeon General, America's chief health educator, provides Americans the best scientific information available on how to improve their health and reduce the risk of illness and injury. The Office of the Surgeon General, under the direction of the Surgeon General, oversees the US Public Health Service and provides support for the Surgeon General in the accomplishment of his/her other duties. The office is part of the Office of Public Health and Science, Office of the Secretary, US Department of Health and Human Services. The Surgeon General is appointed by the President of the United States with the advice and consent of the United States Senate for a four-year term of office. Duties of the Surgeon General as head of the US Public Health Service (USPHS) Commissioned Corps include

- To administer the PHS Commissioned Corps, which is a uniquely expert, diverse, flexible, and committed career force of public health professionals who can respond to both current and long-term health needs of the nation;
- To provide leadership and management oversight for PHS Commissioned Corps involvement in departmental emergency preparedness and response activities;
- To protect and advance the health of the nation through educating the public, advocating for effective disease prevention and health promotion programs and activities, and providing a highly recognized symbol of national commitment to protecting and improving the public's health;
- To articulate scientifically based health policy analysis and advice to the President and the Secretary of Health and Human Services (HHS) on the full range of critical public health, medical, and health system issues facing the nation;
- To provide leadership in promoting special departmental health initiatives (for example, tobacco and HIV prevention efforts) with other governmental and non-governmental entities, both domestically and internationally;
- To elevate the quality of public health practice in the professional disciplines through the advancement of appropriate standards and research priorities; and
- To fulfill statutory and customary departmental representational functions on a wide variety of federal boards and governing bodies of non-federal health organizations, including the Board of Regents of the Uniformed Services University of the Health Sciences, the National Library of Medicine, the Armed Forces Institute of Pathology, the Association of Military Surgeons of the United States, and the American Medical Association.

The US Public Health Service (PHS) Commissioned Corps offers a variety of employment opportunities for professionals throughout the Department of Health and Human Services (HHS) and certain non-HHS Federal agencies/programs. Commissioned corps officer status provides opportunities for mobility, flexibility, and career advancement in diverse work settings. The following list highlights some of the Health and Human Services Agencies/Operating Divisions (OPDIVs)/Programs where PHS Commissioned Officers may serve.

- **Agency for Healthcare Research and Quality (AHRQ)**
  AHRQ supports research designed to improve the outcomes and quality of health care, reduce its costs, address patient safety and medical errors, and broaden access to effective services.

- **Agency for Toxic Substances and Disease Registry (ATSDR)**
  ATSDR's mission is to prevent exposure and adverse human health effects and diminished quality of life associated with exposure to hazardous substances from waste sites, unplanned releases, and other sources of pollution present in the environment.

- **Centers for Disease Control and Prevention (CDC)**
  CDC's mission is to promote health and quality of life by preventing and controlling disease, injury, and disability. CDC seeks to accomplish this mission by working with partners throughout the nation and world to monitor health, detect and investigate health problems, conduct research to enhance prevention, develop and advocate sound public health policies, implement prevention strategies, promote healthy behaviors, foster safe and healthful environments, and provide leadership and training.

- **Food and Drug Administration (FDA)**
  FDA, one of our nation's oldest consumer protection agencies, assures the safety of foods and cosmetics and the safety and efficacy of pharmaceuticals, biological products, and medical devices. Its employees monitor the manufacture, import, transport, storage, and sale of about $1 trillion worth of products each year.

- **Health Resources and Services Administration (HRSA)**
  HRSA directs national health programs that improve the nation's health by assuring equitable access to comprehensive, quality healthcare for all. It works to improve and extend life for people living with HIV/AIDS, provide primary health care to medically underserved people, serve women and children through state programs, and train a health workforce that is both diverse and motivated to work in underserved communities.

- **Indian Health Service (IHS)**
  IHS is the principal federal healthcare advocate and provider for American Indians and Alaska Natives who belong to more than 550 federally recognized tribes in 35 states. It provides comprehensive healthcare services, including preventive, curative, rehabilitative, and environmental.

- **National Institutes of Health (NIH)**
  NIH, with its 27 separate components, mainly Institutes and Centers, is one of the world's foremost medical research centers, and the federal focal point for medical research in the United States. Its mission is to uncover new knowledge that will lead to better health for everyone by conducting research in its own laboratories; supporting the research of non-federal scientists in universities, medical schools, hospitals, and research institutions throughout the country and abroad; helping in the training of research investigators; and fostering communication of medical information.

- **Substance Abuse and Mental Health Services Administration (SAMHSA)**
  SAMHSA works to improve the quality and availability of prevention, treatment, and rehabilitative services in order to reduce illness, death, disability, and cost to society resulting from substance abuse and mental illnesses.

There are non-PHS agencies or programs where Public Health Service Commissioned Officers are sometimes assigned. These include the Federal Bureau of Prisons, the District of Columbia Commission on Mental Health Services, the Environmental Protection Agency, the Centers for Medicare and Medicaid Services, the US Citizenship and Immigration Services, the National Oceanic and Atmospheric Administration, the National Park Services, the US Coast Guard, the US Marshals Service, and the United States Department of Agriculture.

What Are the Entry Criteria for Joining the PHS Commissioned Corps?

To be accepted as an applicant for the Commissioned Corps, you must:

- Be a US citizen;
- Be under 44 years of age (age may be offset by prior active-duty Uniformed Service time and/or civil service work experience in a PHS agency at a PHS site at a level commensurate with the duties of a commissioned officer);
- Have served fewer than eight years of active duty if you are/were a member of another Uniformed Service;
- Be earning or have earned a qualifying degree from an accredited program per the appointment standards for your professional discipline (general duty officers cannot be called to active duty until they have completed their qualifying degree); and
- Meet medical and licensure/certification/registration requirements. For information on licensure/certification/registration requirements specific to your professional discipline, click the hyperlink for your professional category listed on the PHS home page.

In addition, commissioned officers are required to

- Complete a basic suitability clearance. Some officers, such as those hired by the Bureau of Prisons or the Immigration and Naturalization Service, are required to complete a higher level clearance prior to being called to duty. Most officers, however, will actually begin this process after the call to duty.

Depending on an officer's professional category, an applicant must possess a current and unrestricted license or other professional certificates appropriate for his/her profession in any of the 50 States, Washington DC, the Commonwealth of Puerto Rico, or the US Virgin Islands or Guam.

Professional Organizations for Public Health Professionals

The American Public Health Association (APHA)

The American Public Health Association (APHA) is the oldest and largest organization of public health professionals in the world, representing more than 50,000 members from over 50 occupations of public health. APHA has been influencing policies and setting priorities in public health for over 125 years. Throughout its history, it has been in the forefront of numerous efforts to prevent disease and promote health. APHA brings together researchers, health service providers, administrators, teachers, and other health workers in a unique, multidisciplinary environment of professional exchange, study, and action.

The APHA is concerned with a broad set of issues affecting personal and environmental health, including federal and state funding for health programs, pollution control, programs and policies related to chronic and infectious diseases, a smoke-free society, and professional education in public health. APHA actively serves the public, its members, and the public health profession through its scientific and practice programs, publications, annual meetings, educational services, and advocacy efforts. The achievements of APHA are the achievements of the thousands of federal, state, community, and academic health professionals who seek to assure the conditions in which people can be healthy. Whether APHA is proposing solutions based on research, helping to set public health practice standards, or working closely with national and international health agencies to improve health worldwide, its mission is to continue to strive to improve public health for everyone (APHA, 2005). The APHA has a variety of specific sections and special interest groups that have their own unique focus. Members can elect to join specific sections and groups as well as become general members of the APHA.

APHA Sections and Special Interest Groups Sections

- **Alcohol, Tobacco, and Other Drugs** – Promotes public health policy approaches to prevention and treatment of alcohol, tobacco, and other drug problems at all levels.

- **Chiropractic Health Care** – Serves as a vehicle for chiropractic participation in mainstream public health activities and works to enhance chiropractic communications, education, and credibility on public health matters.
- **Community Health Planning and Policy Development** – Influences the design of health systems and policies that are responsive to a changing society, by bringing together technical information and the expertise of communities, health professionals, business, and government.
- **Environment** – Works to focus attention on human health effects of environmental factors; helps to shape national environmental health and protection policies.
- **Epidemiology** – Promotes epidemiological activities; determines optimal immunization policies; analyzes utility of various approaches to disease prevention.
- **Food and Nutrition** – Contributes to long-range planning in food, nutrition, and health policy, which affects the nutritional well-being of the public.
- **Gerontological Health** – Works to stimulate public health actions to improve the health, functioning, and quality of life of older persons and to call attention to their healthcare needs.
- **Health Administration** – Concentrates on improvement of health service administration, including cost-benefit and operations research, program activities, finances, standards, and monitoring the organization of health services.
- **HIV/AIDS** – Provides a professional base for members of diverse disciplines to combine talents and interests to help in the struggle with the HIV-AIDS pandemic; provides leadership to members on HIV-AIDS issues and needs.
- **Injury Control and Emergency Health Services** – Serves as a forum for professionals committed to the control of injuries and the delivery of emergency health care; addresses both intentional and unintentional injuries for all age groups; and encompasses research, education, training, and practice.
- **International Health** – Acts as a focal point for APHA international health activities; encourages consideration of international issues in APHA activities.
- **Maternal and Child Health** – Contributes to policy development in adolescent health, child advocacy, injury prevention, family violence, and perinatal care; keeps members current on related issues.
- **Medical Care** – Encourages research, analysis, and policy development on organization, financing, and delivery of medical care; strives for an affordable, accessible system of high quality.

- **Mental Health** – Promotes public health policy and educational programs dedicated to enhancing the mental health of all persons and to improving the quality of health care for the mentally ill.
- **Occupational Health and Safety** – Strives to promote a healthy and safe working environment by organizing around current issues; contributes to policy development regarding occupational health and safety.
- **Oral Health** – Promotes the importance of oral health and increasing the public's access to oral health preventive and treatment services; monitors and communicates the oral health needs of the public.
- **Podiatric Health** – Advocates a national, preventive foot health strategy; ensures consideration of podiatric concerns in the formation of public health policy.
- **Population, Family Planning, and Reproductive Health** – Addresses issues involving population, family planning, and reproductive health; seeks to ensure that these issues and services remain major domestic and international priorities.
- **Public Health Education and Health Promotion** – Promotes the advancement of the health promotion and education profession and provides a forum for public health educators and those involved in health promotion activities to discuss ideas, research, and training; promotes activities related to training public health professionals.
- **Public Health Nursing** – Advances this specialty through leadership in the development of public health nursing practice and research; assures consideration of nursing concerns by providing mechanisms for interdisciplinary nursing collaboration in public health policy and program endeavors.
- **School Health Education and Services** – Focuses on development and improvement of health services, health education programs, and environmental conditions in schools, colleges, and early childhood care settings; advances public health in all school settings.
- **Social Work** – Establishes standards for social work in healthcare settings; contributes to the development of public health social work practice and research; promotes social work programs in the public health field.
- **Statistics** – Develops and designs effective, uniform statistical programs and studies for recognition, analysis, and solution of emerging health problems and needs.
- **Vision Care** – Promotes recognition of the need for an effective, equitable, and affordable vision care system for the public; advises on organization, delivery, and financing of vision care services.

APHA Special Interest Groups

- **Alternative and Complementary Health Practices** – Works toward the scientific evaluation of methods to promote and restore health not available from conventional medicine. Disseminates knowledge of validated practices and their potential contributions to health care.
- **Community Health Workers** – Seeks to promote the community's voice within the healthcare system through development of the role of new professionals/Community Health Advisors and other community-based professionals; provides a forum to share resources and strategies.
- **Ethics Forum** – Encourages public health officials to deliberately and systematically consider the ethical implications and cultural values behind their decisions.
- **Disability Forum** – Works to broaden the knowledge base and awareness regarding disability and related phenomena among all public health professions, and to provide policy advice to APHA on public health policies and programs for prevention and services to enhance the quality of life of persons with disabilities, including increased public and professional awareness.
- **Health Law Forum** – Encourages recognition and analysis of law's influence on public health programs, access to services, and health outcomes.
- **Laboratory** – Promotes the involvement of laboratory scientists in governmental policies affecting laboratories in the planning, evaluation, and operation of national, state, and local health programs that are dependent upon laboratory data.
- **Veterinary Public Health** – Deals with those diseases or environmental health issues that affect both human and animal populations.

Preparing for a Career in Public Health

Individuals who work in the public health sector have a variety of educational backgrounds and degrees. Many public health professionals do not have a formal degree in public health. Some have degrees in other human services areas such as psychology, sociology, or a clinical degree such as nursing.

There are several different types of graduate degrees in public health at both the masters and doctoral level. A Master of Public Health (MPH) degree is available at a number of institutions of higher education within the United States. MPH degrees range from 36 to 42 credits that can take a minimum of one year to complete. A Master of Science in Public Health (MSPH) is also available. There are a few differences in the two degrees. A MSPH usually requires more course work, for example, 48 credit hours in comparison to 36 credit hours for the MPH degree. In most cases, an MSPH also requires more science base courses and a thesis. While an MPH degree requires science-specific courses such as epidemiology, it also requires courses in administration and behavioral health and usually requires the completion of a practicum and not a formal thesis.

Many schools also offer a Master of Science in Health Studies (MHS) or sciences with a concentration in public health. Some schools offer a Master of Science (SCM) degree also with a concentration in public health. Individuals pursuing an MPH can do a generalist program or chose a specific concentration or area within public health. Some areas of concentration within public health include epidemiology, biostatistics, health policy and management, global or international health, nutrition, behavioral sciences and health education, and environmental or occupational health. Students interested in pursuing an MPH or MSPH degree should take undergraduate courses in the biological sciences and mathematics. Statistics courses are necessary and usually a prerequisite for entrance into master's degree programs within public health.

In addition to master's degree programs, many schools or programs in public health also offer doctoral degrees. Doctoral degrees programs may choose either a doctor of philosophy (PhD) or a doctor of public health (DrPH). The PhD programs tend to be more research based, while the DrPH programs are more focused on leadership and administration. Some academic institutions are now offering certificate programs with a specific emphasis, for example, field epidemiology or public health leadership. The certificate programs are usually 12 credits and are sometimes available via distance learning techniques.

Choosing a Public Health School

There are 36 CEPH accredited schools of public health. All accredited schools meet rigorous accreditation standards and each has unique strengths in research, service, and education. Students of public health come from a variety of educational backgrounds, but there is coursework that can better prepare you for the field of study you choose. For example, coursework in biology and mathematics is highly recommended for students who plan to concentrate in epidemiology or biostatistics. For Behavioral Sciences, Health Education, or Global Health, courses in sociology, psychology, education, or anthropology are beneficial. Health Services Administration students find that a business background is a plus. A biology or chemistry background is helpful for the study of Environmental Health. All schools of public health require competence in effective communication (both verbal and written); therefore, students should try to take advantage of undergraduate opportunities to hone these skills.

While schools of public health look for high graduate entrance exam scores and GPAs, other aspects of an applicant's record, such as career achievement, professional experience, and clarity of career goals also are equally important. Each program or track within a given department may set additional requirements for admission; therefore, applicants should refer to the individual programs for details. A full listing of schools offering accredited degrees in public health can be found at www.asph.org.

SUMMARY: WHY PURSUE A CAREER IN PUBLIC HEALTH?

Public health is an exciting and growing field of study, which challenges its professionals to confront complex health issues, such as improving access to health care, controlling infectious disease, and reducing environmental hazards, violence, substance abuse, and injuries. A diverse and dynamic field, public health draws professionals from varying educational backgrounds and specializations in a wide array of fields. A host of specialists, including teachers, journalists, researchers, administrators, environmentalists, demographers, social workers, laboratory scientists, and attorneys work to protect the health of the public. Public health professionals serve local, national, and international communities, and are leaders who meet the many exciting challenges in public health today and in the future. The field of public health offers great personal fulfillment—working toward improving people's health and well-being is a rewarding day's work.

Public health careers offer something for everyone. Epidemiology and biostatistics involve mathematics and modeling. Environmental health includes a wide range of science skills. Health administration and community health sciences are careers that involve being with people. Health education is a teacher's field. Health policy includes a political component. Perhaps never has there been a more exciting time to pursue a career in public health.

REFERENCES

American Public Health Association (APHA). (2005). *About APHA*. Retrieved October 30, 2005, from http://www.apha.org/about/.
Association of Schools of Public Health (ASPH). (2005). *What is public health?* Retrieved September 5, 2005, from www.whatispublichealth.org.

Blumenthal, D.S. & Rutterber, A.J. (1995). *Introduction to Environmental Health* (2nd ed.). New York: Springer Publishing Co.

Centers for Disease Control (CDC). (1999, April 2). Ten great public health achievements—United States, 1900–1999. *MMWR, 48*(12), 241–243.

Public Health Functions Project. (1995). *Public health in America.* Retrieved September 5, 2005, from http://www.health.gov/phfunctions/public.htm.

Stivers, C. (1991). *The politics of public health: The dilemma of a public profession.* In Litman, T. J. & Robins, L. S. (eds.). *Health Politics and Policies.* Chicago: Delmar Publishers.

The future of public health. (1988). Committee for the Study of the Future of Public Health: Division of Health Care Services, Institute of Medicine. Washington, DC: National Academies Press.

Warwick, M. (2002, July). A public health primer. *Journal of Homeland Security.*

Chapter 19

Health Services Administration

Jon M. Thompson

OBJECTIVES

After studying this chapter, the student should be able to

1. Explain the role of the administrator in the healthcare system.
2. Describe the educational preparation for health services administrators.
3. Identify the various healthcare environments where administrators work and the range of compensation at the entry, middle, and upper levels of administration.
4. Identify resources for additional information on the role of health services administration as a career option.

INTRODUCTION

A leader is not an administrator who loves to run others,
but someone who carries water for his people
so that they can get on with their jobs.
Robert Townsend

Health care is a business and, like every other business, it needs good management to keep it running smoothly. Medical and health services managers, also referred to as *healthcare executives* or *healthcare administrators*, plan, direct, coordinate, and supervise the delivery of health care. The expansion of health services has created increased opportunities for health services administrators who direct these organizations and departments or units within them, so that consumers may receive the healthcare services that they need. These managers include specialists and generalists. Specialists are in charge of specific clinical departments or services, while generalists manage or help manage an entire facility or system. The administrators of health programs, facilities, and organizations do not provide the care directly; rather, they *facilitate* the delivery of care. Administrators lead the way so that the other healthcare providers discussed in this book can do what they do best and provide excellent care to increase the quality and quantity of life for patients.

Description of the Profession of Health Services Administration

Previous chapters highlight the profound changes in the structure, financing, and delivery of health services in the United States over the past two decades. As a result, new health services organizations have emerged and existing ones have reorganized in efforts to provide appropriate, high-quality, and efficient delivery of health care to the people. In addition to the expansion of traditional health services organizations such as hospitals and nursing homes, changes in the industry have led to the development of new organizations such as managed care organizations, retirement communities, ambulatory care centers, and assisted living facilities. Various health professions highlighted in this text perform the primary, secondary, and tertiary prevention procedures for citizens across this country. Little of that care would be possible if not for the efforts of health services administrators. The health services administrator performs those essential tasks to enable the delivery of care to the individuals. Health services organizations such as hospitals, hospital systems, nursing homes, and physician practices need highly skilled administrators or managers to direct the operation of the facility and its services. The complex job of the health services manager includes many responsibilities and duties. Health services administrators carry out several management functions, including planning, staffing, organizing, controlling, directing, and decision-making that affect the health services facility and the care that is provided by the facility (Longest, Rakich & Darr, 2000). The scope of responsibilities depends on the size and internal structure of the facility, as well as the level of the managerial position. The administrator is also concerned with influences and activities that occur outside the facility that affect the facility. These factors include the community and its needs, government organizations that regulate the facility, insurance companies that reimburse the facility, and other facilities and services that may be competitors to the facility. These two domains of management are shown in Figure 19.1.

Health services administrators' primary responsibility is to manage their facility and services in the best way possible to ensure that the patient or consumer receives appropriate, effective, and timely services. Administrators determine appropriate internal structures and lines of reporting (organizing) and determine the best arrangement of staffing for carrying out the work. They hire, evaluate, and terminate staff that work in the facility (staffing). They plan for the future of the facility by making forecasts of needed services and the demand for services (planning). Administrators develop and implement budgets and closely track expenses and revenues to make sure the organization is on sound financial footing (planning). They also monitor and control the overall performance of the facility (controlling) and direct, supervise, and motivate staff to ensure high levels of performance (directing). Finally, administrators make many important decisions on resources, staff, and services to make sure that the facility is providing needed care in the most cost-effective and high-quality manner possible (decision-making).

Because many health services organizations are large, there are opportunities for serving as a manager at different levels within the facility. The top administrator may be called the practice administrator in a physician practice, or the Chief Executive Officer (CEO) or administrator in a large hospital or clinic. The administrator is likely to have several assistant administrators who handle various functions, such as finance, quality, or ancillary services. Also, there are management positions at various department, unit, or service levels within the organization where an administrator may occupy the position

External	*Internal*
Community demographics/need	Staffing
Licensure	Budgeting
Accreditation	Quality services
Regulations	Patient satisfaction
Stakeholder demands	Physician relations
Competitors	Financial performance
Medicare and Medicaid	Technology acquisition
Managed care organizations/Insurers	New service development

Figure 19.1   *Domains of Health Services Administration*

of department head or assistant department head, or supervisor or director of certain functions or activities. Figure 19.2 shows a typical table of organization for a large health services organization and varying levels of managerial positions.

It is important to remember that administrators do not provide clinical services themselves, but rather they facilitate the delivery of services needed by consumers by managing staff and resources. Accordingly, they work with and manage a wide variety of clinical and non-clinical personnel to make sure that appropriate services are being provided, and that there is a means of control over the delivery of care. The administrator must have an understanding of clinical care processes even if the administrator's primary responsibility is to provide the business leadership for the organization. However, there are certain administrative and management positions where the manager may also provide some clinical services to patients. Individuals in these positions, for example, may direct nursing, physical therapy, occupational therapy, and diagnostic services such as radiology (imaging). In these situations, *clinical managers* is a term to describe those individuals.

Where Do Health Services Administrators Administrate?

Health services administrators work in a variety of settings providing health care to patients and communities. The best way to think about health services organizations is to think about their primary focus: Is the organization a treatment facility such as a community hospital or a ambulatory surgery center, a screening or diagnostic facility, a physician practice, a specialized

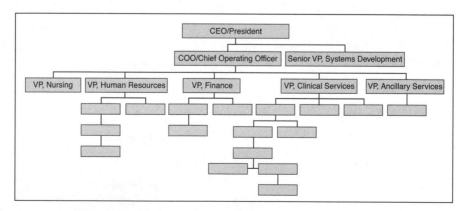

Figure 19.2 *Organizational Chart, Friendly Medical Center*

facility such as a wellness or preventive care facility, or a long-term care facility that provides continuous care to persons with chronic illness? There are many different types of facilities and organizations that require skilled managers who will work in either the top administrative position or some other managerial position within the structure. While the target patient group served by each of these organizations is different, the management functions and responsibilities of the health services administrator are similar across each of these settings. Figure 19.3 provides a listing of settings where health services administrators are employed.

Health services administration is a rewarding, but highly challenging profession. Each workday presents different and challenging issues for the administrator that create opportunities and threats. The role of the health administrator is anything but boring, as administrators have to handle multiple tasks and

---

Inpatient Hospitals
- general, community acute care
- specialty (for example, pediatric, rehabilitation, psychiatric)
- teaching/academic medical centers

Ambulatory clinics/services
- hospital-based
- HMO-based
- freestanding diagnostic/treatment clinics
- ambulatory surgical centers
- mobile clinics

Wellness/Fitness Centers

Physician Practices
- partnerships
- specialty groups
- multi-specialty groups

Skilled Nursing Centers/Nursing Homes

Retirement Communities

Assisted Living Facilities

Home Health Agencies

Public health departments/Community Health Centers

Figure 19.3 *Settings for the Practice of Health Services Administration**

*This listing provides only examples of direct care health care provider organizations where health services administrators are employed.

make many decisions at the same time. Administrators must be skilled in understanding the specifics of health services delivery, particularly the value of new medical and information technology, payment for services by different insurers and government programs, and regulatory and accreditation issues. In addition, administrators must be able to keep the organization running smoothly by motivating and directing staff and continuously meeting the needs of consumers. This requires working with a variety of clinical staff, including physicians, nurses, therapists, and clinical technicians, among others, as well as with different levels of managerial and support staff. At the end of the day, however, each administrator can feel good about his or her role in helping patients receive the services and care they need.

History of the Health Services Administration Profession

Health services administration traces its roots to the 1930s and 1940s when professional programs at universities were first established to prepare administrators. The first of these programs was at the University of Chicago in 1934 (Loebs, 2001). Early educational programs were master's-level programs that used practicing hospital administrators with extensive experience to teach the necessary skills to provide leadership in community hospitals. Later, as professionals received their doctorates in business, health administration, or public administration, professional programs in health administration were developed that were headed by academics. During the mid- to late-1940s, several new graduate programs were established at various universities to meet the need for professionally prepared administrators. This was due to a post World War II boom in hospital construction under the federal Hill-Burton Act and the rise in employer-sponsored health insurance leading to increased revenue for hospitals.

In the period 1960 through 1990, many universities and colleges began offering baccalaureate programs in health administration to prepare health administration professionals for entry-level positions in various health organizations. As health services organizations experienced an increased need for trained managers at all levels, enrollments in both undergraduate and graduate programs increased. This was a time of great expansion in health care, fueled in part by funding for health care made available under Medicare and Medicaid programs established in the mid-1960s. Health services organizations recognized that they needed the expertise and skills of professionally prepared health administrators. Professional associations expanded their efforts to formalize the profession of health administration and to advance the profession's status.

Minimum Education and Certification Requirements for Health Services Administrators

Entry into the profession of health services administration typically begins with a bachelor's degree in health administration or health services administration. In 2005, there were 32 programs that were "Fully Certified" by the Association of University Programs in Health Administration to provide undergraduate preparation in health administration. Programs achieving the designation of Full Certification have met a rigorous set of standards that address curriculum, educational processes, and program outcomes. These programs prepare individuals for entry-level administrative positions such as assistant administrator or director of patient accounts, or positions requiring administrative skills such as contract specialist, marketing coordinator, financial analyst, or quality management/assurance specialist. Because much of the expansion in the health administration field is in entry-level positions, these programs are filling an important gap in the field. Undergraduate programs in health services administration are continuing to address the key competencies needed by entry-level administrators (Thompson, 2005).

In addition, graduates of undergraduate programs in health administration are realizing many opportunities by assuming entry-level jobs in various settings (Shea & Mucha, 1995). For upward movement within an organization, or to start out at a more senior level position, a master's degree in health administration or a master of business administration degree with a healthcare specialty is needed.

To become a CEO, chief operating officer, or other senior level administrator, a master's degree will be required. Most graduate programs require a few years of work experience by applicants as a prerequisite for admission. In 2005, the Accrediting Commission certified 64 graduate programs in health administration in the United States for Education in Health Services Administration (ACHESA).

Administrators are not required to be licensed, except in the case of nursing home administrators. Licensure is granted by individual states for nursing home administrators. Many states are now considering the requirement for licensing of administrators in assisted living facilities. Several professional associations offer credentialing and certification programs for members that promote recognition as meeting the standards of practice established by the respective organizations.

Role of National Professional Organizations/Associations

Because of the diversity of practice settings and different practice foci, there are a number of health administration professional organizations. The largest professional association addressing health administration is the American College of Healthcare Executives (ACHE). The mission of ACHE is to advance member and healthcare management excellence through ethical standards, pertinent knowledge, and a relevant credentialing program. Founded in 1933, ACHE offers professional development programs to its members, access to resources and latest administrative approaches, and credentialing programs that correspond with varying levels of career development. ACHE has over 30,000 members, and has state-level regents as well as university student chapters. Students in health administration programs can join as student members and advance to higher certification levels over time.

The Medical Group Management Association (MGMA), founded in 1926, offers certification for administrators of physician practices and group practices, and addresses the specific management needs of physician practice managers to enhance the effectiveness of medical group practices. MGMA has over 19,000 members, and has student chapters at colleges and universities.

The Healthcare Financial Management Association (HFMA) addresses the needs of healthcare financial management professionals, and has over 30,000 members. HFMA offers educational and professional development opportunities to its members, and provides key information and resources on issues affecting healthcare financial managers. HFMA also offers a certification program for its members, and has state chapters.

The American College of Healthcare Administrators (ACHCA), founded in 1962, focuses on the needs of administrators in nursing homes, retirement communities, and assisted living facilities. ACHCA's mission is to promote excellence in leadership among long-term care administrators, and ACHCA offers members certification in management of long-term care facilities and services. ACHCA has state membership chapters.

Professionals in health administration may benefit from membership in one or more of these professional groups. They offer opportunities for networking with other health professionals, access to association studies, research and literature that offer guidance and suggestions on enhancing practice, certification processes that allow the demonstration of competencies in health administration, and opportunities to serve the profession through various leadership roles. Professional organizations require annual dues and additional fees are charged for other organizational activities such as credentialing and certification, selected information and data, and attendance at conferences and annual meetings. Web sites for these organizations are listed at the end of this chapter.

One additional professional organization that is helpful to students in health administration programs as well as practicing health administrators is the Association of University Programs in Health Administration (AUPHA). AUPHA, founded in 1948, is dedicated to improving the field of health care management and practice by strengthening health administration education. AUPHA has a certification process for undergraduate health administration programs and works closely with ACHESA, which accredits graduate programs in health administration. Health administration students and practicing administrators seeking advanced degrees should consult with AUPHA to determine health administration programs that meet professional certification and accreditation standards. The listing of programs is available at www.AUPHA.org.

Estimated Salary/Earnings

Salaries in the profession of health administration are very good and highly competitive relative to other professional fields. Salaries will vary, of course, by type of position and specific responsibilities (for example, entry-level, mid-level management, and senior management) as well as by geographic area and type of organization (for example, for-profit, not-for-profit, government facility). In 2002, the Bureau of Labor Statistics reported that the median annual earnings of medical and health services managers were $61,370. Earnings for health administrators can vary from $35,000 to over $200,000 per year, with the highest salaries given to experienced administrators with advanced education who head large health services organizations in urban locations. Chief Executive Officers of large hospitals and hospital systems may earn well over $500,000 per year depending on their experience. However, these positions are limited and are made available only to highly select individuals with extensive experience and a track record of accomplishments. Professionals with bachelor's degrees and limited experience are entering the job market in entry-level positions with salary ranges between $25,000 to $50,000 per year. Many health services organizations offer additional pay-for-performance programs that allow administrators to receive additional compensation contingent on the achievement of organizational goals and objectives. Median annual earnings in the sectors employing the largest number of medical and health services managers in 2002 are shown in Table 19.1.

Table 19.1 *Median Annual Earnings of Health Services Managers, Largest Sectors of the Health Services Industry, 2002*

Sector	Median Annual Earnings
General medical/surgical hospitals	$65,900
Home health care services	$56,320
Outpatient care centers	$55,650
Physician offices	$55,600
Nursing care facilities	$55,320
Source: BLM, 2004.	

Trends in the Future of the Profession

The profession of health services administration is forecast to experience significant growth through 2012, and advancement opportunities are excellent as well. The Bureau of Labor Statistics (BLS) of the US Department of Labor predicts that "Medical and Health Services Managers" will be one of the fastest growing fields in this time period, and estimates that an additional 71,300 positions will be created during the period 2002–2012. This represents an average annual growth of just over 7,000 job openings per year. The BLS reports that in 2002, there were about 244,000 jobs in the United States held by medical and health services managers. About 37% of these positions were held by managers working in hospitals, and 17% worked in physician practices and nursing facilities. The remainder worked mostly in home healthcare services, outpatient care centers, community care facilities for the elderly, insurance carriers, and government healthcare facilities.

The BLS reports that employment of medical and health services managers is expected to grow faster than the average for all occupations through 2012, as the health services industry continues to expand and diversify. Forecasted growth is 29% for medical and health services managers during this period. Opportunities are anticipated to be especially good in physician practices (growth in employment is expected to be 55%), home healthcare services, and outpatient care centers, because employment within these sectors is expected to grow the fastest. Much of this growth is due to the shift in locus of care to more convenient and lower cost, non-hospital settings where less specialized healthcare personnel can provide services. Hospitals will continue to employ the most medical and health services managers over the projection period, but the number of new jobs in hospitals is expected to increase at a slightly slower rate than in many other sectors of the health services industry. There are approximately 6,000 hospitals operating in the United States. Additional growth in employment for medical and health services managers is due to growth in opportunities in the insurer and managed care organization market, expansion of healthcare management companies who provide assistance to hospitals and other organizations, and increases in the healthcare consulting business, which provides strategic, operational, and financial assistance to health services organizations. Also, the growth in the elderly population due to aging baby boomers and their growing health needs, as well as longer life expectancy, have prompted additional growth in management opportunities in senior services and long-term care such as assisted living facilities and retirement communities.

Professional health administration groups also forecast strong opportunities for health administrators in the future. Future administrators face a different healthcare world than that of today. The challenges facing the profession require that future administrators have not only technical skills such as computer, finance, budgeting, and planning skills, but also that they possess strong team-building, interpersonal, and leadership skills to motivate staff to higher levels of performance.

Critical Skills/Qualities of Entry-Level Administrators

There are several key skills needed by entry-level professionals in the health services administration field. These skills can be described as technical, conceptual, and interpersonal skills (Katz, 1974). Technical skills are those skills that are used by managers to carry out specific work assignments and manage their completion. These skills include finance, budgeting, computer, and project management skills. These skills are necessary to plan, manage, and evaluate the work of staff who administrators supervise. Health services organizations are service enterprises but also businesses, so business skills are critical to the health services manager's success. A health services administrator would use technical skills in developing and maintaining a budget for a particular hospital unit or department, or by using a computer to track trends in the quality of services by examining customer satisfaction and complaints.

The second set of skills is termed conceptual skills. These skills involve having a detailed understanding of the specific issues that affect the management of health services organizations and personnel, critically analyzing the impact of these issues on the management of the facility and developing sound evaluation of alternatives in making decisions. An example of this skill would be the evaluation of alternatives in expanding the facility and making decisions on the addition of new services.

The third key skill set involves interpersonal skills. This skill set refers to working with and managing others, and includes the ability to communicate effectively with others, serve as part of a team, motivate others, and provide effective leadership. A health services administrator would use interpersonal skills to discuss assignments with his or her staff, meet with staff to determine planning priorities, and evaluate staff through performance appraisals. Health services administrators work with many other individuals who they supervise or with whom they must interact to accomplish the work of the organization. In addition, many activities require working in teams consisting of both clinical and non-clinical personnel.

Entry-level administrators need to be highly motivated to work in this fast-paced field, and enthusiastic about opportunities before them. The supervisor of a new administrative staff member wants to know that their employee is excited about the field and is willing to take on assignments. Therefore, the new administrator must be willing to demonstrate their interest and enthusiasm. Entry-level administrative staff must also recognize that they will be working long hours. Because they are professional employees, new administrators must put in the time it takes to get the job done, which may mean working long days and working some on the weekends. Many healthcare facilities operate on a 24 hour-per-day basis and the job frequently requires that administrators be available to meet with staff or accomplish certain activities at times beyond the normal workday.

Additional skills that entry-level administrators need to possess include organizational skills and a willingness to learn. Being able to manage work tasks and personal time and keep up with all the demands placed on them requires that administrators be organized, keep track of multiple projects, and be timely on assignments and tasks. Finally, health services administrators know that entry-level administrative personnel are still learning and that becoming a good administrator takes time and experience. Experienced administrators may serve as mentors and offer important guidance for new administrators. Entry-level administrators must recognize that they don't have all the answers because they are new to the field; this is understandable, and senior administrators are willing to let them grow through experience and the practice involved in making decisions. Because the healthcare industry is continually changing, health services administrators must engage in life-long learning to stay current with their knowledge.

Challenges Facing Health Services Administrators

The profession of health services administration is complex, dynamic, and rewarding, but it also presents many challenges. These challenges are due to the rapid changes that are occurring in health services delivery, innovations in medical and information technology, intense competition among health services organizations, the pervasive influence of managed care and reduced reimbursements, staffing issues, and pressures for accountability from the community as well as from regulatory and accreditation organizations.

The focus of health services administrators is high performance for their organizations in terms of financial position, quality of service, and customer satisfaction. Administrators are faced with pressures to add the latest medical and information technologies to their organizations so that they can be efficient in the provision of high-quality services. But these advancements often require resources that many health services organizations do not have. Health administrators are also constantly assessing their competitors and deciding how to best compete with, and in some cases, collaborate with, these organizations.

In general, organizations compete on the basis of services offered, quality of care, and cost. Because there are greater numbers of health organizations today than in the past, and due to the fact that many health organizations offer similar services, competition for patients is more intense that in the past. For example, hospitals recognize that their competitors today are not just other hospitals, but include physician practices, freestanding diagnostic centers, and ambulatory surgery centers. Administrators have to develop effective strategies to achieve the necessary treatment volumes for financial performance, strategies which may include competing and/or collaborating with competitors.

Changes in financing and delivery of health services due to managed care and government reimbursement also present a major challenge to health services administrators. In the past 10 to 15 years, the emergence and growth of HMOs, PPOs, and Point of Service plans, and their reimbursement restrictions on health services organizations, have forced administrators of health services organizations to cut their operating costs and to re-think their relationships with health plans. Managed care has shifted the focus of administrators to minimize costs and maximize revenues, while still promoting quality. Also, reimbursement to health services organizations and physicians by Medicare and Medicaid has consistently declined over the past decade, which causes health services organizations to contain services wherever possible to keep operating costs low.

Two final challenges for health services administrators are having appropriate staff and being accountable for the services provided by the institution or organization. Health services administrators face growing concerns with having the appropriate number and types of staff, including physicians, nurses, physical therapists, and other highly specialized personnel. Because some of these staff are in short supply, it is difficult to provide the level of services that are sometimes needed. Pressures to recruit and retain all staff are significant.

Finally, health services organizations are under increased scrutiny by external organizations that regulate and accredit them. State and federal agencies that regulate health services organizations, as well as accrediting organizations, are increasing pressures on health services organizations for accountability. These organizations are advocating for the public interest and are requiring that health services organizations report their performance—in terms of cost and quality, among other indicators—so that the public may make informed decisions about their personal health care and the health services organizations from which they receive services. Pressures on administrators to balance cost and quality of service have never been greater, and health services organizations are in the public eye. Public expectations for good quality, excellent service, and reasonable costs are higher than ever before.

SUMMARY

With the ever-increasing need for healthcare institutions, health services administrators can expect continued employment opportunities and growth. Job opportunities will be especially good in offices of health practitioners, general medical and surgical hospitals, home healthcare services, and outpatient care centers. Applicants with work experience in health care and strong business and management skills likely will have the best opportunities. Career advancement and earnings are high, but long work hours are common in the health services administration field. A master's degree is the standard credential for most senior-level and advanced positions, although a bachelor's degree is adequate for many entry-level positions in smaller facilities and in health information management. Those who choose a career in health services administration enable the medical practitioners who work for them to better care for patients.

ADDITIONAL RESOURCES

American College of Healthcare Executives
Suite 1700
One North Franklin Street
Chicago, IL 60606-4425
Phone: (312) 424-2800
Fax: (312) 424-0023
Web site: www.ache.org or for Health Management Careers (part of ACHE), visit www.Healthmanagementcareers.com

American College of Healthcare Administrators (ACHCA)
300 N. Lee Street
Suite 301
Alexandria, VA 22314
Phone: 703-739-7900 or 888-88-ACHCA (888-882-2422)
Fax: 703-739-7901
Web site: www.achca.org

Association of University Programs in Health Administration (AUPHA)
2000 North 14th Street
Suite 780
Arlington, VA 22201
Phone: 703-894-0940
Fax: 703-894-0941
Web site: www.aupha.org

Healthcare Financial Management Association
Two Westbrook Corporate Center
Suite 700
Westchester, IL 60154-5700
1-800-252-HFMA (4362)
Fax: (708) 531-0032

HFMA DC Office
1301 Connecticut Avenue, N.W., Suite 300
Washington, DC 20036-3417
Phone: (202) 296-2920
Fax: (202) 223-9771
Web site: www.hfma.org

Medical Group Management Association (MGMA)
MGMA Headquarters
104 Inverness Terrace East
Englewood, CO 80112-5306
Phone: (303) 799-1111 or toll-free: (877) ASK-MGMA (275-6462)
Fax: (303) 643-4439

Government Affairs Office
1717 Pennsylvania Ave. N.W. #600
Washington, DC 20006
Phone: (202) 293-3450
Fax: (202) 293-2787
Web site: www.mgma.org

HEALTH SERVICES ADMINISTRATION AND NEW SERVICE DEVELOPMENT: A MINI CASE STUDY

Assume you are a newly appointed Assistant Administrator at a large hospital located in a large urban area that is highly competitive in terms of health services. Your boss has asked you to assess whether or not your facility should establish a Mammography Program as part of your facility's Women's Health Services. This program would be distinct from imaging services that are currently offered at your hospital. A mammography program is a diagnostic breast screening program that is used to detect breast cancer in women.

Identify the actions that you would take as an administrator to carry out this assignment to determine whether or not your facility should move ahead on this new service. Respond to the questions below.

1. What staff members would you need to consult with and why? Should you form a team to address this issue? Why or why not?

2. What would you do to determine the need or demand for this service? What information would you consult and where would you obtain that information?

3. What is the competition for this service? What competitor data should you examine and where will you obtain such data?

4. What steps should you take, and what information should you review, to determine the financial feasibility of this service?

5. What considerations should be given to separate space for this service?

6. What are the implications for managing this service once established? What should the manager of this service focus on once the service has been established?

REFERENCES

Bureau of Labor Statistics, US Department of Labor (BLM). (2004). *Occupational outlook handbook*. Washington, DC: US Department of Labor.

Katz, R. L. (1974, September–October). Skills of an effective administrator. *Harvard Business Review, 52,* 90–102.

Loebs, S. (2001). The continuing evolution of health management education. Special issue: The future of education and practice in health management and policy. *The Journal of Health Administration Education.*

Longest, B. B., Rakich, J. S., & Darr, K. (2000). *Managing health services organizations and systems* (4th ed.). Baltimore, MD: Health Professions Press.

Shea, D. G. & Mucha, L. (1995, Summer). Employment trends and the traditional baccalaureate health administration student. *The Journal of Health Administration Education, 13*(3), 401–419.

Thompson, J. M. (2005, Fall). Competency development and assessment in undergraduate healthcare management programs: The role of internships. *The Journal of Health Administration Education, 22*(4), 417–433.

Chapter 20

Complementary and Alternative Health Professions

Theresa Prodoehl

OBJECTIVES

After studying this chapter, the student should be able to

1. Compare complementary and alternative medicine (CAM) with traditional allopathic medical practice.
2. Explain the historical development process of CAM.
3. Compare the most prevalent methods of CAM used in the United States today.
4. Identify the role of complementary and alternative medicine in the health care system today.
5. Describe the educational preparation and certification required for various forms of CAM.
6. Identify resources for additional information on the role of CAM.

INTRODUCTION

> *To keep the body in good health is a duty . . . otherwise*
> *we shall not be able to keep our mind strong and clear.*
> Buddha (Hindu Prince Gautama Siddhartha, the founder of Buddhism, 563–483 BC)

From ancient Chinese medicine techniques such as acupuncture to naturopathy, complementary and alternative health professions are enjoying a new popularity and respect, even from the medical community.

Complementary and alternative medicine (CAM) includes any therapeutic or preventive services that are used for treating illness or maintaining health that are different from those that are used by traditional Western medicine or conventional medicine as it is practiced in the United States. Conventional or traditional Western medicine, known as *allopathic medicine*, is the system of medical practice that treats disease by the use of remedies that produce effects different from those produced by the disease under treatment. MDs practice allopathic medicine; therefore, medicine that is not the usual Western medicine is non-allopathic. Complementary medicine, gradually becoming included in Western medical schools or hospitals, includes a large number of practices and systems of health care that, for a variety of cultural, social, economic, or scientific reasons are outside mainstream Western medicine. Complementary and alternative medicine, as defined by the National Center for Complementary and Alternative Medicine of the National Institutes of Health (NCCAM), is a group of diverse medical and healthcare systems, practices, and products that are not presently considered part of conventional medicine. While some scientific evidence exists regarding some CAM therapies, for most there are key questions that are yet to be answered through well-designed scientific studies—questions such as whether these therapies are safe and whether they work for the diseases or medical conditions for which they are used. The list of methods considered to be part of CAM changes continually. As those therapies proven safe and effective, new approaches to health care emerge. Integrative medicine, as defined by NCCAM, combines mainstream medical therapies and CAM therapies for which there is some high-quality scientific evidence of safety and effectiveness.

Trends in CAM

The current trend is to encourage the use of non-traditional healthcare services as a supplement to conventional treatments, as opposed to using CAM instead of conventional care. It is becoming preferred and more accepted to complement or integrate traditional care with alternative forms of care in an attempt to have the best of both worlds when maintaining health. At times this kind of care is referred to as Integrative Medicine or Complementary Medicine. The purpose of this chapter is to review the career opportunities in the areas that are the predominant non-allopathic, non-traditional therapeutic healthcare systems practiced in the United States. In addition to the variety of systems of medicine, there are careers available to practitioners of specific techniques used as part of a system of medicine or utilized by consumers independently.

The techniques that will be addressed in this chapter include acupuncture, chiropractic care, naturopathy, homeopathy, massage therapy, and herbal medicine.

Therapies and treatments considered CAM in the United States are often mainstream medicine in other areas of the world. Americans will view any medicine that is not taught by our medical schools or used in our hospitals as non-traditional or CAM. Some of our medical schools and hospitals are integrating non-allopathic modalities into their curricula and in time the use of the terminology of CAM may become obsolete or confusing as integration of alternative systems into mainstream medicine continues. There are other CAM therapies practiced in the United States and in the world, such as Ayurveda, which will not be covered in this chapter due to the overwhelming number of techniques and the fact that many are not as accepted as health care or are not as popular in the United States at this time.

CAM is one of the fastest growing sectors of American health care. This will mean that there will be increasing demands for CAM providers in the future, providing a promising career outlook. Presently, only chiropractic warrants attention from the United States Bureau of Labor Statistics as a health career. However, there is a growing interest in CAM in the United States. The National Institutes of Health developed the National Center for Complementary and Alternative Medicine (NCCAM) to oversee research and to be a resource for accurate information.

Established in 1998, the National Center for Complementary and Alternative Medicine (NCCAM) is one of the 27 institutes and centers that make up the National Institutes of Health (NIH). The NIH is one of eight agencies under the Public Health Service (PHS) in the Department of Health and Human Services (DHHS). NCCAM is dedicated to exploring complementary and alternative healing practices in the context of rigorous science, training complementary and alternative medicine (CAM) researchers, and disseminating authoritative information to the public and professionals.

Hippocrates (460–377 BC) is credited with saying "Prayer indeed is good, but while calling on the gods a man should himself lend a hand." This concept appears to fit the current trends seen in CAM over 2300 years later. There are many alternative ways to "lend a hand" when seeking health. For example, many individuals feel that prayer can help, and certainly will not hurt. In 2004, the NCCAM and the National Center for Health Statistics reported that more than 36% of all Americans have used some form of alternative medicine (Barnes, Powell-Griner, McFann, & Nahin, 2004). When prayer specifically for health reasons is included, that figure rises to 62%. Prayer was the therapy most commonly used among all the CAM therapies included in the survey; 43% had prayed for their own health, almost 25% had others pray for them, and almost 10% had participated in a prayer group for their health. While prayer is a significant component to CAM, because it is highly personal and not actually a profession, details on this method are not provided in this chapter. However, if you are interested, you are encouraged to seek additional information beginning with the http://nccam.nih.gov Web site.

Americans spent more than 36 billion dollars on alternative therapies in 1997, exceeding out-of-pocket spending for all US hospitalizations. The Journal of the American Medical Association reports a 47.3% increase in total visits to alternative medicine practitioners between 1990 and 1997 (Astin, 1998). The Astin study showed that people turn to alternative healing not so much as a result of dissatisfaction with conventional medicine, but largely because the health care alternatives more closely mirror their own values, beliefs, and philosophical orientations toward life.

Nearly three fourths of US medical schools offer elective courses in alternative and complementary medicine or include it in required courses. Many doctors and nurses now seek information and continuing education in natural medicine modalities. Collaborative healing arts centers and integrative medicine clinics are opening up across the United States to address the needs of the whole person from a variety of healing arts perspectives. Moreover, patient demand for health insurance coverage for natural therapies is increasing, as people want improved access to alternative therapies (Natural Healers, 2006).

To provide more information on the use of CAM in the United States, NCCAM conducted a survey to provide the most comprehensive and reliable findings to date on Americans' use of CAM (Barnes et al., 2004). The 2002 edition of the NCHS's National Health Interview Survey (NHIS), an annual study of over 31,000 adults, interviewed tens of thousands of Americans regarding their health- and illness-related experiences, and included detailed questions on CAM. Excluding megavitamins, 74% of respondents report using complementary or alternative medicine at least once, and 64% used some method within the past 12 months. When you remove prayer for health, 49% reported using CAM at any time, 36% in the past 12 months. CAM use spans people of all backgrounds. However, according to the survey, some people are more likely than others to use CAM. Overall, CAM use is greater by women than men, and seen more frequently in people with higher educational levels, especially with people who have been hospitalized in the past year.

NCCAM Domains of Care

To organize the overwhelming amount of therapies considered as CAM in the United States, NCCAM created five broad categories of CAM interventions, which include at least 600 specific therapies. This taxonomy is expected to evolve over time, but presently the five categories include: (1) Biologically based practices; (2) Energy medicine; (3) Manipulative and body-based practices; (4) Mind-body medicine; and (5) Whole medical systems. When prayer is included in the definition of CAM, the domain of mind-body medicine is the most commonly used domain (53%). When prayer is not included, biologically based therapies (22%) are more popular than mind-body medicine (17%).

Brief Description of Domains

Biological Practices

Biologically based therapies in CAM use substances found in nature, such as herbs, foods, and vitamins. The domain of biologically based practices includes, but is not limited to, botanicals, animal-derived extracts, vitamins, minerals, fatty acids, amino acids, proteins, prebiotics and probiotics, whole diets, and functional foods. Biological practices performed by herbalists and others make up 21.9% of CAM use according to the 2004 survey (Barnes et al., 2004).

Energy Medicine

Energy medicine is a domain that deals with energy fields. Vital energy, believed to flow throughout the material human body, is difficult to measure

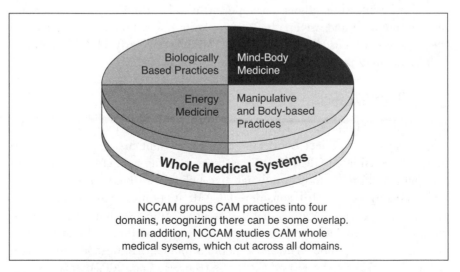

NCCAM groups CAM practices into four
domains, recognizing there can be some overlap.
In addition, NCCAM studies CAM whole
medical sysems, which cut across all domains.

Figure 20.1 *Domains of CAM*
Source: NCCAM, 2004b

by means of conventional instrumentation. Nonetheless, therapists claim that they can work with this subtle energy, see it with their own eyes, and use it to effect changes in the physical body and influence health. Practitioners of energy medicine believe that illness results from disturbances of these energies. Herbal medicine, acupuncture, and acupressure, for example, are all believed to act by correcting imbalances in the internal biofield, such as by restoring the flow of Qi (pronounced "chee") through meridians to reinstate health. Only 0.5% of CAM use falls in this domain according to the NCCAM survey.

Manipulative and Body-Based Practices

Manipulative and body-based practices include a mixture of CAM interventions and therapies. A short list includes chiropractic and osteopathic manipulation, massage therapy, reflexology, rolfing, Alexander technique, Feldenkrais method, and a host of others. Currently the most utilized CAM treatments in the United States include chiropractic care and massage therapy. In 1997, US adults made an estimated 192 million visits to chiropractors and 114 million visits to massage therapists. Visits to chiropractors and massage therapists combined represented 50% of all visits to CAM practitioners (Eisenberg et al., 1998).

Manipulative and body-based practices focus primarily on the structures and systems of the body, including the bones and joints, the soft tissues, and the circulatory and lymphatic systems. Some practices derived from traditional systems of medicine in other countries, such as those from China, India, or Egypt, while others developed within the last 150 years (for example, chiropractic and osteopathic manipulation). Combined, these make up the bulk of body-based practices (NCCAM, 2004). Nearly 11% of CAM use falls in the manipulative and body-based domain.

Mind-Body Medicine

Mind-body medicine uses a variety of techniques designed to enhance the mind's capacity to affect bodily function and symptoms. Some techniques that were considered CAM in the past have become mainstream (for example, patient support groups and cognitive-behavioral therapy). Other mind-body techniques are still considered CAM, including meditation, prayer, mental healing, and therapies that use creative outlets such as art, music, or dance. Mind-body interventions constitute a major portion of the overall use of CAM by the public. The most popular domain, mind-body medicine, accounts for 52.9% of reported CAM use (Barnes et al., 2004).

Whole Medical Systems

A healthcare system includes a variety of modalities or techniques used together to heal or maintain health as practiced by a particular culture. The number of different systems reflects the variety of healthcare techniques as practiced by different cultures that have evolved over time from ancient civilizations through modern times. Some techniques used by the systems are similar but will have variations based upon cultural differences. Whole medical systems make up approximately 2.7% of CAM use.

The predominant systems of care that will be discussed later in this chapter include:

1. Traditional Chinese Medicine (TCM), also known as Oriental Medicine (OM) or Traditional Oriental Medicine (TOM);
2. Naturopathic medicine, developed in the United States over 100 years ago using ancient natural healing techniques;
3. Homeopathic Medicine, founded by a German physician, Dr. Samuel Hahnemann, in the 1800s;
4. Chiropractic medicine, also developed in the United States in the late 1800s;
5. Massage therapy, which encompasses a variety of practices and techniques;
6. Herbal medicine, which draws upon the traditions of a variety of cultures.

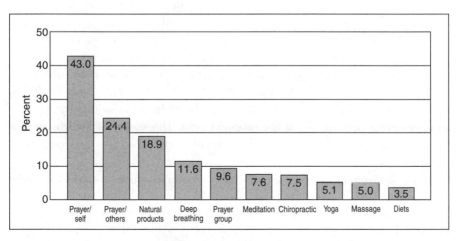

Figure 20.2   *10 Most Common CAM Therapies—2002*
Note: The therapies listed were measured in terms of the percentage of adults who used CAM.
Source: Barnes et al., 2002.

The 2004 survey of CAM use asked people to select from five reasons to describe why they used CAM. The survey found that most people use CAM along with conventional medicine rather than in place of conventional medicine. Results were as follows (people could select more than one reason):

- CAM would improve health when used in combination with conventional medical treatments: 55%
- CAM would be interesting to try: 50%
- Conventional medical treatments would not help: 28%
- A conventional medical professional suggested trying CAM: 26%
- Conventional medical treatments are too expensive: 13%

What Is the Difference Between Conventional Western Medicine and CAM?

Currently, the main difference between conventional medicine and alternative medicine is the approach toward the patient and the illness. Traditional medicine, as we know it, typically has tried to enhance or replace the body's natural healing system with a variety of physiological, physical, and chemical reactions that are measurable by modern science. Techniques to encourage healing aim at a specific problem or dysfunction after identifying it using a variety of laboratory testing techniques. Treatment often includes using a medication to control or destroy the offending organism or using surgery to eliminate or circumvent the problem. Alternative methods try to work with a body's natural healing system. Techniques that are used boost the body's own healing capabilities as well as restore a balance within the whole person as opposed to isolating a specific area. The focus includes finding the imbalance that allowed the problem to begin and correcting it, as opposed to just attacking the problem only. The vision of health care in the future includes the use of both of the approaches in the best combination possible.

Many alternative healing modalities incorporate more contact time per patient than the Western medical model. The practitioner often takes more time to learn about the person, conduct the assessment, and provide treatment. A natural health practitioner may ask questions that delve into other aspects of the patient's life beyond the physical symptoms. Overall, there is a greater emphasis on the importance of the patient/practitioner relationship. Natural health practitioners often look at a patient's diet, lifestyle, exercise habits, energy, emotions, dreams, and much more to get the complete picture of one's health. Often, a combination of factors affect one's health: nutritional deficiencies, poor digestion, food allergies, toxicity from environmental pollutants, or mental or emotional stress, overuse of antibiotics, etc. Treatments may last from one half hour to 50 minutes for a massage, or 1.5 to 2 hours for a first visit to a naturopath or acupuncturist, compared with 7 to 15 minutes for a conventional medicine office visit.

Career Opportunities in Complementary and Alternative Medicine

Some students of the healing arts find themselves in private practice or in practitioner groups after several months of schooling, while other natural healing careers require three to five years of preparation and training. Potential students, as well as practitioners already in the field, are seeing training programs (and continuing education) become more standardized; more schools are gaining accreditation and many modalities are experiencing increased regulations and licensing requirements in their fields.

Overall, practitioners trained in the natural healing arts are experiencing tremendous career opportunities in a climate of support, growth, collaboration, and integration. While some practitioners have a private practice, others work for clinics, wellness centers, and other companies. Some healing modalities, once considered fringe, are now "mainstream," and other ancient healing traditions are enjoying newfound interest, curiosity, and acceptance. Natural health is an area to watch as more healing modalities continue to emerge and become an integral part of how we heal ourselves (Natural Healers, 2006).

Traditional Chinese Medicine

Traditional Chinese medicine (TCM) is the current name for an ancient system of health care developed in China at least 2,000 years ago. TCM is a system of healing that dates back to 200 BC in written form. Korea, Japan, and Vietnam have all developed their own unique versions of traditional medicine based on practices originating in China. TCM is based on a concept of balanced *qi*, or vital energy, believed to flow throughout the body to regulate a person's spiritual, emotional, mental, and physical balance and influenced by the opposing forces of yin (negative energy) and yang (positive energy). Achieving health requires maintaining the body in a "balanced state" and disease is attributed to an internal imbalance of yin and yang. This imbalance leads to blockage in the flow of *qi* (or vital energy) and of blood along pathways known as meridians. TCM utilizes acupuncture, herbology, massage, and lifestyle changes through diet, exercise, and meditation to re-create a balance of *qi* within the body to promote healing and restore health (NCCAM, 2006).

Acupuncture ("AK-yoo-pungk-cher") is a method found within traditional Chinese medicine. Today, acupuncture describes a family of procedures involving stimulation of anatomical points on the body by a variety of techniques. American practices of acupuncture incorporate medical traditions from China, Japan, Korea, and other countries. The acupuncture technique that has been most studied scientifically involves penetrating the skin with thin, solid, metallic needles that are manipulated by the hands or by electrical stimulation (NCCAM, 2006).

A well-trained practitioner of acupuncture may choose to enter into private practice, join other healthcare practitioners at a wellness center, teach public education classes, and conduct workshops, seminars, or retreats. Many traditional medical doctors and chiropractors are adding acupuncture to their skills and using it within their established practice. The state requirements for practice are inconsistent as they are for most of CAM treatment modalities. For example, some states require applicants to graduate from an accredited college or fulfill an English language requirement. Some states require an apprenticeship while others do not. Individuals interested in this career path should check on their state regulations concerning education requirements before selecting a program for traditional Chinese medicine or acupuncture. In states that do not recognize acupuncturists as licensed medical practitioners, the acupuncturist may be required to work under the supervision of another medical person such as a medical or osteopathic doctor. In a few states, the practice of acupuncture is restricted to medical doctors or their equivalent.

Many acupuncture schools do not require candidates to have an undergraduate degree. However, all American College of Acupuncture and Oriental Medicine accredited schools require at least two years of undergraduate study, such as community college, prior to entry. Many programs prefer applicants to have a bachelor's degree. Most acupuncture programs last three years. Several medical schools now include acupuncture courses. There are currently over 22,671 licensed acupuncture practitioners in the United States. Forty-one states and the District of Columbia either license, certify, or register practitioners.

Professional Organizations for Traditional Chinese Medicine and Acupuncture

- *American Association of Oriental Medicine* – The American Association of Acupuncture and Oriental Medicine (AAAOM) was formed in 1981 to be the unifying force for American acupuncturists who are committed to ethical, high educational standards, and a well-regulated profession to ensure the safety of the public (http://www.aaom.org/).
- *American Academy of Medical Acupuncture and Medical Acupuncture Research Foundation* – AAMA/MARF, with a membership of licensed acupuncturists, integrates traditional and modern acupuncture with Western medical practice creating a comprehensive approach to health care. Research projects, training, and referrals are promoted (http://www.medicalacupuncture.org/).
- *National Certification Commission for Acupuncture and Oriental Medicine* – The NCCAOM is a nonprofit organization established by the profession to promote nationally recognized standards of competence and safety in acupuncture and Oriental medicine, in the United States (http://www.nccaom.org/).

Naturopathic Medicine

Naturopathy or naturopathic ("nay-chur-o-PATH-ic") medicine, is an alternative system of healing that views disease as the result of changes in the processes by which the body naturally heals itself. The basic theoretical principle and treatment modalities relate to the healing traditions from a variety of cultures. The term "naturopathy" literally translates as "nature disease." Today naturopathy, or naturopathic medicine, is practiced throughout Europe, Australia, New Zealand, Canada, and the United States. It is thought to have originated in Europe, although some resources credit development in the United States 100 years ago (Morton & Morton, 1997). Naturopathic medicine believes that there is a healing power in the body that establishes, maintains, and restores health. Practitioners work with the patient to encourage this power using modalities such as herbal medicine, nutritional therapy, traditional Chinese medicine, acupuncture, homeopathy, hydrotherapy, counseling, behavioral and lifestyle modifications, and minor surgery (NCCAM, 2006).

As primary healthcare practitioners, the majority of naturopathic doctors (NDs) practice privately. Some work alone, while others share their practice with complementary and conventional practitioners. Additional opportunities exist in teaching, research and development, marketing, public education, and consulting for industry and government. Licensed naturopathic doctors work as primary care physicians. Like most physicians, the majority of their day is spent seeing patients in a medical office. A typical patient visit lasts for 30 minutes (a first visit may run between 60 and 90 minutes depending on the complexity of the case). A patient visit usually includes diagnosis, discussion of possible treatments, counseling about lifestyle or nutrition, prescription of natural remedies, or referral to other medical specialists if necessary. When appropriate, the ND may also perform treatments in their office, such as hydrotherapy.

The average income of naturopathic doctors tends to fall in the low to mid-range of family practice doctors, according to a survey done by the AANP. Naturopathic education is structured and detailed. Naturopathic medical school itself is a four-year, full-time program in which the first two years resemble the basic science and pathology training that takes place in medical schools. Years three and four, however, are considerably different, for this is when naturopathic students learn various natural therapies, of which homeopathy is one of the most popular. Approximately 1,000 hours of clinical training are required. Currently, eleven states license naturopathic doctors as primary care physicians, and several other states are considering granting a medical license for naturopathic doctors. Upon graduation, students take the Naturopathic Physicians Licensing Exams (NPLEX). The NPLEX serves the same purpose as any medical board exam, testing the student's proficiency in the skills and knowledge necessary for a physician.

Similar pre-med requirements to get into medical school are required to get into naturopathic school. Schools require that the undergraduate degree include a minimum of 20 semester credits of standard pre-medical classes such as chemistry, biology, botany, and anatomy/physiology. Other than that, they encourage students to come from a well-rounded academic background.

Professional Organizations for Naturopathic Physicians

- *American Association of Naturopath Physicians* – Founded in 1985, the American Association of Naturopathic Physicians (AANP) is the national professional society representing naturopathic physicians who are licensed or eligible for licensing as primary care providers. This association's Web site offers resources and information regarding disease prevention and health restoration, as well as curricula for naturopathic medical schools (http://www.naturopathic.org).

- *American Holistic Medical Association* – Founded in 1978 to unite licensed physicians who practice holistic medicine, the mission of AHMA is to support practitioners in their evolving personal and professional development as healers and to educate physicians about holistic medicine (http://www.holisticmedicine.org).
- *Association of Accredited Naturopathic Medical Colleges* – The Association of Accredited Naturopathic Medical Colleges (AANMC) was established in February 2001 to propel and foster the naturopathic medical profession by actively supporting the academic efforts of accredited and recognized schools of naturopathic medicine (http://www.aanmc.org).

Homeopathic Medicine

Homeopathy or homeopathic ("home-ee-oh-PATH-ic") medicine is a system of medicine that is based on the Law of Similars. The term homeopathy comes from the Greek words *homeo*, meaning similar, and *pathos*, meaning suffering or disease. Homeopathy seeks to stimulate the body's defense mechanisms and processes to prevent or treat illness. Treatment involves giving very small doses of substances called remedies that, according to homeopathy, would produce the same or similar symptoms of illness in healthy people if given in larger doses. Treatment in homeopathy is individualized (tailored to each person). Homeopathic practitioners select remedies according to a total picture of the patient, including symptoms, lifestyle, emotional and mental states, and other factors. This approach is utilized worldwide, particularly in Europe, Latin America, and Asia, where homeopathy is considered more mainstream than alternative medicine. Because of their long use in the United States, the US Congress passed a law in 1938 declaring that homeopathic remedies are to be regulated by the FDA in the same manner as nonprescription, over-the-counter (OTC) drugs, which means that they can be purchased without a physician's prescription. Today, although conventional prescription drugs and new OTC drugs must undergo thorough testing and review by the FDA for safety and effectiveness before they can be sold, this requirement does not apply to homeopathic remedies. Remedies are required to meet certain legal standards for strength, quality, purity, and packaging. In 1988, the FDA required that all homeopathic remedies list the indications for their use (that is, the medical problems to be treated) on the label. The FDA also requires the label to list ingredients, dilutions, and instructions for safe use.

Rarely does one have a practice using only homeopathic remedies. There are a variety of other professionals who use remedies within their practice. Some use it as a primary modality and others use it sporadically. In the United States, licensed professionals who are likely to prescribe homeopathic remedies include naturopathic physicians, chiropractic doctors, acupuncturists, physician assistants, nurse practitioners, nurses, and dentists.

Commonly, training programs in homeopathy are three- or four-year programs, usually consisting of extended weekend (three- or four-day) courses that meet every month or every other month. Currently there are three states that license homeopaths who are also physicians: Arizona, Connecticut, and Nevada. California, Rhode Island, and Minnesota have new Health Freedom laws that allow unlicensed practitioners to practice homeopathy. Homeopathy is not regulated in any state so anybody can use it in the legitimate course of his or her business. However, using the term "homeopathic doctor" implies that individual is practicing medicine; such practitioners then fall under the laws governing the practice of medicine in that state. In all states, you cannot practice medicine without a license. You can "counsel" people on their health and suggest homeopathic remedies as long as you do not state or even imply that you can diagnose or treat illness.

Prerequisites vary by homeopathy school. Some courses are only for medical practitioners. These professional seminars require students to have a medical degree/license or to be enrolled in a recognized college. Other courses are open to any interested student and have no formal prerequisites. In the United States, the Council on Homeopathic Education reviews educational programs. This organization is a private nonprofit group.

Professional Organizations

- *The National Center for Homeopathy* – Provides research synopses, membership information, introductions to homeopathy/media kit, how to find a homeopath, and more resources (http://www.homeopathic.org/).
- *North American Society of Homeopaths* – An organization of professional practitioners in North America dedicated to developing and maintaining high standards of homeopathic practice (http://www.homeopathy.org/).
- *The American Association of Homeopathic Pharmacists* – An alliance of homeopathic manufacturers, pharmacists, and other qualified parties, promoting excellence in the practice of homeopathic pharmacy, manufacturing, and distribution (http://www.homeopathyresource.org/).

Chiropractic Medicine

Chiropractic ("kie-roh-PRAC-tic") is a manipulative, body-based form of alternative care. The word "chiropractic" combines the Greek words *cheir* (hand) and *praxis* (action) and means "done by hand." Chiropractic is a form of spinal manipulation that is one of the oldest healing practices. Hippocrates in ancient Greece described spinal manipulation. Daniel David Palmer founded this system in 1895 in Davenport, Iowa. According to chiropractic theory, the health of the body is dependent upon the balance of the autonomic and peripheral nervous systems that relate to the spinal column. The basic concepts of chiropractic can be described as follows:

- The body has a powerful self-healing ability.
- The body's structure (primarily that of the spine) and its function are closely related, and this relationship affects health.
- Chiropractic therapy is concerned with the goals of normalizing this relationship between structure and function and assisting the body as it heals.

Chiropractors, also known as *doctors of chiropractic* or *chiropractic physicians*, diagnose and treat patients whose health problems are associated with the body's muscular, nervous, and skeletal systems, especially the spine. The overall approach is holistic, taking into consideration exercise, diet, and sleeping habits. Chiropractors use manipulative therapy for spinal adjustments as a primary treatment tool. Treatment protocol may include water, light, massage, ultrasound, electric, and heat therapy as well. Braces, tape, and supports as part of therapy may accompany recommendations for changes in lifestyle related to stress, diet, and exercise. Chiropractic treatments alleviate musculoskeletal conditions—problems with the muscles, joints, bones, and connective tissue such as cartilage, ligaments, and tendons. Chiropractic treatments have been reimbursed by health insurance and some hospitals allow chiropractors practice privileges. Chiropractic treatment is one of the more utilized of the CAM treatments by Americans. In 1997, it was estimated that Americans made nearly 192 million visits a year to chiropractors. Over 88 million of those visits were to treat back or neck pain. Conditions commonly treated by chiropractors include back pain, neck pain, headaches, sports injuries, and repetitive strains. Patients also seek treatment of pain associated with other conditions, such as arthritis.

All states and the District of Columbia regulate the practice of chiropractic and grant licenses to chiropractors who meet educational and examination requirements established by the state. Chiropractors can practice only in states where they are licensed. Some states have agreements permitting chiropractors licensed in one state to obtain a license in another without further examination, provided their educational, examination, and practice credentials meet state specifications. Most state boards require at least two years of undergraduate education; an increasing number are requiring a four-year bachelor's degree. All boards require the completion of a four-year program at an accredited chiropractic college leading to the Doctor of Chiropractic degree.

Job prospects are expected to be good for persons who enter the practice of chiropractic medicine. Employment of chiropractors is expected to grow faster than the average for all occupations through the year 2012 as consumer demand for alternative health care grows. Approximately 70% of active chiropractors have a private practice. The remaining chiropractors work in a group medical practice or work for other chiropractors. A small number teach, conduct research at chiropractic institutions, or work in hospitals and clinics. Chiropractors emphasize the importance of healthy lifestyles and do not prescribe drugs or perform surgery. As a result, chiropractic care is appealing to many health-conscious Americans. Chiropractic treatment of back, neck, extremities, and other joint damage has become more accepted as a result of recent research and changing attitudes about alternative health-care practices. Some insurance plans cover chiropractic services, although the extent of such coverage varies among plans. Median annual earnings of salaried chiropractors were $65,330 in 2002. The middle 50% earned between $44,140 and $102,400 a year. Self-employed chiropractors usually earn more than salaried chiropractors do. According to the American Chiropractic Association, in 2000, the average income for all chiropractors, including the self-employed, was about $81,500 after expenses.

Professional Organizations for Chiropractic Physicians

- *American Chiropractic Association* – The ACA is a professional organization representing Doctors of Chiropractic. Its mission is to preserve, protect, improve, and promote the chiropractic profession and the services of Doctors of Chiropractic for the benefit of patients they serve. The purpose of the ACA is to provide leadership in health care and a positive vision for the chiropractic profession and its natural approach to health and wellness (http://www.amerchiro.org/).
- *The National Association for Chiropractic Medicine* (NACM) – NACM is a consumer advocacy association of chiropractors who confine their scope of practice so as to fall within specified scientific parameters and seek to make legitimate the utilization of professional manipulative pro-

cedures in mainstream healthcare delivery. The NACM offers consumer assistance in finding member practitioners (http://www.chiromed.org/).

- *The Association of Chiropractic Colleges* – This organization provides worldwide leadership in chiropractic education, research, and service. The Association includes and represents all CCE accredited colleges and programs that serve its institutions and their students, the profession and its patients, and the public by advancing chiropractic education, research, and service (http://www.chirocolleges.org/).

Massage Therapy

Massage therapy is the manipulation of the soft tissues of the body including muscles, connective tissue, tendons, ligaments, and joints. Manipulation includes rubbing, stroking, kneading, or tapping with the hand or an instrument for therapeutic purposes. It is considered an alternative health option to help alleviate the soft tissue discomfort associated with everyday and occupational stresses, muscular overuse, and many chronic pain syndromes. It can also greatly reduce painful muscular patterning following overuse or trauma to musculature. There are a variety of traditions or styles in massage therapy. Most varieties can be broken down into the following broad categories:

- Traditional European Massage
- Contemporary Western Massage
- Structural/Functional/Movement Integration
- Oriental Methods/Energetic Methods (Non-oriental)

Traditional European massage includes methods based on conventional Western concepts of anatomy and physiology and soft tissue manipulation. There are five basic kinds of soft tissue manipulation techniques: effleurage (long flowing or gliding strokes, usually toward the heart, tracing the outer contours of the body), petrissage (strokes that lift, roll, or knead the tissue), friction (circular strokes), vibration, and tapotement (percussion or tapping).

Contemporary Western massage includes methods based primarily on modern Western concepts of human function, anatomy, and physiology, using a wide variety of manipulative techniques. These may include broad applications for personal growth, emotional release, and balance of mind-body-spirit in addition to traditional applications. These approaches go beyond the original framework or intention of Swedish massage. They include Esalen or Swedish/Esalen, neuromuscular massage, deep tissue massage, sports massage, and manual lymph drainage. Most of these are American techniques developed from the late 1960s onward.

Structural/Functional/Movement Integration approaches organize and integrate the body in relationship to gravity through manipulating the soft tissues, and/or through correcting inappropriate patterns of movement. These methods bring about balanced use of the body structure, movement, and the nervous system. They create greater integration and more ease of movement. The most common approaches include Rolfing, Hellerwork, the Rosen Method, the Trager approach, the Feldenkrais Method, the Alexander Technique, and Ortho-Bionomy.

Oriental methods are based on the principles of Chinese medicine and the flow of energy or *qi* through the meridians with the ultimate goal being restoration of harmony or balance in the flow of *qi*. Acupuncture meridians determine points for applying the massage techniques. Herbs and acupuncture may accompany these massage techniques. Application of strong or light pressure by finger or thumb tips to predetermined points is characteristic of oriental massage, rather than by the sweeping broad strokes of Western style massage. There are over a dozen varieties of oriental massage and bodywork therapy, but the most common forms in this country are acupressure, shiatsu, and Jin Shin Jyutsu.

The oriental massage methods are energetic methods in that they are working with energy according to principles of Chinese medicine. There are other energetic methods that are not based on Chinese principles. The most prominent of these are Therapeutic Touch, polarity therapy, and Reiki.

According to the American Massage Therapy Association (www.amta massage.org), some practitioners work for other healthcare professionals such as chiropractors and physical therapists, and others work in physical fitness facilities, such as health clubs, day spas, resorts, hair salons, and cruise ships, while still others practice in hospitals. Other massage therapists work for themselves in a private full-time or part-time business. Massage therapy can be an excellent part-time career. The pay is good and the work is enjoyable, as well as flexible, depending on how therapists schedule clients. Salaries for massage therapists fall within wide ranges, depending on the facility and number of hours worked.

In 2004, 33 states and the District of Columbia regulated the practice of massage. In addition to state regulation of massage, cities, towns, and counties may also have their own laws regulating the practice of massage (BLS, 2006). There is a national certification exam (NCE) available which is a standardized entry-level test for massage practitioners. Some states will require practitioners to graduate from an accredited massage therapy program as well as pass the NCE. Typically, the only prerequisite for beginning massage school is simply to have a high school diploma.

Professional Organizations

- *The American Massage Therapy Association* (AMTA) – Represents massage therapists and works to establish massage therapy as integral to the maintenance of good health and complementary to other therapeutic processes; to advance the profession through ethics and standards, certification, school accreditation, continuing education, professional publications, legislative efforts, public education, and by fostering the development of members. The American Massage Therapy Association requires that its professional members graduate from a minimum 500 in-class-hour massage therapy training program, or pass a national certification exam, or possess a current AMTA-accepted license to practice. Members are expected to earn continuing education credits and uphold the AMTA Code of Ethics (http://www.amtamassage.org/).
- *Associated Bodywork and Massage Professionals* – A professional association representing massage education, bodywork, somatics practitioners, and estheticians (http://www.abmp.com/home/index.html).
- *The International Massage Therapy Association* – Professional association for the empowerment of massage therapists through tools, support, and knowledge needed to enhance effectiveness and business success (http://www.internationalmassage.com/).
- *National Certification Board for Therapeutic Massage and Bodywork* (NCBTMB) – An organization dedicated to fostering high standards of ethical and professional practice in the delivery of services through a recognized credible credentialing program that assures the competency of practitioners of therapeutic massage and bodywork (http://www.ncbtmb.com/).

Herbal Medicine

Herbal medicine is the art or practice of using herbs and herbal remedies to maintain health and to prevent, alleviate, or cure disease—called also *herbalism*. It has been practiced by a variety of cultures since the beginning of time. Europe and other areas of the world conduct research, regulate, and utilize this area of healing far more than the United States at this time. Currently, the Federal Food and Drug Administration does not regulate the use of herbal remedies. It is important to have knowledgeable and qualified herbalists to assist in the use of herbs for effective use and protection of the consumer. There is no national or state system of licensure or certification for herbalists. Professional groups may grant certification to members that have reached a certain level of training as an herbalist. Some herbalists concentrate on growing or wildcrafting (picking) herbs. Others manufacture herbal products. Still others teach or counsel people about the use of herbs as medicine.

One branch of anthropology, called ethnobotany, studies the use of plants in other cultures, particularly their use as medicine. Ethnobotanists, who receive their training through the standard university system, have classified a number of medicinal herbs. Their work helps preserve the traditional folk medicine of indigenous people around the world. The American Botanical Council Web site lists some current ethnobotanical expeditions.

Legally, in the United States, the practice of medicine is restricted to those professionals who have a license. Practice is generally defined as both diagnosis and prescription, with a focus on the treatment of disease (the laws vary from state to state). There are no restrictions, however, on teaching people how to take better care of their health. Most herbalists define themselves as teachers, healers, or counselors rather than as medical practitioners. Several complementary medical professions are licensed and do use herbal medicine as part of their practice. Herbalists who want to practice medicine generally choose to do so under the license of another profession such as acupuncturist or naturopathic doctor.

Careers in herbalism include working within the herb industry as an herb buyer, formulator, researcher, consultant, retailer, grower, medicine maker, writer/journalist, or educator. Some herbalists have found positions working in practices with physicians or other practitioners. While there are opportunities for working in an integrative setting, this is not a solid career path because it is still illegal to practice herbal "medicine" as a non-licensed practitioner.

Based on a review of salaries published by the American Herbalists Guild, herbalists' annual incomes range from $20,000 to $120,000. A large number of working herbalists were interviewed and asked how much money they make. The most common answer was "as much as you want." Some choose to live very Spartan lives, "off the grid," and away from civilization. Others make comfortable wages as counselors, teachers, manufacturers, or writers.

Herbalists generally fall under the state regulations governing a small business owner rather than under the laws concerned with the practice of medicine. If an herbalist is growing herbs for other people's use, or manufacturing a product from raw herbs, regulations pertaining to the safe production of foods or food supplements may apply. Some states do restrict the sale of certain herbs considered potentially harmful, such as ephedra (ma huang). Many herbalists started their training by taking correspondence courses and then going onto more "one-on-one" training with other professionals. There are a wide variety of correspondence courses offered, and very few have any eligibility requirements. Programs exist for most styles and disciplines of herbal medicine and range from introductory to advanced, earth-based to scientific, some offering a blend of approaches. There are many well-established programs in traditional Chinese medicine and a wide variety of programs in Western botanical medicine. However, currently there is no formal system of accreditation for herbal schools. Generally, when picking a school, the student wants to look at the experience of the teacher. Both the American Herbalists Guild and the American Botanical Council provide information on schools.

Professional Organizations

- *The American Botanical Council* – Established in 1988, the American Botanical Council (ABC) is the leading independent, nonprofit, international member-based organization providing education using science-based and traditional information to promote the responsible use of herbal medicine. ABC serves the public, researchers, educators, healthcare professionals, industry, and media, and has been a highly respected source and an innovative force for many years (http://www.herbalgram.org/).

- *American Herbalist Guild* – Professional organization for herbalists, offering membership and certifications to trained herbalists. The American Herbalists Guild was founded in 1989 as a nonprofit, educational organization to represent the goals and voices of herbalists. It is the only peer-review organization in the United States for professional herbalists specializing in the medicinal use of plants. AHG membership consists of professionals, general members (including students), and benefactors (http://www.americanherbalistsguild.com/).

SUMMARY

Complementary and alternative therapies are now in demand by health consumers throughout the developed world. They have had an impact on every facet of the healthcare system and all specialties of medicine. In 2002, the National Health Interview Survey (NHIS) included questions on CAM therapies commonly used in the United States. Women and those with higher education levels report greater use of CAM therapies, with 36 percent of US adults aged 18 years and over using some form of complementary and alternative medicine (NCCAM, 2004a). Within that survey, 55% of adults said they were most likely to use CAM because they believed that it would help them when combined with conventional treatments, and 26% used it because a conventional medical professional suggested they try it. Further research by NCCAM and others will provide the scientific validity to confirm or debunk claims of a wide array of complementary and alternative medical therapies. Findings such as these indicate CAM is perhaps becoming more complementary than alternative to traditional medicine.

DISCUSSION QUESTIONS

1. What is the definition of complementary and integrative health care?
2. What types or categories of care are considered CAM?
3. What are the differences between traditional Western medicine and CAM?
4. What CAM careers require education similar to traditional medical schools?
5. What CAM career schools have prerequisites similar to traditional medical schools?
6. What CAM treatments are the most popular in the United States?
7. What CAM treatments are the least accepted in the United States?
8. Which CAM treatments have more credibility in Europe than they do in the United States?
9. What is the current status of legislation concerning the practice of CAM in the United States?
10. What CAM modalities have you used? Why?
11. What CAM modalities would you be least likely to use? Why?
12. Do you think career opportunities in CAM in the United States will improve? Explain.

REFERENCES

Astin, J. (1998, May 20). Why patients use alternative medicine: Results of a national study. *Journal of the American Medical Association, 279*(19), 1548–1553.

Barnes P. M., Powell-Griner, E., McFann, K., & Nahin, R. L. (2004). Complementary and alternative medicine use among adults: United States, 2002. *CDC Advance Data Report, 343*. Retrieved August 29, 2005, from nccam.nih.gov/news/report.pdf.

Credit, L. P. & Hartunian, S. G. (1998). *Your guide to complementary medicine.* New York: Avery Publishing Group.

Eisenburg, D. M., Davis, R. B., Ettner, S. L., Appel, S., Wilkey, S., Van Rompay, M., et al. (1998, November 11). Trends in alternative medicine use in the U.S. *Journal of the American Medical Association, 280*(18), 1569–1575.

Michael, A. M. & Morton, M. (1997). Excerpted from *Five steps to selecting the best alternative medicine.* Novato, CA: New World Library.

National Center for Complementary and Alternative Medicine, National Institutes of Health (NCCAM). (2004, May 27). (2004a). More than one-third of US adults use complementary and alternative medicine, according to new government survey. Retrieved February 12, 2006, from http://nccam.nih.gov/news/2004/052704.htm.

National Center for Complementary and Alternative Medicine, National Institutes of Health (NCCAM). (2004, September). (2004b). The use of complementary and alternative medicine in the United States. Retrieved April 1, 2006 from http://nccam.nih.gov/news/camsurvey_fs1.htm.

National Center for Complementary and Alternative Medicine, National Institutes of Health (NCCAM). (2006). Factsheets: CAM. Retrieved November 22, 2006 from http://nccam.nih.gov.

National Center for Homeopathy Web site. (2002). What is homeopathy? Retrieved April 1, 2006 from http://www.homeopathic.org/whatis.htm.

Natural Healers Web site, NaturalVillage.com, Inc. (2006). Careers in natural healing. Retrieved November 22, 2006 from http://www.naturalhealers.com/qa/careers.html.

Pelletier, K. R. (2000). *The best alternative medicine*. New York: Simon & Schuster.

Sale, D. M. (2005). Overview of legislative development concerning alternative health care in the United States. A research project of the Fetzer Institute. Retrieved November 28, 2006, from http://www.healthy.net/public/legal-lg/regulations/fetzer.htm.

United States Bureau of Labor Statistics (BLM). (2006). US Department of Labor Statistics, Occupational Outlook Handbook, 2006–07 Edition, Massage Therapists. On the Internet at http://www.bls.gov/oco/ocos295.htm. Visited November 29, 2006.

Chapter 21

Creative Arts Therapies

Erika Leeuwenburgh
Ellen Goldring
Ann Nancy Fogel
Theresa M. Lynch
John Mondanaro
Stephanie Omens
Mizuho Kanazawa

OBJECTIVES

After studying this chapter, the student should be able to

1. Explain the role of creative arts therapies in the healthcare system.
2. Explain the historical development process of creative arts therapies.
3. Describe the educational preparation and certification required for creative arts therapists.
4. Explain the role of the child-life specialist in the care of children and their families.
5. Identify resources for additional information on the role of creative arts therapies and child life specialists.

INTRODUCTION

Art, in its broadest sense, is the expression of creativity or imagination, or both. Whether through song, dance, drawing, photography, poetry, or any other form of artistic expression, the arts are the mechanisms by which individuals express their thoughts, feelings, and emotions. Works of art have the ability to communicate ideas, create a sense of beauty or pleasure, and generate strong emotions. Creative arts are a collection of disciplines whose principal purpose is the output of material that reflects a message, mood, and symbolism for the viewer to interpret. Creative arts therapists work with individuals of all ages to help them heal, cope with, and understand a wide array of physical and mental health conditions.

What Is Creative Arts Therapy?

Therapy encompasses a variety of treatments especially of bodily, mental, or behavioral disorders. "Therapy," derived from the Greek word "therapeia," means "to serve or help medically." The objective of therapy is to help individuals with physical, mental, or social handicaps to regain their capacity for self-help and independence. This chapter illustrates how *creative arts therapies* in conjunction with medical and other allied health professionals, aid patients across the lifespan in a variety of health concerns.

Art, music, drama, and dance/movement therapists incorporate creative expression of feelings through a myriad of materials within a therapeutic relationship in order to address physical, psychological, cognitive, emotional, and social needs of children and adolescents. Creative arts therapies provide a dynamic, action-oriented treatment utilizing symbolic expression and metaphor that embrace a wealth of meaning. Carefully selected materials and directives purposefully elicit self-expression and meet the needs of the patient. Therapists focus on the patients' creative process and product—both of which are equally significant as the patient communicates through both means. In addition, the creative process has inherent qualities that influence the autonomic system of the body, which can decrease stress and stimulate the mind. Healing qualities in the act of playing music, writing lyrics, dancing, painting, reenacting an event, and other creative arts experiences can provide a meditative, peaceful, and life-affirming experience that positively affects the body, mind, and spirit, thus promoting an overall sense of well-being.

Creative arts therapies include art therapy, dance/movement therapy, drama therapy, music therapy, poetry therapy, and psychodrama. These therapies use arts modalities and creative processes during intentional intervention in therapeutic, rehabilitative, community, or educational settings to foster health, communication, and expression; promote the integration of physical, emotional, cognitive, and social functioning; enhance self-awareness; and facilitate change. According to the National Coalition of Creative Arts Therapies Associations (NCCATA), participation in all the creative arts therapies provides people with special needs ways to express themselves that may not be possible through more traditional therapies. Individuals with artistic interests who are drawn to the helping professions or the health care field might consider some of these professional options.

Art Therapy

*Art is the desire of a man to express himself, to record
the reactions of his personality to the world he lives in.*
Amy Lowell (1874–1925)

Art therapy is a human service profession utilizing art media, images, and the creative art process. It focuses on patient/client responses to the created art productions, as they reflect an individual's development, abilities, personality, interests, concerns, and conflicts. Art therapy practice is based on knowledge of human developmental and psychological theories. It encompasses the full spectrum of current models of assessment and treatment, including educational, psychodynamic, cognitive, transpersonal, and other therapeutic means of reconciling emotional conflicts, fostering self-awareness, developing social skills, managing behavior, solving problems, reducing anxiety, aiding reality orientation, and increasing self-esteem.

Art therapy is an effective treatment for the developmentally, medically, educationally, socially, or psychologically impaired. Art therapists also work with individuals dealing with psychological issues such as bereavement, divorce, or general life changes. Art therapists may practice in mental health, rehabilitation, medical, educational, and forensic institutions with populations of all ages, races, and ethnic backgrounds, working in individual, couples, family, and group therapy formats.

The American Art Therapy Association, Inc. (AATA) regulates educational, professional, and ethical standards for art therapists. The Art Therapy Credentials Board, Inc. (ATCB), an independent organization, grants the postgraduate credential of Registered Art Therapist (ATR) after reviewing documentation of completion of graduate education and postgraduate supervised experience. The ATR who successfully completes the written examination administered by the ATCB is qualified as Board Certified (ATR-BC), a credential requiring maintenance through continuing education credits (ATCB, 2005).

Music Therapy

*After silence, that which comes nearest to
expressing the inexpressible is music.*
Aldous Huxley (1894–1963), *Music at Night,* 1931

Music Therapy is an established healthcare profession that uses music to address physical, emotional, cognitive, and social needs of individuals of all ages. Music therapy improves the quality of life for well individuals, and meets the needs of children and adults with disabilities or illnesses. Music therapists use both instrumental and vocal music strategies to facilitate changes that are non-musical in nature. After assessment of the strengths and needs of each client, qualified music therapists provide indicated treatment and participate as members of the interdisciplinary team to support a vast continuum of outcomes. Individuals of all ages can benefit from music therapy.

A music therapist might work in psychiatric hospitals, rehabilitative facilities, medical hospitals, outpatient clinics, day care treatment centers, agencies serving developmentally disabled persons, community mental health centers, drug and alcohol programs, senior centers, nursing homes, hospice programs, correctional facilities, halfway houses, schools, or in private practice. Music therapy is beneficial with children, adolescents, adults, and the elderly with mental health needs, developmental and learning disabilities, Alzheimer's disease and other aging related conditions, substance abuse problems, brain injuries, physical disabilities, and acute and chronic pain, including mothers in labor.

The 20th century discipline of music therapy began after World War I and World War II when community musicians of all types, both amateur and professional, went to Veterans hospitals around the country to play for the thousands of veterans suffering both physical and emotional trauma from the wars. The patients' notable physical and emotional responses to music led the doctors and nurses to request the hiring of musicians by the hospitals. It was soon evident that the hospital musicians needed some prior training before working with patients and so the demand grew for a college curriculum. The first music therapy degree program in the world was founded at Michigan State University in 1944 (AMTA, 2005a).

Research in music therapy supports the effectiveness of interventions in many areas such as overall physical rehabilitation and facilitating movement, increasing motivation to become engaged in treatment, providing emotional support for clients and their families, and creating an outlet for expression of feelings. Music therapists work in many different settings including general hospitals, schools, mental health agencies, rehabilitation centers, nursing homes, forensic settings, and private practice. Music therapists design interventions to

- promote wellness
- manage stress
- alleviate pain
- express feelings
- enhance memory
- improve communication
- promote physical rehabilitation.

Qualified music therapists provide indicated treatments including creating, singing, moving to, and/or listening to music. Musical involvement in the therapeutic context strengthens clients' abilities and can transfer to other areas of their lives. Music therapy also provides avenues for communication that can be helpful to those who find it difficult to express themselves in words. Research in music therapy supports its effectiveness in many areas such as overall physical rehabilitation and facilitating movement, increasing people's motivation to become engaged in their treatment, providing emotional support for clients and their families, and providing an outlet for expression of feelings. Music therapy functions as a multidimensional intervention across the spectrum of diagnoses within a medical setting. Sessions can occur with individual patients, patients and their friends or family members, and/or support groups of all ages. Such sessions can provide impetus for understanding and communicating the impact of hospitalization, a new diagnosis, and living with a life-threatening or chronic illness.

Music therapists actively work within multidisciplinary teams which can include doctors, nurses, physical therapists, social workers, and other creative arts team members. This therapy offers patients and their family members qualities that the other creative arts cannot—soothing music that can relax tensions in the environment or specific cultural music related to the patient's family of origin. Patients on life support machines, or near death, can be joined through song and sound. When patients are non-verbal and unable to interact, the therapist may engage family members by asking them to identify music for the patient that the therapist can play on a guitar. Improvisational music played by the therapist can reflect the mood and connect in a non-verbal fashion. This profound intervention includes everyone in the room from staff, patient, and family members to visitors, transforming the environment from a sterile, sad, and foreign one to a soothing and soulful space.

One example of the benefit of music therapy is in the care and support of infants and mothers of the Neonatal Intensive Care and General Pediatric Units (Leeuwenburgh, 2000; Abromeit, 2003). The music therapist provides comfort, positively impacts the neonates' sound environment, and enriches parent-child bonding through the healing and soothing qualities of the lullaby's rhythm, lyrical tone, and musical qualities. Parents can use their voices while working with a music therapist who is playing various melodic instruments. This can foster a profound sense of connection between parents and their infants whose bonding experiences are compromised within the NICU.

Professional members of American Music Therapy Association hold bachelor's degrees or higher in music therapy from accredited colleges or universities. The credential "MT-BC" (Music Therapist-Board Certified) is issued upon successful completion of (1) an AMTA-approved academic and clinical training program and (2) a written objective national examination (AMTA, 2005b).

Drama Therapy

Drama is life with the dull bits cut out.
Alfred Hitchcock (1899–1980)

Drama therapy is a health and human services profession that seeks to facilitate physical integration and personal growth for individuals, couples, families, and various other groups using theatrical and dramatic processes. Using role-play, theater games, mime, puppetry, and other improvisational techniques, drama therapists help the client to tell his or her story in order to:

- Solve a problem.
- Achieve a catharsis.
- Extend the depth and breadth of inner experience.
- Understand the meanings of images.
- Strengthen the ability to observe personal roles while increasing flexibility between roles.

Drama therapy benefits many client populations and is used in a variety of settings. These include psychiatric hospitals, mental health facilities, day treatment centers, nursing homes, centers for the physically/developmentally/learning disabled, substance abuse treatment programs, schools, businesses, and correctional facilities. Some populations served include children with learning and social difficulties, the developmentally delayed, psychiatric patients, the disabled, substance abusers, AIDS patients, and those with disorders associated with aging.

Registered Drama Therapists receive training in theater arts, psychology, and psychotherapy. Training includes improvisation, puppetry, role-playing, pantomime, mask work, and theatrical production. Training in psychology and psychotherapy includes theories of personality, group process, and supervised clinical experience with a broad range of populations. The Registered Drama Therapist (RDT) has a master's degree, and additional varying hours of drama/theater experience. The National Association for Drama Therapy (NADT), established in 1979 to uphold the ethical standards and professional competencies among drama therapists, monitors the criteria for training and registration of drama therapists. There are two ways of becoming a registered drama therapist (RDT): (1) completion of a master's degree from an NADT approved drama therapy program or (2) completion of criteria for alternative training (NCCATA, 2005a).

Dance/Movement Therapy

Dance is the hidden language of the soul.
Martha Graham (1893–1991)

Based on the assumption that body and mind are interrelated, the American Dance Therapy Association (ADTA, 2005) defines **dance/movement therapy** as "the psychotherapeutic use of movement as a process which furthers the emotional, cognitive, and physical integration of the individual." Dance/movement therapy effects changes in feelings, cognition, physical functioning, and behavior. Dance/movement therapy emerged as a distinct profession in the 1940s, through the pioneering efforts of Marian Chace. Psychiatrists in Washington, DC, found that their patients were deriving benefits from attending Chace's unique dance classes. As a result, Chace was asked to work on the back wards of St. Elizabeth's Hospital with patients who had been considered too disturbed to participate in regular group activities. A nonverbal group approach was needed and dance/movement therapy met that need.

Dance/movement therapy is an effective treatment for people with developmental, medical, social, physical, and psychological impairments. Dance/movement therapy is practiced in mental health rehabilitation, medical, educational, forensic, nursing homes, day care, and disease prevention settings, and in health promotion programs. Dance/movement therapy is used with people of all ages, races, and ethnic backgrounds in individual, couples, family, and group therapy formats. Today, in addition to those with severe emotional disorders, people of all ages and varying conditions receive dance/movement therapy. Examples of these are individuals with eating disorders, adult survivors of violence, sexually and physically abused children, dysfunctional families, the homeless, autistic children, the frail elderly, and substance abusers.

An evolving area of specialization involves using dance/movement therapy in disease prevention and health promotion programs and with those who have chronic medical conditions. Many innovative programs provide dance/movement therapy for people with cardiovascular disease, hypertension, chronic pain, or breast cancer. Research has been undertaken on the effects of dance/movement therapy in special settings (such as prisons and centers for the homeless) and with specific populations, including the learning disabled, frail elderly, emotionally disturbed, depressed and suicidal, mentally retarded, substance addicted, visually and hearing impaired, psychotic, and autistic. Those with physical problems (such as amputations, traumatic brain injury, stroke, and chronic pain) and with chronic illnesses (such as anorexia and bulimia, cancer, Alzheimer's disease, cystic fibrosis, heart disease, diabetes, asthma, AIDS, and arthritis) have also been studied.

The American Dance Therapy Association, formed in 1966, maintains a code of ethics and established standards for professional practice, education, and training. There are dance/movement therapists in 43 states and US territories and 21 countries. Entry into the profession of dance/movement therapy is at the master's level. The title "Dance Therapist Registered" (DTR) is granted to entry-level dance/movement therapists who have a master's degree that includes 700 hundred hours of supervised clinical internship. The advanced level of registry, "Academy of Dance Therapists" (ADTR), is awarded only after DTRs have completed 3,640 hours of supervised clinical work in an agency, institution, or special school, with additional supervision from an ADTR (ADTA, 2005).

Poetry Therapy/Bibliotherapy

One ought, every day at least, to hear a little song,
read a good poem, see a fine picture, and if it
were possible, to speak a few reasonable words.
Johann Wolfgang von Goethe (1749–1832)

Poetry therapy and **bibliotherapy** synonymously describe the intentional use of poetry and other forms of literature for healing and personal growth. The term "biblio" means books and, by extension, literature. Bibliotherapy is the use of literature to promote mental health. Developmental interactive bibliotherapy refers to the use of literature, discussion, and creative writing with children in schools and hospitals, adults in growth and support groups, and older persons in senior centers and nursing homes. In these community settings, bibliotherapy is used to not only foster growth and development, but also as a preventive tool in mental health. Clinical interactive bibliotherapy refers to the use of literature, discussion, and creative writing to promote healing and growth in psychiatric units, community mental health centers, and chemical dependency units. Poetry therapy began in the United States when Pennsylvania Hospital instituted creative writing as a treatment modality over 200 years ago. Today poetry therapy is widely practiced in a variety of diverse settings with various populations. Poetry therapy is a holistic approach that respects the various links of wellness, with its attentiveness to body, mind, and spirit. It may be a primary or an ancillary therapy. A trained poetry therapist actively engages people to identify issues and express feelings, and empowers clients to transform life issues using the language arts (NAPT, 2005d).

Bibliotherapy has a broad range of applications with people of all ages and is useful for health maintenance, as well as for its treatment of various illnesses and conditions. Examples of the populations served are veterans, substance abusers, adolescents, and the learning disabled, families with problems, prisoners in rehabilitation, the frail elderly, the physically challenged, and survivors of violence, abuse, and incest. The literature and case studies provide evidence that poetry therapy is an effective and powerful tool with many different populations.

Poetry therapy is an interactive process with three essential components: the literature, the trained facilitator, and the client(s). A trained biblio/poetry therapist selects a poem or other form of written or spoken media to serve as a catalyst and evoke feeling responses for discussion. The interactive process helps the individual to develop on emotional, cognitive, and social levels. The focus is on the person's reaction to the literature, never losing sight of the primary objective—the psychological health and well-being of the client. The poetry therapist creates a gentle, non-threatening atmosphere where people feel safe and are invited to share feelings openly and honestly. The facilitator chooses literature that will be effective therapeutically; this requires training, knowledge of literature, and clinical skills.

The National Association for Poetry Therapy (NAPT), incorporated in 1981, confers professional credentials to biblio/poetry therapists who have met its rigorous standards. The poetry therapist today is a professional who is well grounded in psychology and literature, as well as group dynamics. NAPT maintains a registry of biblio/poetry therapy practitioners in educational, medical, geriatric, therapeutic, and community settings (NAPT, 2005a). The only persons authorized to call themselves poetry therapists are those who have fulfilled the necessary training requirements and have been awarded (or who are eligible to be awarded) the designation of either Certified Poetry Therapist (CPT) or Registered Poetry Therapist (RPT) by the Federation for Biblio/Poetry Therapy (formerly NAPT) through its Certification Committee.

The CPT is trained to facilitate groups and work with individuals in developmental settings such as schools, libraries, recreational facilities, and similar growth and development oriented organizations. The CPT may also work in a mental health setting as an adjunct therapist in cooperation with a primary therapist. In clinical settings, the CPT works under the clinical supervision of an RPT or other qualified mental health professional.

The CPT brings a unique background to the healthcare setting, blending a love of literature and creative writing with an understanding of basic psychology and group dynamics. Although the CPT's training is geared to working in developmental settings with healthy populations, the CPT must be able to recognize the difference between "normalcy" and pathology, and must be able to determine when a distressed individual needs to be referred to another mental health professional. A bachelor's degree and appropriate knowledge of psychology and literature plus 440 hours of additional training with a mentor/supervisor are required for certification (NAPT 2005b).

The RPT has trained more extensively and in greater depth than the CPT and works with more difficult and troubled populations. Because the RPT has previously earned an advanced clinical degree in psychotherapy, counseling, psychiatry, or social work, the RPT is qualified to work with clients of all types in settings such as clinics, hospitals, prisons, and similar institutions, as well as with mentally healthy populations. RPTs also work with individuals having adjustment problems brought about by developmental or life crises or disabilities. A Master's Degree or higher in a clinical field, along with appropriate knowledge of psychology and literature, and up to 975 hours of additional training are required to be a registered poetry therapist (NAPT, 2005c).

Psychodrama

I made some mistakes in drama. I thought the drama was when the actors cried. But drama is when the audience cries.
Frank Capra, American film director (1897–1991)

Psychodrama seeks to use a person's creativity and spontaneity to reach his or her highest human potential. With its perspective on the social network in which an individual lives, it promotes mutual support and understanding. Psychodrama is a therapeutic discipline that uses action methods, sociometry, role training, and group dynamics to facilitate constructive change in the lives of participants. Psychodrama is effective in mental health programs, business, and education. Psychodramatists provide services to diverse groups—from children to the elderly, and from the chronically mentally ill to those seeking understanding and learning in their work settings. By closely approximating life situations in a structured environment, the participant is able to re-create and enact scenes in a way that allows both insight and an opportunity to practice new life skills. In psychodrama, the client (or protagonist) focuses on a specific situation to be enacted. Other members of the group act as auxiliaries, supporting the protagonist in his or her work, by taking the parts or roles of significant others in the scene. This encourages the group as a whole to partake in the therapeutic power of the drama. The trained director helps to re-create scenes that might otherwise not be possible. The psychodrama then becomes an opportunity to practice new and more appropriate behaviors, and evaluate their effectiveness within the supportive atmosphere of the group. Because the dimension of action is present, psychodrama is often empowering in a way that exceeds the more traditional verbal therapies (NCCATA, 2005b).

There are several additional branches of psychodrama. Sociometry is the study and measure of social choices within a group. Sociometry helps to bring to the surface patterns of acceptance or rejection and fosters increased group cohesion. This surfacing of the value systems and norms of a group allows for restructuring that will lower conflicts and foster synergistic relationships. Sociodrama is a form of psychodrama that addresses the group's perceptions on social issues. Rather then being the drama of a single protagonist, this process allows the group as a whole to safely explore various perceptions. Members might address problems such as teenage pregnancy or drug abuse, and together arrive at understanding and innovative responses to these difficult issues.

The American Society of Group Psychotherapy and Psychodrama was founded in April, 1942. The American Board of Examiners in Psychodrama, Sociometry, and Group Psychotherapy is a national organization that sets and promotes standards for this discipline. Requirements for certification include a master's degree from an accredited university in a field relevant to the applicant's areas of practice, a minimum of 780 training hours under a board certified trainer, and supervised experience. Passing both a written and on-site examination are part of these requirements. There are two levels of certification. A Certified Practitioner (CP) has been: a) professionally trained and supervised in psychodrama, sociometry, and group psychotherapy by a Board certified Trainer, Educator, Practitioner (TEP); b) has met established standards of the profession; and c) has successfully fulfilled the requirements of the Board of Examiners. A Trainer, Educator, Practitioner (TEP) is a Certified Practitioner who has: a) received a minimum of three years additional supervised training, education, and experience in the design and implementation of professional training programs; and b) has successfully fulfilled the requirements of the Board of Examiners.

Child Life and the Creative Arts Therapies

The remainder of this chapter will present and illustrate the field of Child Life and Creative Arts Therapies. The Child Life / Creative Arts Therapy Services clinicians of the Joseph M. Sanzari Children's Hospital in Hackensack, New Jersey, explain how Art, Music, Drama, and Dance/Movement Therapists improve health care experiences for children and their families. When children are ill or injured, it is essential to remember that the family also becomes the patient. Parents, siblings, and even grandparents may have fears, concerns, and worries about the child who is not well. The creative therapies highlighted in this chapter are also beneficial when working with other populations and in other healthcare settings.

Child Life and Creative Arts Therapy Services present a comprehensive psychosocial approach to treating pediatric patients and their siblings. The authors work in a New Jersey-based medical center's Child Life / Creative Arts therapy program, established in 1987, that incorporates both child life practices and creative arts in one service. The clinicians are child life specialists, art therapists, music therapists, drama therapists, and dance/movement therapists working within medical teams where children's and adolescents' minds, bodies, and spirits are equally cared for and treated. The clinicians' goals are to optimize children's growth and development while increasing their ability to cope with potentially stressful experiences, a traumatic event, a life-threatening illness, or the death of a loved one. The child life staff tries to meet these goals through evidence-based practices and interventions, which increase communication, understanding, self-expression, and self-esteem. The primary objective is to enable the patient and family to become active participants in the health and healing of the pediatric patient.

A *Child Life Specialist* is a specially trained professional who helps children and their families understand and manage challenging life events and stressful healthcare experiences. Child Life Specialists are skilled in providing developmental, educational, and therapeutic interventions for children and their families under stress. Child Life Specialists support growth and development while recognizing family strengths and individuality, and respecting different methods of coping (Child Life Council, 2005b).

Certified Child Life Specialists (CCLS) have earned a bachelor's or master's degree; their educational background includes human growth and development, education, psychology, and counseling. They are required to complete an internship program and a rigorous application and examination process. Child Life Specialists are certified through a program administered by the Child Life Council (CLC).

The Mission Statement of The Child Life Council

We as Child Life professionals strive to reduce the negative impact of traumatic life events and situations that affect the development, health, and well-being of infants, children, youth, and families. We embrace the value of play as a healing modality as we work to enhance the optimal growth and development of infants, children, and youth through assessment, intervention, prevention, advocacy, and education (Child Life Council, 2005a).

Child Life began in 1922 when Mott's Children's Hospital in Michigan and Babies and Children's Hospital of Columbia Presbyterian in New York established the first Early Childhood Play programs. They were among the first to recognize the importance of normalizing the hospital experience for children by offering play and educational services. They recognized a need for someone within the healthcare team to focus exclusively on the emotional, developmental, and educational aspects of hospitalized children. This would provide a bridge between psychiatry and nursing and offer a novel approach to childcare.

Child Life Programs blossomed throughout the United States and Canada and the Child Life Specialist became firmly established within the healthcare system. Medical play areas and educational programs including pre-admission tours, individual support groups for patients, parents, and their siblings, and preparation for procedures through play were defined. The Child Life Council (CLC), formed in 1982 to address the specific needs within the profession, created official guidelines and standards for the universal acceptance of the Child Life profession. Today's Child Life standard practice of care is recognized by the American Academy of Pediatrics. In 1998 the professional certification process was refined to incorporate a written exam following the previously accepted academic preparation of a minimum of a baccalaureate and mastery of successful practical experiences in a variety of healthcare settings supervised by a certified Child Life Specialist. Presently, the accepted level of practice for a Certified Child Life Specialist is to hold a master's-level degree in Child Life or a related field of study and be multi-licensed/certified accredited in counseling, human-services-related field such as social work, or one of the creative arts (Art, Music, Dance, Drama, Poetry). The Child Life Council has established an official "Child Life Week," celebrated the third week of every March worldwide. At last count, there were 2800 members of The Child Life Council working in over 460 accredited Child Life programs throughout the world.

Normalization of the Hospital Environment

The health care industry has come to recognize the needs of children in hospitals. The goal of creating a child-friendly environment is to create an atmosphere that reflects the needs of the patients, from both aesthetic and developmental standpoints. As opposed to the bland and under-stimulating décor of earlier times, the current trend allows children to heal in an attractive and positive atmosphere.

Only a few decades ago, the concept of a hospital playroom did not exist. Children admitted for treatment were separated from their caregivers (parents and family) and ordered to remain in their hospital beds. The changes that have taken place since those times are remarkable. Today, the walls of pediatric units are adorned with bright colors and murals. Child Life specialists are at the forefront of this effort, helping to decorate their respective units, decreasing the perceived harshness of the medical environment. Children visiting these areas become involved in making the hospital more comforting by creating and contributing their artwork. It is their way of leaving an imprint on the healthcare world for doctors, clinicians, and other patients to see.

Playrooms create an inviting space for children to play with toys and engage in activities with siblings, parents, peers, and Child Life Specialists/Creative Arts Therapists. While "fun" is the focus, one cannot ignore the other benefits involved with having a dedicated space for play and artistic expression. Playrooms provide a safe, non-medical atmosphere that serves as a meeting ground for patients and their family members. Children have the opportunity to socialize and support each other, as some patients may be dealing with similar medical conditions. Caregivers and parents readily use the playroom as a hub to interact with other adults while watching their children. In addition, it is a haven for those who wish to engage in typical activities in a normally unpredictable medical environment.

Medical play sessions, music jam sessions, and creative art experiences are individual or group experiences. The child life specialist may coordinate group medical play incorporating the use of actual medical supplies to normalize these materials and make them less threatening. Children safely explore and increase their understanding of medical procedures within this child-friendly environment.

What Is the Role of the Child Life Specialist?

A Child Life Specialist addresses the emotional, social, and cognitive needs of the ill or well children visiting the medical center. The specialist observes and assesses the pediatric patient's development and ability to cope within the hospital milieu. Specialists foster children's growth and ability to adjust and adapt through age-appropriate activities; child-friendly playrooms which use stress reduction techniques and verbal, and non-verbal communication; and other specific interventions. Play opportunities are instrumental to optimize development and promote a sense of mastery and understanding of the hospital and medical procedures. In addition, the specialist is responsible for creating a safe and child-oriented playroom—an environment for children and their families to engage in non-medical and familiar activities.

This innovative approach to child life programming offers verbal and non-verbal psychosocial services that are a universal form of communication not limited or restricted by age, language, and cognitive abilities. Each Child Life / Creative Art Therapist works within multidisciplinary medical teams. They function closely with other healthcare professionals in different units, including: the Pediatric Emergency Room, Pediatric Intensive Care, Inpatient General Pediatrics, Pediatric Ambulatory Care Services, The Neonatal Intensive Care, Pediatric Nephrology Program, and Pediatric Day Surgery. Child life specialists also work within The SIDS Center of New Jersey and the Tomorrows Children's Institute for Children with Cancer and Blood Disorders, The Pediatric Neuroscience Institute, The Molly Center for Children with Diabetes and Endocrine Disorders, and The Steven Bader Institute, where patients with infectious diseases receive treatment. In addition, adult units refer the Child Life clinicians to work with children whose parents are critically ill, near death, or have recently died.

Art, Music, Drama, Dance/Movement Therapists: Certified Child Life Specialist

Child Life Specialists and Creative Arts Therapists establish goals based upon a patient's specific need, diagnosis, age, ability, interest, and culture. Therapeutic goals may include helping the patient address his or her medical condition or treatment, developing positive coping skills, or dealing with bereavement issues. Pediatric inpatient and outpatient services are provided for both individual and group therapies. Suppose groups gather children and adolescents with cancer, diabetes, rheumatological and other illnesses, and individuals facing bereavement issues to offer peer support, thereby decreasing their sense of isolation and helping them to cope. The clinician's individualized interventions focus upon enhancing coping; decreasing stress; providing an understanding before, during, and after a medical treatment; or providing crisis intervention with a child anticipating or grieving the death of a loved one. Along with other members of the healthcare team, Child Life Specialists seek to reduce the stress experienced by pediatric patients. It is important to communicate age-appropriate information—about the often hectic medical environment and the procedures taking place—in a manner understandable for the patient.

Child Life Specialists explain, in a developmentally appropriate, engaging, and empathic manner, the equipment and personnel the child encounters, such as blood pressure monitors, pulse oximeters, physicians, etc. When an invasive procedure occurs such as an intravenous catheter insertion, the specialist provides pre-procedural education, using a specialized medical play doll. This helps the child to understand the goals of the procedure and the sequence of events. Such intervention integrates a visual tool specifically geared toward a child, who has not developed abstract thinking and thus requires additional forms of communication to conceptualize and cope with procedures. It provides a sense of control and understanding of the beginning, middle, and end of the process. Therapists use dolls to demonstrate and explain diagnostic procedures such as ultrasounds and CT scans. Child Life Specialists utilize coping skills such as guided imagery techniques, breathing exercises, and developmentally appropriate activities to enhance the child's capacity to self-soothe and tolerate unfamiliar and sometimes uncomfortable experiences.

Siblings of pediatric patients are important in any pediatric area. Siblings of patients will react to medical conditions and seek support and reassurance from caregivers. Providing services to these children can reduce feelings of resentment and exclusion as well as subsequent relational problems within the family that may last for quite some time. Education, relevant discussion, and expressive activities help a sibling focus and process feelings regarding the medical condition or emergency. By guiding these children toward taking a more active role in the care of their brothers and sisters, they feel a greater sense of inclusion and empowerment. The following case studies highlight the role of the Child Life Specialist at the Joseph M. Sanzari Children's Hospital. Similar programs are available in the over 460 accredited Child Life programs throughout the world.

Case Study One: A Trip to the ER

A four-year old female presented in the trauma unit with a head injury. According to paramedic reports, the child pulled a television set down onto her as she watched her favorite cartoon. The television landed directly on her face, causing a head injury. As pediatric trauma physicians and surgeons made assessments, she began to de-compensate. Her blood pressure and heart rate began to fall and she was no longer reactive. In order to stabilize this patient, the physician decided to intubate (to insert a tube into the larynx). The tension in the environment was high as the medical team hurriedly provided the care necessary to save her from further injury. Just outside her room, her 11-year-old brother witnessed these events—his mother crying inconsolably and begging the physicians to help her daughter—and he had no understanding of the situation.

At this moment, the Child Life Specialist entered the trauma area. With the patient in a non-responsive state, she introduced herself and escorted the brother to a waiting area after obtaining parental consent. He remained in close proximity to his sister, but without exposure to the treatment area. The clinician calmly explained the role of each staff member in the treatment area, helping the boy feel less intimidated. As the healthcare providers called out treatment orders in the trauma room, the clinician translated the medical terminology into terms understandable by the child.

The child life specialist offered the boy arts-and-crafts supplies to create colorful items for his sister, quelling his anxiety. Her brother got busy making items to decorate her hospital room in the Pediatric Intensive Care Unit (PICU). Along with these, he used fabric markers to draw pictures on a pillowcase and even wrote a hand-written "Get Well" message.

Meanwhile, results of diagnostic tests showed that the little girl sustained bruising to the frontal brain area. According to the doctors, her chances for recovery were excellent but they remained cautious and kept her intubation tube in place. She was taken to the PICU for observation. Before entering the PICU, the Child Life Specialist educated the patient's sibling about the environment in which his sister would be cared for. Age appropriate, non-threatening details about his sister's physical appearance and responsiveness level, the monitoring devices, IV Poles, and ventilator were given. He was encouraged to ask as many questions as necessary for him to have a reasonable grasp of the experience.

After the patient settled in her room, her brother placed the pillowcase over the upper body of his sister where, according to him, it would be closest to her heart. The Child Life Specialist then assisted him in hanging the decorations he created on the walls, filling the space with loving and positive creations. There was a noted change in the brother's affect as he actively participated in his sister's care, after having been helpless while witnessing the trauma. The intervention minimized his fear, comforted him, and provided him with a specific role. Interacting with a Child Life Specialist helped transform this young boy's experience in several ways. The emotions that he might have been hiding were given their place on the construction paper and pillowcase. By decorating his sister's room, he helped make her environment less "medical-looking" and increased its warmth. Finally, the education received during his experience empowered him with knowledge and increased his sense of control over a situation in which he initially felt powerless.

The ability to communicate with other members of the multidisciplinary team is essential to providing optimum patient care in the Emergency Department. Utilizing the resources available within that team of professionals helps to ensure a positive outcome for patients and staff. Child Life Specialists advocate for services offered by various disciplines that help meet the medical and/or psychosocial needs of patients and families such as social work, consumer affairs, and pastoral care. These teams of professionals arrange family care meetings, crisis intervention counseling, religious guidance, transportation arrangements, and specialized service preparations.

Case Study Two: Art Therapy with Pediatric Oncology Patients and Their Siblings

Mary was 13-years-old when diagnosed with cancer. The Art Therapist / Child Life Specialist worked with Mary for two years. Mary's intensive treatment included long hospital stays. Mary loved art, and the themes she chose were highly decorative. Working on her art seemed to give her a sense of order and control. She shied away from art experiences that were clearly expressive. Her focus was solely on the finished product, preferring her art to be well structured, neat, and organized. Her younger sister by three years, Bianca, described Mary's room at home as being meticulous and noting, "everything has a place in Mary's room; in my room everything is just thrown wherever."

Mary received daily art therapy while hospitalized and weekly outpatient sessions when she was home. Bianca became involved in art therapy sessions on a regular basis to address issues related to being a sibling of a patient with a life-threatening illness. Siblings, profoundly affected by the many changes within the family structure due to the impact of the illness, have a variety of emotional responses to the change in family member's roles and routines. Bianca witnessed her sister change physically and emotionally during frequently hospitalized periods.

The two sisters were as different from each other in temperament as in their creative style. Mary was confident about her artistic skills and oriented toward realistic imagery. She chose art interventions such as a dried flower arrangement within a container, painting a picture of a bird, turning medical supplies into people using fabric, yarn, and googly eyes. When she created an abstract design, it was planned by color and pattern. While in the hospital for a long stay, she asked to organize the art therapy supply boxes, her favorite one being the bead box. Lying in bed, Mary would painstakingly make sure that every bead was in its designated section. At home, Mary had her craft supplies maintained in this scrupulous manner. During her battle against cancer, feeling ill and tired from the chemotherapy, the act of carefully placing a bead in its proper place gave Mary a sense of control and allowed her to feel purposeful and her normal self.

Conversely, Bianca expressed that she did not enjoy art and lacked both talent and creative ideas. She compared her creativity to her sister's. Mary was neat and her work well thought out. Bianca was more physical, impulsive, and questioned whether she could make art; it would never look "good." The challenge was to help her see the validity of her own imagination; there were different styles and purposes of art. One of the first directives with Bianca was to make an "angry" painting and a "happy" painting. With color and brushstroke, she allowed herself to create two distinct and expressive pieces clearly representing each emotion. This was an accomplishment for a girl convinced that her art was meaningless and that she felt no emotions.

Strong emotions were overwhelming for these sisters. Mary avoided them while creating decorative art. However, she carefully chose when to share her feelings about being ill, physical changes she was undergoing, missing school, and her sibling relationship. Carefully, with tears and in a safe environment, Mary was able to open the door to these painful emotions. By returning to the art, she would return to a different state and regain composure. She was able to manipulate the art medium and could predict the outcome. Bianca, on the other hand, would not approach the subject of her emotions or responses to her sister's illness. However, art therapy would gradually move her into a freer expressive mode.

At age 15, Mary was admitted to the pediatric intensive care unit. There was no more treatment available and her body systems were failing. Her parents welcomed support for Bianca, since they were completely absorbed in the critical care of Mary. Before Bianca entered the PICU room, she was prepared for all she would see. Her sister was connected to machines and unable to speak. Bianca remained in the room for a short while and then requested to go to the art room. She discussed her sister's condition and was hopeful about recovery. It was evident she had not processed all she had been told her about sister's condition. Mary had been seriously ill for two years, and Bianca had adjusted to life with her sister going to the hospital and returning home. She wanted to believe that the situation was status quo. Her parents were unable to help Bianca understand that it was likely Mary would die, for they too were having trouble accepting this possibility. Amidst their pain they were able to see that it would be best if Bianca were included and asked the therapist to help.

The actual process of anticipatory grief for this family began the day of Mary's diagnosis. Although remaining positive to the end, there is an unavoidable experience of loss when a loved one becomes ill. It ebbed and flowed during different times of her treatment, but now it was unavoidable and the parents were powerless in the struggle to have their daughter cured. "The illness and loss of the child will have a direct impact on the siblings, depending on their own capacity to give meaning to its occurrence and to mourn the loss effectively" (Fanos, 1996). At 12 years old, Bianca was able to understand the body's functions and that death is permanent. Mary's doctor, in a sensitive and age-appropriate manner, informed Bianca that her sister might die, and no other medicine could cure her cancer. He reassured her that there were medicines to ease Mary's pain and that the healthcare team would continue to keep her comfortable. In spite of this information, Bianca remained in denial until the therapist encouraged her to communicate with her sister, a chance to say goodbye. In Mary's room Bianca held her sister's hand and sat by her bedside. Everyone left so the sisters could have their time together and that evening Mary died.

Bianca and her mother came weekly after Mary's death for bereavement counseling while her father declined support. The mother met with the oncology/hematology social worker while Bianca met with the Art Therapist/Child Life Specialist. Inspired by an art piece in the room, Bianca wanted to make a mold of her hand. She then made a mold of her foot. The therapist followed the child's lead as the art therapy process advanced. Bianca decided to paint a box. The next session she placed the hand and foot in the box, closed the lid and said, "I will never be able to touch my sister again, to feel her, to hug her."

Bianca had poignantly moved through a critical task of bereavement, acknowledging the loss on cognitive, emotional, and even physical levels. The sculptures of Bianca's hand and foot inside a box are symbolic for important tasks. Bianca moved through her grief while using the art to connect with her sister through their hands and feet. Having only experienced life as a younger sister, Bianca defined herself through this relationship. Bianca lost her "identification figure" that is "instrumental in leading the younger child out into the world" (Fanos, 1996). The therapeutic relationship continued while Bianca proceeded to move through her own adolescence. The family entered family therapy and continued bereavement counseling, as their family constellation had changed dramatically with Mary's death. When Bianca faced her 15th birthday she began to display physical symptoms and fears related to her sister's death. Courageously, the members of the family faced another difficult bereavement phase.

Mary and Bianca found unique ways to benefit from art therapy within the medical setting. The former created pleasing products and was able to do so throughout most of her arduous treatment. "Hence, the role of Creative Arts Therapists in this setting is to provide a rich and varied creative arts environment in which the children and their families can shape and form their lives and their style and make their own mark through their illnesses" (Rode, 1995). Painful emotions can be expressed visually when utilizing art therapy with a bereaved sibling. The process of creating concretizes an experience that is hard to fathom and put words to. Bianca used the art for personal exploration, as a springboard. "Creative arts therapy helps to promote communication so that the child can become effectively involved in his or her mourning process (Zambelli et al., 1988). Art therapy was a source for self-identification, affirmation, and expression and was able to meet the individual needs of two very different sisters.

Case Study Three: Two Tales of Drama Therapy and Child Life

The drama therapist helps children adjust to the hospital milieu. Drama therapists advocate for children to be the main characters in their stories of hospitalization. Children come to the inpatient floor for diverse reasons. Whether hospital admission occurs after a dog bite, attempted suicide, pneumonia, or chronic illness, these events are one of the prime dramas of these children's lives. Everyone has a story to tell. We develop our physicality, our view and attitude toward life, how we talk, and who we are, based on our experiences, and our understanding of them. Such a process, although abstract, is a tangible one. The safest and most human way to have access to a person's life is through a story. The drama therapist facilitates this story telling and provides a safe space, a haven in which stories can blossom. Children need to express, cultivate, and mentally "digest" the hospital setting, and then gain experience coping with it.

Matthew's Tale

Matthew was a delayed seven-year-old boy having difficulty with urination. A urinary catheter needed to be in place before discharging him from the hospital. Matthew had a great imagination. Through play, the therapist learned that he regularly enjoyed telling stories about dinosaurs killing other animals. The drama therapist developed a rapport during consecutive sessions by providing Matthew with dinosaurs and other figures. He immediately entered the realm of play, inviting the therapist into his world, moving the figures and creating a story. Usually a scared and withdrawn child in the hospital setting, Matthew displayed considerable energy in his play. The theme of the play was the dinosaurs' battle with other animals. Matthew identified with dinosaurs. In his dramatic play, dinosaurs became strong, outnumbering other animals, and then weak to the point that the species was in danger of extinction. Each story's theme repeated this battle.

Matthew's mother frequently discouraged and minimized his imaginative stories. Matthew had strong feelings about physical boundaries and was fearful of touch. The drama therapist educated his parents about children's developmental needs and play as a mode of communication, expression, and coping to foster greater understanding and compassion towards their son.

Matthew failed to cope well with realistic information. The sight of medical staff and objects such as needles or tubes produced overwhelming anxiety. The drama therapist attempted to prepare Matthew for a catheterization. Using a doll and non-threatening medical props, the therapist communicated essential information by providing the sequence of events of the procedure, and their reason. In discussing methods to cope with the procedure, Matthew suggested to the therapist his desire to be an invisible superhero in the treatment room and chose a red cape from the therapist's scarf bag. Prior to the procedure, Matthew expressed that he wanted to remain in the dramatic realm during the procedure. The drama therapist's job was to support his coping style and to communicate this to the medical staff and his mother. The drama therapist and the patient agreed on the telling of a dinosaur's story for the entire time the catheter was inserted in the boy's penis. Matthew threw a magic powder around him and hid behind the therapist so that no one could see him. Matthew entered the treatment room as the invisible superhero, announcing aloud that he was present. The medical staff played along with him and gave the child control. The drama therapist directed medical personnel to make sure Matthew was safe to continue using his imagination as a coping mechanism during the procedure.

As soon as Matthew, the invisible superhero, lay down, the ritual of creating the dinosaur's story began between the therapist and the child. Therapist: "Once upon a time . . ." Child: "There were many, many, dinosaurs . . ." The child continued the tale with the therapist's support by reflecting and asking questions. When Matthew felt he was coping well, the dinosaurs' numbers increased. While the medical staff was placing the catheter into his penis, the most invasive part of the procedure, the dinosaurs were in danger of being outnumbered by other animals. The therapist quickly encouraged Matthew to recall the magical powers of dinosaurs and utilize them. His story reflected the fear and anxiety he was experiencing in the present and through making interventions within his own story, he was mastering the situation. At the end of the procedure, Matthew decided to "show" himself, no longer the invisible superhero. At the procedure's completion and surrounded by medical staff and his mother, he declared that he was Matthew again. Matthew stood in the treatment room with a confident and proud face.

In individual drama therapy work, the child is allowed to project himself or enact events as in a safe space in the play language that he often prefers. He can project his story, through play, onto toys—using masks, puppets, music, and characters. Matthew projected his fears onto characters and used his imagination to cope. The experience of play enabled this child to be in control and gain perspective through the distancing of play. This is a crucial experience in the inpatient setting where children have minimal control over medical procedures. A child becomes playwright, actor, and director. As dinosaurs conquered the other animals, Matthew's affect grew; he conveyed confidence in his body and strong tone of voice. He was able to express a range of emotions, thus allowing him to release, express, and cope in a safe manner.

Human development continues from birth throughout adulthood. The drama therapist's strong hope is to contribute to each child's healthy emotional development and self-growth process while hospitalized. In order to meet a child and promote such a process, it is imperative that the therapist listen to each story— adapting, guiding, and advocating for the child's unique coping style.

Case Study Four: Psychosocial Care for Pediatric Diabetes Patients

Drama therapists are certified Child Life Specialists, integrating child life theory and practice with their modality. Treatment is available to children in both an individual and group setting, depending on specific needs of the child. At the Molly Center for Children with Diabetes and Endocrine Disorders, the psychosocial needs of children are assessed by the drama therapist.

The following is a description of a group that meets regularly with the drama therapist for psychosocial support, to address issues related to their diabetes. Psycho-educational needs, interpersonal skills, and personal issues related to diagnosis, medication management, and overall coping with diabetes are goals for this group of school age children. At the start of this and each group, the children meet with their parents, the drama therapist, and a social worker. The social worker facilitates the parent support component separately, while the drama therapist meets with the children's group. All the children test their blood sugar levels. There is no nurse present during the support group and parents meet for their own support group facilitated by a social worker separately from the children.

Eight children, ranging from 8 to 10 years of age, participate in a 45-minute session. They know each other well from previous group participation. This is the 5th group in a 12-week group cycle. The children join the drama therapist in the center of the room in a circle, seated on the floor. The children have a great deal of energy at the start of this group. They are excited to be together and eager to engage in the drama therapy group. They are familiar with the modality and understand and participate well within the norms of the group. They stand and go around the room and say their names. Each child adds his or her own gesture to the saying of his/her name and the group repeats it back to each child. Sally starts. She says, "My name is Sally." "Add a gesture to that name, Sally," the drama therapist requests. "Sally," the girl repeats and adds a waving motion with both her arms. "Sally..." the group repeats to the girl and they mimic her arm movements. The mirroring and the physical gesture bring an energy and greater relatedness to the group. All members of the group take turns, saying their own names and adding their own gestures. As with Sally, the group picks up and repeats each gesture and name.

"Now that we are all here," says the therapist, "are we ready to enter into a world of our imagination?" The group responds that they are. "Well then, let's reach up and pull down our drama therapy curtain and we can step into this world of our imagination and play together here with the images and stories that we create. We can play here as long as we want, and then we can let it go and play again with something else," says the therapist. The group reaches up and pulls down an imaginary curtain. "Take a hold of this magic drama therapy curtain and we will all step into it on the count of three," instructs the therapist. "This will symbolize that we are entering our imaginary world and we will leave the hospital behind us while we play together with each other and with diabetes, One – two – three!" The group members all part the curtain and step toward the center of the circle, saying their names.

"Okay, here we are together. Where are we?" asks the therapist. Bobby says, "We are in a boat." The group begins swaying back and forth in motion, indicating they are all on the same boat together in the water. The therapist understands that all these children are in the same boat; they all have diabetes and can commonly relate around this issue. "Who is the captain of the boat?" she asks. "I do not have diabetes; you need another captain," the therapist says. "I am the captain," Andy says. Many of the group members take on roles of the crew and passengers on the boat. Some members do this spontaneously, while others need assistance from the group's leader. When necessary, the leader casts members into roles. The boat begins to sway with greater intensity and it is clear the water is no longer calm. "Oh no! There is a storm coming in!" The group notes this change in the weather, plays with this transition and the therapist asks if anyone brought enough supplies along to survive a shipwreck. "No, we didn't bring anything with us today; we are not prepared to be lost at sea," one of the members cries. "Did anyone bring any insulin?" Other members of the group call out the everyday items that must be remembered by a child with diabetes. Insulin syringes, blood sugar meters, something to treat a low blood sugar, and other items are named. Someone looks down and points to something in the water. "What is that? Is it a shark?" The group members all react to this image of the shark and many members enjoy playing with this frightening image. "The boat is sinking," Andy says. "We will all need to jump out and swim to save our lives!" On the count of "one – two – three" the group decides they will all jump into the water and swim to safety. They reach an island and someone says, "We are on the Diabetes Island, but we do not have anything to treat our diabetes!"

"What do we need on this island?" the therapist asks and members individually name their requirements. "Together let's reach up and take down some insulin," the therapist instructs. All the members raise their arms and pull down the insulin. Together the group brings down a blood sugar meter and test strips. The group continues like this in a structured role play, testing their blood sugar, drawing up insulin, and giving themselves their injections. "Wow," the therapist remarks, "you are all very good at surviving on this island and you really know how to be resourceful in managing your diabetes. It is time for us to return to the hospital and end our drama therapy group for today." The group is instructed to bring down the drama therapy box, open the box, and place inside all the images and stories that were included in the day's group. This image is one the children are accustomed to using with the drama therapist. They bring down the box and place inside the image of the boat, the characters played by each child, the shark, and the props related to diabetes that they used during the session.

"Now we will bring down the curtain and step out, saying our names. This symbolizes that we are leaving our imaginary world and going back to the hospital. It also means the end of the group for today." The therapist leads the members through this closing monologue and the session ends.

As seen in this case study, a drama therapy group uses abstraction and metaphor to play out many of the children's fears and daily interactions with their illness. The structure unifies the members and allows them freedom to explore. It also safely contains their interactions through the therapist's ability to engage and maintain the group's focus. The energy of the group is high as they connect to one another through shared fear, anxiety, and common experiences. The image of the shark can be interpreted as the looming fears and anxieties they face daily to manage their diabetes. These metaphors are readily accessed, and played with by every member of the group. The real and imaginary worlds are analogous on many levels. The children have a life-threatening experience. They encounter a dangerous entity—one which has painful and sharp "teeth" analogous to the insulin syringes used to administer life-sustaining medications. The image of the boat and the island symbolize being together with the other members as well as the sense of isolation patients often feel. This drama therapy group facilitates the children's shared experience, which decreases their stress and sense of isolation. Most important, the group enhances the children's ability to cope and provides them with positive peer relationships, enriching their self-esteem.

SUMMARY

A Child Life Program in a medical center requires the professional and financial support of administrators and medical clinicians. It has been the authors' good fortune to work in a progressive institution receptive to non-revenue-producing services that noneleless improve patients' quality of life. The process of transforming the medical model to utilize Child Life services with these modalities takes a significant amount of commitment, time, and teamwork. It is often necessary to validate our professions through presenting standard practices of care, documenting research, and educating parents, staff, and the public about the efficacy of these services. The disciplines of Child Life and Creative Arts Therapy provide a psychosocial complement to medical care and are essential to treating the "whole" child while improving patient satisfaction and the quality of life for pediatric patients.

ADDITIONAL RESOURCES

The Child Life Council, Inc.
11820 Park Lawn Drive, Suite 240
Rockville, Maryland 20852
Telephone Number: (301) 881-7090
Web site: www.childlife.org

The National Coalition of Creative Arts Therapy Associations (NCCATA)
c/o AMTA
8455 Colesville Road, Suite 1000
Silver Spring, Maryland 20910
Web site: http://www.nccata.org/

The American Art Therapy Association (AATA)
1202 Allanson Road
Mundelein, Illinois 60060
Telephone: (847) 949-6064
Web site: www.arttherapy.org

The American Dance Therapy Association, Inc. (ADTR)
2000 Century Plaza, Suite 108
Columbia, Maryland 21044
Telephone: (410) 997-4040
Web site: www.adta.org

The American Music Therapy Association (AMTA)
8455 Colesville Road, Suite 1000
Silver Spring, Maryland 20910
Telephone: (301) 589-3300
Web site: http://namt.com/

The National Association for Poetry Therapy (NAPT)
525 South West 5th Street, Suite A
Des Moines, Iowa 50309
Telephone: (515) 282-8192
Web site: www.poetrytherapy.org

The American Society of Group Psychotherapy and Psychodrama
(ASGPP)
301 North Harrison Street, Suite 508
Princeton, New Jersey 08540
Telephone: (609) 452-1339
Web site: www.asgpporg.org

The National Association for Drama Therapy, Inc. (NADT)
15 Post Side Lane
Pittsford, New York 14534
Telephone: (585) 381-5618
Web site: www.nadt.org.

The American Society of Group Psychotherapy & Psychodrama
(ASGPP)
301 N. Harrison St., Suite 508
Princeton, NJ 08540
Telephone: (609) 452-1339
Web site: http://www.asgpp.org

RECOMMENDED READING

1. *Working With Children In Hospitals: A Professional Guide,* Emma Plank, reprinted 2nd edition, 1965, Chicago Year Book Medical Publishers, Inc.
2. *Protecting The Emotional Development Of The Ill Child: The Essence Of The Child Life Profession,* 1965, Evelyn Orland, Psycho Social Press, Madison Ct.
3. *What's In A Name? Child Life And The Play Lady Legacy,* Stefi Rubin, Children's Health Care, Winter 1992, Vol. 21, No. 1.
4. *Playing and Reality,* Winnicott, D. W., 1971, Harmondsworth, Middlesex: Penguin.
5. *Earthtales,* Gersie, A. (1992). London: Green Print.
6. *Playing for Real: The World of a Child Therapist,* Richard Bromfield, Ph.D., Dutton, 1992.
7. *Medical Art Therapy with Children,* Edited by Cathy Malchiodi, Jessica Kingsley Publishers, 1999.
8. *Supervision in the Helping Professions.* Second Edition, Peter Hawkins and Robin Shohet, Open University Press, Maidenhead, Philadelphia, PA., First Publication 2000, Reprinted 2002, 2003.

REFERENCES

Abromeit, D. (2003). The newborn individualized developmental care and assessment program as a model for clinical music therapy interventions with premature infants. *Music Therapy Perspectives, 21*(2), 60–68.

American Academy of Pediatrics (AAP). (1993). Policy statement. *American Academy of Pediatrics, 91*(3), 671–673.

American Dance Therapy Association (ADTA). (2005). Dance/movement therapy fact sheet. Retrieved August 5, 2005, from http://www.adta.org/about/factsheet.cfm.

American Music Therapy Association (AMTA). (2005a). Frequently asked questions about music therapy. Retrieved August 10, 2005, from http://www.musictherapy.org/faqs.html.

American Music Therapy Association (AMTA). (2005b). What is music therapy? Retrieved August 5, 2005, from http://www.musictherapy.org/.

Art Therapy Credentials Board (ATCB). (2005). What is art therapy? Retrieved August 5, 2005, from http://www.atcb.org/whatis.htm.

Child Life Council. (2005a). *Mission Statement.* Retrieved August 9, 2005, from http://www.childlife.org/About/profession_mission_vision.htm.

Child Life Council. (2005b). What is a child life specialist? Retrieved August 9, 2005, from http://www.childlife.org/About/what_is_specialist.htm.

Fanos, J. (1996). *Sibling loss.* Mahwah, NJ: Lawrence Erlbaum Associates.

Leeuwenburgh, E. (2000). Music therapy in the neonatal intensive care unit: A family-centered care approach. In J. V. Loewy (Ed.), *Music therapy in the neonatal intensive care unit* (pp. 39–50). New York: Beth Israel Medical Center.

National Association for Poetry Therapy (NAPT). (2005a). How do I become a poetry therapist? Retrieved August 5, 2005, from http://poetrytherapy.org/training.html.

National Association for Poetry Therapy (NAPT). (2005b). Training and education. Training requirements for CPT. Retrieved August 9, 2005, from http://poetrytherapy.org/training.html.

National Association for Poetry Therapy (NAPT). (2005c). Training and education. Training requirements for RPT. Retrieved August 9, 2005, from http://poetrytherapy.org/training.html.

National Association for Poetry Therapy (NAPT). (2005d). What is poetry therapy? Retrieved August 5, 2005, from http://poetrytherapy.org/training.poetrytherapy.html.

National Coalition of Creative Arts Therapies Associations (NCCATA). (2005a). Drama therapy. Retrieved August 5, 2005, from http://www.nccata.org/drama.html.

National Coalition of Creative Arts Therapies Associations (NCCATA). (2005b). Psychodrama. Retrieved August 5, 2006, from http://www.nccata.org/psychodrama.html.

Rode, D. (1995). Building bridges within the culture of pediatric medicine: The interface of art therapy and child life programming. *Art therapy: Journal of the American Art Therapy Association, 12*(2), 104–110.

Zambelli, G. C., Clark, E. J., Barile, L., & deJong, A. F. (1988). An interdisciplinary approach to clinical intervention for childhood bereavement. *Death Studies, 12*, 41–50.

Index

---

page numbers followed by *f* denote figures; those followed by *t* denote tables